SENT TO HEAL

A Handbook on Christian Healing

D0771737

SENT TO HEAL

A Handbook on Christian Healing

HAROLD TAYLOR

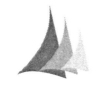

Speedwell Press

Sent to Heal: A Handbook on Christian Healing
Second Edition
By Harold Taylor

Editor: Paul Nockleby
Cover: Dawn Mathers Design

FOREWORD

Every now and then one comes across a book that is destined not only to find a place in one's library, but to become an indispensable reference text that always lies close at hand. Such is this book. It will certainly fulfill its role of being a "handbook" to all involved in healing ministries.

The author has combined together in this book a wonderful blend of information about the healing ministry in general and teaching that is both comprehensive and enlightening. He has approached the topic with an openness that is itself healthy, yet with discernment that is quite rare.

John Stott once wrote that life is a "pilgrimage of learning," and in this book Harold Taylor has allowed us to share in the insights of his own spiritual pilgrimage. The product is a work that comes from an academic perspective due to the author's background as a Bible College lecturer. However, it also has the added benefit of a warm pastoral approach that seeks to bring the insights of the spiritual truths gained over the years, to the deepest needs of people today. Harold Taylor's emphasis upon "wholeness", rather than upon physical or emotional healing alone, reflects the growing awareness of all those involved in healing ministries that God is concerned with every aspect of our lives.

Much of the value of this book lies in the ability of the author to research the historical background to healing through the ages, and to assess the contribution of the various approaches. Thanks to this book the reader is able to look at what is happening today generally, both inside and outside the churches, and in this book receives valuable guidelines for becoming involved in Christian healing.

These guidelines will help those who read this volume from developing wrong attitudes about healing, and will encourage practice that will be beneficial to those receiving healing ministry, and will also be glorifying to God.

Rev. Jim Holbeck
St. Andrew's Healing Ministry, Sydney, Australia

PREFACE

Sent to Heal is a very valuable gift to the Order of St. Luke in North America but also to the church at large. It is not only a valuable resource for anyone wanting to learn about the Christian ministry of healing and how it developed throughout the ages but also gives information about how one might respond in one's own life to Jesus' mandate to the church "to heal the sick."

As one responsible for and dedicated to the growth of the Christian healing ministry in North America I am always looking for valuable resources that I think will help both the members of the Order of St. Luke and also members of the church to be more effective in the Christian healing ministry. *Sent to Heal* is just such a book that I would highly recommend not only to those beginning in the healing ministry but also those seasoned and experienced in this ministry.

I hope and pray that you will find this book a useful resource in helping you to understand what Jesus meant when he gave his mandate to the church as recorded in Luke's Gospel to preach the Gospel and to heal sick and to tell people that when healing occurs the Kingdom of God is in their midst. The exciting thing is that this ministry is both yours and mine and this book will help us all to respond more effectively Christ's call to us to be healers of the sick.

Yours in Christ's Healing Love,
Ven. Lawrence W. Mitchell, Saskatoon, Saskatchewan, Canada
North American Director, The International Order of St. Luke

CONTENTS

INTRODUCTION

The first edition of this book was well received and used in Australia and New Zealand as a source of information about the healing ministry and as important reading for involvement and membership in the Order of St. Luke. The book is now being offered to a wider audience, and is recommended by OSL in North America and throughout the world as a valuable resource. While there are many additions and changes, the purpose of the book remains the same — to provide a reasonably in-depth presentation of some of the significant issues relating to the healing ministry.

As in the first edition, the second edition attempts to offer a broad understanding of healing and wholeness which addresses the whole person — our thinking, emotions, relationships with others and the world in which we live, and our relationship with God the creator Lord. The book acknowledges different approaches to healing found in different churches and groups, and seeks to understand these, whilst also offering an interpretation of the healing ministry which enables Christians to cooperate in this ministry rather than "trying to push their own barrow." The general aim of the book is to serve as one resource among many to help and encourage Christian people to be effectively involved in the healing mission given by Jesus Christ to the church.

There is an enormous amount of literature on the healing ministry especially on the "how to" and experiential level of ministry, and often offering a particular perspective, and ignoring or downplaying other healing ministries which have different emphases. The ministry of healing is practiced in many churches, with some seeing it as central to all ministry. In other churches, the healing ministry remains on the sidelines, and involves only "those who are into it." Despite the large amount of literature available, the subject of healing is often not studied in many churches. Few theological colleges and Bible colleges offer concentrations or programs in the healing ministry. In the Australian scene, healing is often treated as a minor discipline within general pastoral care & counseling or as an elective along with many other practical ministry courses. In some colleges the subject does not appear in the curriculum at all, because it is regarded as not worthy of serious theological study. There are some notable exceptions to this, but it remains true that few colleges take the subject of healing as seriously as other biblical, theological, historical, and counseling subjects.

Therefore, there is great need for a comprehensive textbook which takes the healing ministry seriously within general theological training for those preparing for ministry. This book offers a broadly based approach to the major issues of the healing ministry, and is meant for those who wish to understand and become involved in this ministry. This book is intended both for those who are involved in ministry, as professionals and especially as lay members of the church, and in particular members of healing and prayer groups within the church, such as the Order of St. Luke.

How to Use This Book

This book is designed as a study handbook to encourage a deeper understanding of the healing ministry. It aims to give a general overview rather than a detailed analysis of the chapter topics.

Most chapters begin with *a human situation or event*, and the reader is asked to interact with that situation, and respond to the questions raised. It is important to complete these questions, as the situation is offered as a way to open up the issue addressed in the chapter.

Sharing and Discussion questions are designed to help you think about each particular topic, and to apply the material to your own life and situation. You can discuss the questions in a group with others, or you can use them as a basis for your own reflection. You may find it helpful to write some notes as you reflect on the various topics. If you are sharing with others in a regular meeting, do not try and discuss all the questions in one session; each chapter has sufficient material for more than one meeting. You may decide to spend several discussions just on one chapter. Some people may find it helpful to read the book right through, to gain a broad overview of the contents, and then commence discussions on the various chapters. Again it may be helpful to read each chapter two or three times before you commence discussions with others. All of these various arrangements would be subject to the make-up and decision of the group involved.

References for Further Reading at the end of each chapter have been revised and updated in the light of recent new material. These references provide extra sources of information if you wish to pursue any topic in greater depth. Most of the books listed should be available in Christian bookshops. Some of the older books may be out of print, or may be available through theological and Bible college libraries. References to particular articles in magazines and journals should also be available through these colleges.

The *Endnotes* give the source of material from other authors, and also offer suggestions where further information can be found on particular topics. There is also an abundance of material available on the internet, but no attempt has been made to include references to these resources.

It is very important to keep on growing in knowledge, faith, and prayer. This can be done by regular participation in the Order of St. Luke, and other healing groups; through sharing in training courses; and by a program of reading.

Being a loner in the healing ministry can be dangerous, as we are prone to wander off along our own paths and very quickly lose an informed and balanced understanding and practice of healing. If the reader is not involved with the Order of St. Luke, then a regular meeting with others is an important aspect of training, and the reader is encouraged to become part of a disciplined functioning group. There are a wide range of training courses available to equip people for effective involvement in the healing ministry, and the reader should contact his or her local church or chapter of the Order of St. Luke for more information.

About the Order of St. Luke

The Order of St. Luke derives its name from St. Luke "the beloved physician" (AV); "our dear friend Luke, the doctor" (NIV). It was founded in the USA in 1947 by Rev. Dr. John Gayner Banks, a priest of the Episcopal Church. The Order is now an international and inter-denominational organization involving Christians in many churches on six continents: Africa, Asia, Australia, Europe, North America, and South America.

The aim of the Order is to promote the understanding and practice of the healing ministry according to biblical teaching, and to help to restore this ministry as a normal part of church life. It seeks to work with all churches and to offer a disciplined fellowship which focuses on healing as an essential part of the gospel and integral to the church's mission.

Membership of the Order is open to all Christians, clergy and laity, who believe in the healing ministry of Christ and who are committed to the furtherance of this ministry. Groups of OSL members from the same area meet in chapters which may be formed by a minimum of seven people who are recognized as members in good standing in their local church, with one of the number being an ordained minister. Each chapter meets regularly for teaching, prayer, and regular healing services as arranged in local churches. In North America there are nearly 300 chapters organized into fourteen regions, each region looked after by a regional director.

The Order of St. Luke affirms the church's faith as contained in the accepted creeds of the church, especially the Apostles' and Nicene Creeds, and recognizes the various statements of faith from different denominations.

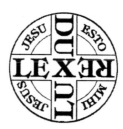

The emblem of the Order of St. Luke consists of a cross within a circle, with the Latin words, "Jesu Esto Mihi Jesus" meaning "Jesus be to me my Savior." Each arm of the cross has a three-letter Latin word reflecting attributes of Jesus Christ: Lux (Light), Rex (King), Dux (Leader), and Lex (Law). The emblem taken as a whole, is a prayer: "O Jesus be to me my Savior, my Light, my King, my Leader, and my Law."

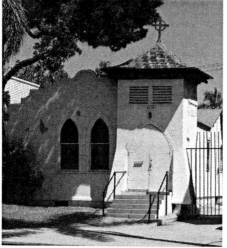

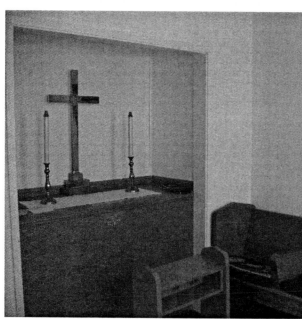

The Rev. John Gayner Banks, founder of OSL, was rector at St. Luke Episcopal Church in San Diego, California, from 1937-1944, where he organized the first healing ministry. St. Luke Church has a chapel (left) set aside for prayer and healing ministry.

The overall aim of the Order of St. Luke is to promote a deeper knowledge and acceptance of the healing ministry as a normal part of a balanced presentation of the gospel. To achieve this, it encourages the study of scripture, and provides the opportunity for members and interested people to meet together for study, prayer, sharing and ministry. It encourages cooperation between the ministry of the church and the healing professions, and seeks to be an avenue whereby this cooperation can be achieved and maintained.

Each member of the Order seeks to be effective in his or her healing ministry, through regular prayer, fellowship, Bible reading, the cultivation and use of the special gifts and talents given by God, and commitment to a lifestyle that is healthy in body, mind and spirit.

Acknowledgments

The author and publisher wish to thank copyright holders for granting permission to reproduce copyrighted material. Unless otherwise indicated, scripture references and quotations are from the *New International Version of the Bible,* copyright International Bible Society, 1978, and used with permission. Quotations from other versions are acknowledged and used with permission: *The Holy Bible—Knox Version,* copyright Macmillan, 1955; *The Jerusalem Bible,* copyright Darton, Longman, and Todd, 1968; *The Living Bible,* copyright Tyndale Publishing, 1971; *The New American Standard Bible,* copyright Lockman Foundation, 1977.

All sources used in the text are acknowledged in the Endnotes. Special acknowledgment is made of the following: *Healing and Wholeness,* Crowborough, East Sussex: for permission to reproduce excerpts from the following material: A. Arbuthnot and B. Green, Number 1, January/March, 1991; G. Tuckwell and D. Flagg, Number 8, October/December, 1992; R. Parker, Number 11, July/September, 1993.

Thanks also to Hodder and Stoughton, London, for permission to reproduce diagram and written material from F. MacNutt, *Healing*, 1988; and for permission to reproduce excerpts from the following: M. Cole (ed.), *What is the New Age*, 1990; J. Glennon, *Your Healing Is Within You*, 1978; *How Can I Find Healing*, 1984; R. Green, *God's Catalyst*, 1991; J. Gunstone, *The Lord is Our Healer*, 1986; M. Maddocks, *A Healing House of Prayer*, 1987. Acknowledgment is made to J. Richards, for permission to reprint illustrations, *Faith and Healing*, Network, Number 6, Floreat Flame Books, Mirrabooka, WA.

Excerpts from the following publishers and publications are also acknowledged: ABC Enterprises, Melbourne: D. Milliken and N. Drury, *Worlds Apart*, 1991. Baker Book House, Grand Rapids: D. Benner (Ed), *Baker Encyclopedia of Psychology*, 1985; G. Collins, *Your Magnificent Mind*, 1988; E. Miller, *A Crash Course on the New Age Movement*, 1989; M. A. Pearson, *Christian Healing*, 1990. IVP, Leicester, material from D. Huggett and P. Hacking, in J. Goldingay, *Signs, Wonders, and Healing*, 1989; J. A. Motyer, *The Message of James*, 1985. Arthur James, London: A. Sanford, *The Healing Light*, 1949, Australian Edition, 1986. Kingsway Trust Group Ltd., Eastbourne: K. Logan, *Close Encounters with the New Age*, 1991; S. Hughes, *God Wants You Whole*, 1984. Presbyterian and Reformed, New Jersey: C. S. Storms, *Healing and Holiness*, 1990. SPCK, London: M. Maddocks, *The Christian Healing Ministry*, 1990. Victor Books, Wheaton: D. Seamands, *Healing of Memories*, 1985. CWR, Waverley: S. Hughes, *The Christian Counsellor*, Volume 1, Number 1-4, 1991. Word, Melbourne: S. Pfeifer, *Healing at any Price*, 1988. G. Collins, *Christian Counselling*, 1989. World Council of Churches, Geneva: *International Review of Missions*, Volume 53, Number 311, July 1964; *Healing and Wholeness*, (Christian Medical Commission), 1990.

1

WHAT IS HEALTH AND HEALING?

The Order of St. Luke is a worldwide, interdenominational body of Christians, who believe that the healing of the body and mind was an important part of the total ministry of Jesus Christ, and that he commissioned his followers to continue this ministry. The ultimate aim of the Order is the restoration of the healing ministry as a normal part of church life.

Today, the phrase "the healing ministry of the church" is widely used. Although this is not a biblical phrase, Paul does describe healing amongst the ministries and gifts that God has given to His church (1 Corinthians 12:28, 30). The actual phrase "the ministry of healing" has been used from about 1880 onward to describe the involvement of the Christian church in healing. But what is health and healing? And what sort of ministry do we want to see restored as a normal part of church life?

Tom, Merle and Fred are all members of a local health club, and regularly participate in the club's programs. Each day, they have a fairly strenuous work-out, with regular exercises and proper diet, in order to keep fit and healthy. When they were asked what being healthy really means, they gave the following answers:

- For Tom, being healthy is having all engines on the go and running smoothly, with no breakdowns.

- For Merle, being healthy is being fit and able to enjoy life without being sick, or under a cloud. It is a general feeling of "okayness."

- Fred sees "healthy" as feeling good inside himself, feeling well, and ready to face things.

When they were asked what are the opposites of health, they included such words as, "sickness," "laziness," "anxiety," "sloppiness," "brokenness," "diseased" and "damaged."

Enrico and his wife, Gabriella, live with their six children in a slum area in Manila. Their home consists of discarded timber, cardboard, and plastic sheeting, which they have scavenged from the rubbish dump. They are part of a village of more than three thousand people, who share two water taps among the entire village. They have no toilet system, and they cook their meals on a small stove in their house. For these amenities, they pay rent to the local landlord, who is supposed to care for them and provide medical and educational help. However, little or no medical or educational help is ever available.

As members of the local Christian fellowship, Enrico and Gabriella try to bring their neighbors to an understanding of Jesus Christ, and help to organize the village to work for better conditions. When they were asked about health and being healthy, they said:

> To be healthy is to be without sickness. It is to be recognized and treated equally; it is to be free from these terrible conditions. It is to be able to organize our own lives and also, to have some good food, and good access to medical help, and schooling for our children.

Reflect on these two situations and their understanding of health and healing, and then write down your own definition of health and healing, as you understand it at this particular time. As you do this, consider the question: "To what extent is our understanding of health and healing determined by our living conditions, and our affluence or poverty?"

This chapter aims to:

- Gain an understanding of the meaning of health and healing from a Christian perspective;

- Consider how this understanding affects the healing ministry of the church.

Healing and Health

The word *healing* relates to the idea of health. In medical terms, healing or health usually refers to the cure of some sickness, or the repair of a wound, or ulcer, or fracture and the like. It is the restoration, or repair of something which has been damaged. In ordinary conversation, it usually has the meaning of restoring a sick person to being well again, or making the person better, or someone recovering after being injured or damaged; so that the person, or the situation, or even the animal, can be described as being healthy, rather than sick.

But what is health?

The English word, "health," comes from an Old English word *hal,* meaning whole. From this, we get words like whole, hale, holy, and also healthy. All these words originally had the idea of whole-ness, or soundness. One contemporary definition of health, which emphasizes the idea of wholeness, is given by the World Health Organization (1948):

> Health is a state of complete physical, mental and social well-being, and not merely the absence of disease or infirmity.

This definition describes health as more than just a description of the physical body. Health also refers to the person's mind, and to the situation in which the person lives. It is more than just the absence of disease, but is a state of complete physical, mental and social well-being, in all areas of life. (This definition was later expanded to include the word "spiritual" in its description of well-being — see Endnote 1.)

A wider definition of health is given by the Christian Medical Commission of the World Council of Churches:

> Health is a dynamic state of well-being of the individual and society, of physical, mental, spiritual, economic, political and social well-being; of being in harmony with each other, with the material environment and with God.[1]

Since 1980, the Christian Medical Commission has been involved in many discussions with people from different countries and cultures on the meaning of health and healing from a Christian perspective. One of the results of these discussions is the realization that health and healing cannot be limited to one area of life, but relates to all areas where there is "dis-ease," whether it be physical, mental, emotional, spiritual or social. Health and healing are therefore affected by such things as war, poverty, prejudice, and injustice; by attitudes of anger, guilt, resentment, and hopelessness; as well as the presence of physical disease and sickness.[2]

Two words often used in these discussions are **"harmony"** and **"wholeness."** Both words are commonly used today, and are not necessarily interpreted in a Christian way. Often "harmony" and "wholeness" are used to explain ideas in "New Age," Buddhist, and other health/spirituality perspectives, for example, in alternative/complementary medicine. So we speak of "harmony" of body, mind, and spirit, living in "harmony" with nature, and so forth. "Wholeness" is commonly used to refer to the totality of each person, for example.

Some Christians reject using words like "harmony" and "wholeness" because of possible non-Christian associations and connotations. But there is no need to reject them — rather we should ask whether they contain ideas which may help us to understand more clearly Christian and biblical perspectives on healing. Indeed, many writers on Christian healing ministry use these words because they point to valid ideas about health and healing, and use of contemporary language can help people understand more clearly what Christian healing is all about.

"Harmony" is from a Greek word "harmonia/harmos" which means "a fitting together of parts to form a smoothly connected whole." It can refer to musical harmony, when all the various parts of a musical score, or orchestra, or song, are in tune together, and are not discordant. It can also describe an agreeable understanding in thinking and action, which is free from dissent, strife, and conflict. It is also sometimes used in a medical sense to describe joints fitting and working together smoothly, for example, knee and elbow joints. When joints are damaged, they cause pain and discomfort, and can be thought of as "disjointed" or "out of harmony".

"Wholeness" refers to well-being in all aspects of life, which includes physical, emotional, intellectual, and spiritual health; and includes good relationships with other people in community and society. Wholeness is often defined by words such as "peace" and "integrity". Wholeness suggests a moving forward toward a greater harmony and well-being in every aspect of our lives. One writer comments on what it means to experience wholeness:

> Becoming whole does not mean being perfect, but being completed. It does not necessarily mean happiness, but growth. It is often painful, but fortunately, it is never boring. It is not getting out of life what we think we want, but it is the development and purification of the soul.[3]

If we use these words to describe health we could say that *being healthy* is to be whole and in harmony in all aspects of life, and *to be healed* is being restored to this state of wholeness and harmony.

These definitions are different from the popular understanding of health as relating primarily to physical health and fitness.

Many Christians use these words because they offer this comprehensive understanding, and also because they reflect the biblical understanding that a person can only be described as truly healthy when his or her *whole* being, including all their relationships, is functioning harmoniously.

But why refer to the Bible, the Christian scriptures, at all? If some contemporary words provide a good understanding of health and healing, why not use them, rather than going back to ancient scriptures? Are we not more advanced in our understanding of healing in the 21st century than ancient scriptures, which were written many hundreds of years ago?

The Christian perspective begins with the scriptures because Christians believe that they show or reveal God's purposes for all people. The scriptures explain and demonstrate God's desire that all people would experience the life and love of His kingdom; for God "wants all to be saved, and to come to a knowledge of the truth" (1 Tim 2:4), which includes a healing of body, mind, and spirit. The scriptures have authority for our understanding of healing ministry, because they are the written revelation of God's purposes for all people.

As the written revelation of God's purposes, the scriptures also provide a standard or benchmark offering perspectives and guidelines which help in evaluating many popular ideas about health, healing, relationships, and so forth. This is important and essential if Christians are to understand and relate in any meaningful way to the great numbers of people who accept and practice and base their lives on the great smorgasbord of popular therapies and theories which are available in the contemporary marketplace.

A further question is: If it is important to understand and examine the scriptural teaching about health and healing, where do Christians start? With the Old Testament or with the teaching of Jesus? Many Christians start with the work and teaching of Jesus, because healing was an essential aspect of his ministry, and the church's involvement in the healing ministry is based on his example and command. However, it is important to note that Jesus' teaching and practice was based on his understanding of God's presence and work among all peoples, especially the people of Israel, as this is revealed in the Old Testament scriptures. It was from this understanding that Jesus developed his own perspectives and expressions of healing, which affirmed, changed and expanded the Old Testament witness to God's healing power and presence. The Old Testament was "the Bible that Jesus read." The Old Testament perspectives formed a foundation for the New Testament.

But we must also keep in mind that the words and ideas of the Old Testament are expanded and fully expressed or "fulfilled" in the New Testament, especially in the life and ministry of Jesus. He fulfilled or "brought out the deeper meaning" of the Old Testament (see Matt 5:17). This means we must read the Old Testament scriptures in the light of Jesus, who affirms, critiques, and deepens their meaning. One of the church leaders in the second century gave a valuable principle of how to interpret the Old Testament: "We read and accept [the Old Testament], provided it is Jesus who reads it to us." (See Chapter Two for more discussion on the authority and interpretation of the scriptures in relation to the healing ministry.)

Health and Healing in the Scriptures[4]

The definition of *health* as "harmony" and "wholeness" is similar to the perspectives outlined in the scriptures, where the meaning of health depends on what we believe about the nature and destiny of men and women. The Christian faith has a definite and clear view of people as having been made in the image of God. And so the *overall* quality of health and well-being depends on the quality of the relationship between creator and creatures. The biblical understanding of health and healing is much more comprehensive than some modern concepts of health. A person can only be described as truly healthy when his or her whole being, including all relationships, is healthy. The most significant relationship is with God, and where this is fractured or disturbed, all other relationships are affected, whether within ourselves, with others, or with the environment in which we live. Both Old Testament and New Testament use a variety of words to express these ideas.

In the scriptures, the actual word "health" is not mentioned very much, but the idea of health is found throughout both the Old Testament and the New Testament.

Old Testament

Several words are used to describe the different aspects of sickness and healing. Some of the main words are:

"halah" is a common word for sickness or being ill, for example, 1 Sam 19:14; 1 Kings 14:1. It refers to feeling weak or failing, as in Gen 45:1. It also describes general discomfort, the weakness of old age, being bruised and wounded (compare with "feeling poorly").

"nagap/naka" means to be stricken with some disability or sickness, for example, blindness (Gen 19: l), crippled feet (2 Sam 4:4), tumors (1 Sam 5:12), plague (1 Chron 21:14).

"sapo" refers to the cure of physical sickness, leading to recovery and normal functioning, that is, "to get better" (2 Kings 5:3, 6, 7, 11).

"rapha" is one of the most frequently used words in the Old Testament, and is used to describe the character of God as healer. The Lord is "Jehovah Rophe" (Exodus 15:26). It means to patch up,

to mend, and to unite something which has been torn apart, to restore something which has been broken to its original condition. The word is applied to many different situations, for example, restoration from physical disease (Exodus 15:26); repairing an altar (1 Kings 18:30); sweetening water (2 Kings 2:21-22); healing the hurts of the nation (Hosea 6:11); healing damaged emotions (Psalm 147:3-4); restoring land to productivity (2 Chron 7:14); and the cure of specific diseases, for example, leprosy (Numbers 12:13).

Note that these biblical words usually are used in a literal way to describe physical and emotional healing. But sometimes these words are also used as metaphors to describe emotional, spiritual, social, and national healing and recovery, including the restoration of the land to good production.

"shalom" is sometimes regarded as the golden word, as it combines many of these Old Testament ideas. It is often translated as peace, health, well-being, and is used in three main ways:

- It describes general physical well-being, being in good health, being OK, being "all right" (2 Kings 5:21-22); being in a state of "rightness" including inward peace (Numbers 6:24-26). In Psalm 38:3 there is no health, or soundness, no shalom, because of the feelings of sin and guilt. It also has the idea of overflowing abundance (Jeremiah 33:6-9). These references suggest a positive, active presence of health and well-being, not just the absence of conflict and illness. (Compare this abundance and presence with the WHO definition, quoted above.)

- It refers to positive social relationships, for example, peaceful relations between nations 1 Kings 5:12; a covenant of peace and harmony between God and his people (Ezekiel 34:23-26, Isaiah 54:10); a peace expressed in justice and right relationships in society (Isaiah 32:16-17).

- It describes attitudes of honesty and integrity in moral and ethical living — to seek peace and to act with integrity (Psalm 34:11-15); for example, a man of peace is one who is "upright and of good character" (Psalm 37:37).

So *shalom* suggests well-being, completeness, soundness, harmony, and well-being in physical, emotional, social, national, and even international relationships, affecting the earth itself.

When these Old Testament words are taken together, it is clear that "health" has a very wide meaning — referring to all aspects of a person's life. But it is more than just fine ideas. Health never exists in a vacuum, but must be shown in daily living. Health involves lifestyle choices, obedience to God's law, ethical and moral decisions, and integrity in all relationships. And overarching all these aspects is the foundation of a right relationship with God. When people are "right," in "harmonious relationship" with God and obedient to his law and covenant, then they are truly healthy (for example, Psalm 1, 24:3-5), even though they may be physically sick and in some form of distress. If this God-ward relationship is broken or damaged or is non-existent, then there is profound spiritual ill health which flows over into all other areas of life, causing "dis-ease," which may manifest itself in many different ways.

To sum up, the basic idea of health in the Old Testament is of sound and healthy relationships. Healing includes the whole person in all their relationships — to God, to others, to themselves, and to the physical environment in which they live.

New Testament

The New Testament builds on the Old Testament understanding of health, with several words which give a wide understanding and show the variety of meaning used in the idea of health.

Hugies/hugieia is derived from Hygieia, the Greek goddess of health, and has the basic idea of soundness. In the New Testament, the word refers to the soundness or wholesomeness of teaching (Titus 2:8). When used in relation to health, it means physical soundness or completeness, and includes the idea of freedom or release from any limitation; for example, the lame man at the pool of Bethsaida, whose limbs were made sound for him to take up his bed and walk (John 5:1-9). Jesus' question to the man, "Do you want to be whole?" could be translated, "Do you want to be *sound*, or freed from your limitations?" (Compare Mark 5:34 — "Be freed from your suffering.") *Hugieia* is also used to translate the Hebrew word, *shalom*.

Eirene describes the state of peace, harmony and rest, as opposed to a state of conflict, war and disturbance. It is the most common translation of *shalom*, and includes the idea of wholeness, and is especially applied to man's relationship with God, which is described as "peace through Jesus Christ" (Romans 5:1). This harmonious relationship between God and man is also to be expressed in all human relationships (2 Corinthians 13:11; 1 Thessalonians 5:13). Jesus pronounces this peace to the woman healed from severe bleeding (Mark 5:34).

Zoe refers to life in its highest and fullest sense: it is "life in all its fullness," "abundant life," "eternal life" (John 10:10, 17:2). *Bios* is the normal human life in which we all share, but Jesus offers *zoe*, the highest form of life, as the gift of God. It consists of the true knowledge of God, which comes from a true relationship with God. *Zoe* as described in the New Testament is concerned not only with human physical life, but with a higher, eternal quality of life, which is not only temporal and physical, but also spiritual and eternal. The truly healthy person is the one who has *zoe*.

Teleios has the meaning of maturity, and is sometimes translated as "perfect". Something is perfect when it attains the purpose for which it was created; it is moving toward maturity and completeness, with the incomplete being left behind (Matthew 5:48; Ephesians

4:13). The healthy person is the person growing to maturity in spiritual and moral understanding.

Sozo means being "safe" and "sound", and is connected with the idea of freedom and deliverance from some danger, or disease, to a safe, sound and healthy condition. It is sometimes translated as salvation, at other times as wholeness, or as health. Whenever it is used, *sozo* always refers to the whole person, whether the disease is physical, spiritual, mental or emotional. So Jesus says to the woman with the flow of blood, "Your faith has healed you" (Mark 5:34), and to the woman who is a sinner, "Your faith has saved you" (Luke 7:50). In each situation, it has the idea of the healing of the body along with the healing of the whole person.

Therapeuo is the root of words like "therapy" and "therapeutic". It originally meant to give some service to someone; for example, giving medical treatment to a person to restore them to health. *Therapeuo* is used for many of the miraculous healings of Jesus, both physical healings and also exorcism. Jesus often used this word to describe his own healing activity (Matthew 8:7; Luke 14:3). Jesus also used the word when the disciples were commissioned for their ministry (Matthew 10:8; Luke 10:9).

Iaomai/iatros is the word for physician and refers to healing or cure from disease and sickness. It is the word which Luke uses often, probably because he was a physician, and it refers almost exclusively to physical healing (Luke 9:2).[5]

When we turn from these biblical meanings to our modern understanding we find a significant difference. There are very few English words which convey the deep and comprehensive meaning of the Hebrew and Greek words for health and healing. Often the words "health" or "healing" or "whole" in English are used in limited ways to refer to physical or perhaps emotional well-being or fitness, but our usage tends to ignore the wider meanings involving social relationships and attitudes, and there is often no reference to any spiritual dimension at all. We settle for a popular but narrow understanding of health and healing, and allow ourselves to be shaped by modern-day attitudes and assumptions, rather than wider biblical perspectives.

These modern-day attitudes and assumptions also affect the way many Christians think about the healing ministry. For example, many healing services focus primarily, if not entirely, on physical healing. If prayer is sought or offered, most expect that it will be directed to individual physical healing, with perhaps some minor references to emotional healing; and to spiritual healing, usually in the area of deliverance and demonic oppression. Much of the literature on the healing ministry focuses on individual and personal wellness, that is, being free from disease and sickness afflicting the human body, or on overcoming and releasing a person from the power of evil. These are important aspects of the total healing ministry, but should not be so emphasized as to cause serious neglect of other wider social meanings of healing. (See Chapter 14 for a discussion of the wider social dimensions.)

So it is important to understand health and healing in a *comprehensive* way and to resist the temptation to interpret the biblical understanding according to our (often) limited contemporary understanding and isolated experiences of health and healing. It should be the other way round — that is, we bring our contemporary emphases and evaluate them in the light of the biblical material.

When these ideas from Old Testament and New Testament are taken together, they give a very broad understanding of health, which can be summarized in these statements:

• The meaning of health is to be in right relationships, of men and women to God, to themselves, to the neighbor and to the environment. The most important of these relationships is with God. If this relationship is right, then the others will flow from this. However, if the relationship with God is fractured or neglected, then all the other relationships will be out of harmony and will lack shalom.

- Health is God's will. God wants all people to be "healthy," in a true relationship with Him. When men and women are in this relationship, this becomes the foundation for being truly healthy.

- Health is the gift of God. Life and health cannot be demanded, but accepted as God's gift and used accordingly. The contemporary demand to recognize health as a basic right for all people is good, in that it seeks to care for the total well-being of people, but it is inadequate insofar as it ignores any relationship with God, for true health cannot exist independently of God.

- Health is of the whole person; spirit, soul and body belong together and cannot be separated. People cannot be broken into parts which exist in isolation, but all are interlocked together. Thus Paul speaks of spirit, soul and body being kept blameless, because it is the whole person who is involved (1 Thessalonians 5:23).

- Because true health is concerned with all our human relationships, it is to be measured by the standard of Jesus Christ. As perfect man, he was truly healthy in all aspects of his life — physically, mentally, socially and spiritually — and thus Jesus is the standard for the Christian disciple of what it means to be truly healthy in all aspects of life and in our relationship with God.

A Christian Understanding of Healing

From this biblical understanding, it is now possible to emphasize some important aspects of Christian healing.

All people need healing. The Christian understanding of men and women is that their relationship with God has been fractured and broken by sin and disobedience and this relationship needs to be restored. All people need restoration to well-being, in body, mind, and spirit because all have sinned and turned away from God (Romans 3:23).

All healing is from God. We are not able to heal ourselves, and healing occurs because of the activity of God in His creation and in our lives and situations. The insights and skills of medicine make use of what God has provided in His creation and in His providential care. The church gives thanks to God for this provision and seeks to work with the medical profession in using the good gifts which God has given; but the church also believes that God has provided special resources in His act of salvation through Jesus Christ, and these resources are essential for a true understanding of the healing which God offers.

Healing is God's purpose for all people, so that they may experience fellowship with Him, in which all brokenness and alienation is overcome.

Healing relates to the whole person. Sickness or ill health may be physical, mental, emotional, social and spiritual, and all of these may need healing. One aspect may be predominant in some situations — for example, physical sickness, social conflict, spiritual maladjustment — but healing refers to the well-being of the *whole person*; so a healing ministry should address matters which cause dis-ease in *all* areas of life. This may include such issues as poverty, injustice and war, as these are some of the basic causes for physical, emotional and spiritual sickness.

Healing is more than physical cure. Often the words "healing" and "cure" appear to have the same meaning; however a distinction can and should be made between them. *Cure* refers to the removal of some disease, or the restoring of something lacking in the body; whereas *healing* has a much wider meaning, referring to the wholeness of body, mind and spirit.

It is possible for people to be cured without being truly healed and also to be substantially healed without necessarily being cured. In the New Testament the story of the ten lepers illustrates the difference between cure and healing (Luke 17:11-19). All ten were cured of their leprosy, but only one of them returned to give thanks. The failure of nine lepers to return to give thanks indicated to Jesus a lack which called into question the quality and extent of their healing.

In the same way, it is possible for a person to receive surgery and excellent medical care and to be cured from a physical problem, but not to have grown in any other way in his or her life. The person cured of a physical illness may not experience healing in their deeper relationships. In the New Testament, many instances of healing refer to the cure or healing of a person's physical ailment, and so physical healing is an essential part of the total ministry given by Jesus to the church; but physical healing is only one part of the wholeness which is God's purpose for us.

Healing is not complete in this life. We remain part of a creation marked by decay and frustration, and our minds and bodies are witness to this fact (Romans 8:18-25). Our bodies, minds, and spirits need constant nutrition, rest, and renewal to rebuild and to prevent decay. We are all subject to disability and death, and complete healing and health is not possible in this mortal life. We may be able to experience "substantial healing" in this life, but only in the future life will we find complete well-being of body, mind and spirit.

Healing is the concern of the church. If health and healing are God's purpose for men and women, then it is the task of the church to be involved in helping to achieve this purpose. The message of the gospel is that healing and salvation are available in Jesus Christ, and the church is commissioned to share this Good News.

Some Contemporary Definitions

The comprehensive understanding of healing given above is seen in the following statements from different authors. As you read each statement, note and underline what you see as the most significant ideas and words.

- Healing is the process of restoring the broken harmony which prevents personality, at any point of body, mind or spirit, from its perfect functioning in its relevant environment; the body in the natural world, the mind in the realm of ideas, and the spirit in its relation to God.[6]

- The purpose of the healing ministry is to help people maintain a healthy balance among body, mind and spirit, and to assist in correcting any imbalance and in making whole that which is broken or not functioning properly. Wholeness does not necessarily mean perfect physical health.[7]

- Healing is a pastoral function that aims to overcome some impairment by restoring a person to wholeness and by leading him (or her) to advance beyond his (or her) previous experience. The wholeness which pastoral healing seeks to achieve is not simply restoration of circumstances that prevailed before impairment began. Rather . . . it is hoped that the person will become integrated on a higher spiritual level than previously experienced. Healing is more than mere restoration, for it includes a forward gain over the condition prevailing before illness.[8]

- Health is a dynamic state of well-being of the individual and society, of physical, mental, spiritual, economic, political and social well-being — of being in harmony with each other, with the material environment and with God.[9]

- Good health is harmony of relationships, harmony within

ourselves and with ourselves, with other people, with things, and with God. Sickness is disharmony in any or all of these.[10]

- Because Jesus Christ is at the center of the healing ministry and health is to be measured by his standard, then any definition must include this emphasis. Thus, Bishop Morris Maddocks defines Christian healing as: "Jesus Christ meeting you at your point of need." He explains the definition in these words:

Christian healing is, first and foremost, about Christ. It follows the pattern he set in his own ministry, and the commission he gave to his disciples, and the fact that it happens at all is the fruit of his work, both in the creation, and in the salvation of mankind. In both these mighty works, humankind has been created and recreated in the image of God — has been made whole. This is what distinguishes Christian healing from other types of healing. It is the whole work of Christ, in a person's body, mind and spirit, designed to bring that person to that wholeness which is God's will for us all.[11]

Conclusion

If the aim of the Order of St. Luke is the restoration of the healing ministry as a normal part of church life, the following ideas should be part of such a ministry:

- The aim of any healing ministry will be to restore an individual to a dynamic sense of well-being and to bring wholeness to a person's body, mind and spirit, so that all their relationships are being made whole.

- The healing ministry should be directed to the community and society, as well as to the individual, because social relationships need to be healed also. This suggests a wider understanding of healing than is often practiced in many churches, where the focus is often only on the individual person and any social factors and social illness is ignored. This means that healing must be concerned with social conditions and issues like justice, oppression, economic and political exploitation, all of which affect the well-being of people.

- The healing ministry should be firmly based on a biblical understanding of health and healing and focused on Jesus Christ as the true Healer.

The chapters that follow will take up many of the particular issues contained in this chapter. There will be a consideration of healing as related to physical, emotional and spiritual healing, as this is the ministry in which the Order of St. Luke is most directly engaged, but the wider aspects of healing will also be considered, to gain a comprehensive understanding of this ministry.

Sharing and Discussion

1. What are some of the ideas about health which are common in our society today? How did you form your ideas of health? — from your education in school? from your family situations? from the media? from your culture and society?

2. Compare the commonly accepted ideas about health with the biblical understanding of health and healing. In what ways does our contemporary understanding of health need to be corrected? Do the biblical ways of understanding need to be re-evaluated and corrected in the light of today's discoveries and insights into health problems?

3. Reflect on the various definitions of health and the healing ministry provided above in this chapter. Which emphases do you find helpful in clarifying your own understanding of the healing ministry?

4. Morris Maddocks distinguishes between "Christian healing and

other types of healing." Do you think this is a valid way of thinking, or do you think that "Christian healing" is just the same as other types of healing which do not claim to be Christian in their understanding?

5. Think about the words of J. A. Sanford concerning wholeness: "It does not mean being perfect, but being completed. It does not necessarily mean happiness, but growth. It is often painful but fortunately, it is never boring . . . "

How do you respond to this understanding of wholeness as it relates to your own life experience? Is it a valid way to think about wholeness, or do you have some problems with it?

6. What does the understanding of health and healing as wholeness mean for:

(a) Your individual life?

(b) The life of a congregation in a local church situation?

(c) The role of the congregation and church in the community?

References for Further Reading

Brown M., *Israel's Divine Healer*, Zondervan, Grand Rapids, Michigan, 1995.

Christian Medical Commission, *Healing and Wholeness, The Church's Role in Health*, WCC, Geneva, 1990.

Maddocks, M., *Twenty Questions about Healing*, SPCK, London, 1981.

Maddocks, M., *The Christian Healing Ministry*. SPCK, London 1990.

Health, Faith and Healing, International Review of Mission, WCC Geneva, Vol. 90, Nos. 356/357, Jan/April 2001.

Sanford, J. A., *Healing and Wholeness*, Paulist, N.Y., 1977.

Wagner, J. K., *Blessed to be a Blessing*, The Upper Room, Nashville, 1980.

Wellock, P., *In Search of Wholeness — A Christian Perspective*. OSL Australia, 2005.

Wilkinson, J., *Health and Healing*, Handsel Press, Edinburgh, 1980.

Wilkinson, J., *Healing and the Church*, Handsel Press, Edinburgh, 1984.

Wilkinson, J., *The Bible and Healing*, Eerdmans, Grand Rapids, 1998.

2
THE AUTHORITY AND COMMISSION TO HEAL PART I — THE OLD TESTAMENT AND THE GOSPELS

Today there are many conflicting voices and claims to authority, so the question: "What is the authority for the healing ministry in the church today?" is of fundamental importance.

Three people who are all into the healing ministry were discussing the reasons why they are involved.

Reg is a member of a healing group because he feels he has a natural gift of healing. Whenever he lays hands on people something seems to happen and the people are often healed or very much better. He believes this "power" is part of the universal energy and he is able to use it because he simply accepts it, and is open to this energy. He is not a religious person, in the sense of belonging to any church, but believes that when he opens himself to this energy he then has the right to lay hands on people for their healing. Reg believes it is a natural right and a natural gift available to anyone. The authority for his healing work is in his own understanding of the natural power of the universe in which he shares and which he is using.

Evelyn is a health technician, trained in the field of medicine and psychology, but also with an awareness of some of the areas of alternative healing therapies. Evelyn is skeptical of the claims made by alternative therapies, but nevertheless she does not dismiss them entirely. Evelyn is a very competent, caring person who is constantly seeking to bring healing to people and to meet their total health needs. She is skeptical of those who claim to have any special healing gift, and she does not respond eagerly to the idea that prayer, meditation and other methods are valid ways of healing. When Evelyn is asked about her authority for her work as a health technician, she responds by listing all the training she has received, the experience of actually dealing with patients, and the technical skills and other professional qualifications of the medical workers in her community. The authority by which Evelyn works is in the profession to which she belongs and stems from the training she has received.

Phil is a Christian who believes he has a role to play in the healing ministry simply because he is a disciple of Jesus Christ. He believes that Jesus Christ commissioned his followers to heal the sick. Phil has no medical degree or training, nor does he feel he has any particular gift of healing, but he believes that he ought to be involved in the healing ministry because the Bible tells him to do so. Phil believes the Bible to be the book which reveals and shows clearly God's purpose for people. In the Bible it is clear that God is the healer (Exodus 15:26), that Jesus Christ healed the sick (Matthew 4:23), and that the church is commissioned to continue this ministry today (Luke 9:1; James 5:13-16). When asked where his authority comes from, Phil quickly responds, "From the words of Jesus in the Bible. Without those words in the Bible, I would have no authority to be involved."

Here are three different sources of authority among many others. There is authority within ourselves; there is authority as part of a professionally trained system; there is authority in the words of Jesus in the Bible.

- Are all these sources of authority of equal value and what is the authority for the modern church to be involved in the healing ministry?

- Respond to this question and share your ideas with others.

This chapter aims to:

- Understand the Christian claim that the authority for the healing ministry is found in understanding God's purpose far His people, as this is shown in the scriptures, especially in the ministry of Jesus.

- Understand the Old Testament perspectives on of sickness and healing;

- Study the healing ministry of Jesus and see how his understanding and practice of healing related to the Old Testament understanding.

What is Authority?

A simple definition is: "Authority is the right to command belief, or practice." There are different types of authority.

- Authority may be given in a formal position which is recognized by others. This can be called an *extrinsic* authority; that is, something outside the person. For example, a police officer has authority because of his position and can therefore command a particular action. The Prime Minister or President has authority because of the office that he holds.

- There is another kind of authority – called *intrinsic* authority — which is inward or inherent within a person or thing by virtue of knowledge or lifestyle or skill. Someone can be recognized as an authority on a particular subject because of his (or her) knowledge. Also, a book may be accepted as an authority on a given subject because of the breadth of knowledge it contains. For example, the Guinness Book of Records possesses an authority which has been built up over the years. In relation to people, someone like Mother Theresa speaks with authority, because of her lifestyle and commitment to the poor.

- Jesus spoke with an inherent authority, even though he was not one of the official scribes and teachers of the law (Matthew 7:28, 29). This was not an official authority, but rather what can be called a *charismatic* authority, as a result of being filled with the Holy Spirit. People were impressed with his authority and they responded with awe and humility (Mark 5:6, 22; Luke 7:1-10). His sense of purpose and presence imparted an authority to his words and actions. It was a spiritual authority given from God and not dependent on any official position recognized by society.

Where, then, is the authority for the belief in, and practice of, the healing ministry today? Is it given as part of an official position; for example, as with the leader of a church, or is the authority within each person, or only within those with special healing gifts? This question is part of a larger issue on the nature of religious authority in general. Where do the various religious systems get their authority for belief and practice? Some derive their authority from a particular set of writings, which are believed to be supernaturally given; some from the traditions which have been built up over many centuries; some from the writings of particular people; and some from the sense of the divine within each person. How can we evaluate the truth of these authorities and decide which are to be accepted over all others, or whether all authority carries equal validity, be it from a human or divine source? The basic question is: Is there a Supreme Being higher than anything or anyone in the created order who has the right (authority) to determine what we are to believe and how we are to live?

For the Christian, God is the supreme authority because He is the creator and redeemer of all people and is not dependent on others for His existence. As the eternal God, He continues to sustain and provide for the needs of the created order, and for all people who share in the life of the world. Because of who He is and what He does, He has a rightful authority to prescribe belief and behavior.

If God is the ultimate authority, can we know His purpose and intention for our human lives and for the life of the world? Can we know what is the true belief and practice? The Christian response is: "Yes, we can know God, His providence, love, mercy, forgiveness, holiness, strength and His purposes for us." This knowledge is the true wisdom and is greater than any other knowledge or power (Jeremiah 9:23, 24). But from where do we get this treasured knowledge?

Is our human reason sufficient to give us this knowledge? The power of human reason is wonderful, but it cannot give a complete understanding, because God is beyond and deeper than our ability to reason and think. Also, our human powers of reasoning have been infected by our disobedience and sin and there is often a moral resistance to the truth. Human intelligence is a great gift, but by itself it cannot give the true knowledge of God (1 Corinthians 1:21). But can we gain this true knowledge of God through spiritual experiences which are part of our human experience and are found in every religious system? Such experiences may claim to show the true way and bring illumination and meaning into our lives. However, these experiences can also be very subjective and lack any objective reality; and are affected by our twisted thinking and disobedience and can distort the truth and make God in a human image, which is idolatry. Paul explains this universal human dilemma in Romans 1:18-31, especially Romans 1:21-23. So the questions remain: Can you fathom the mysteries of God? Can you probe the limits of the Almighty (Job 11:7)? The answer is "No." Neither human reason nor spiritual experience can give complete certainty in our knowledge of God.

The Christian answer is that God cannot be truly known as the result of people's search for Him (either through reason or spiritual experience), but only through God's self-revelation or self-disclosure to men and women, that is through divine revelation.

How does God reveal His purpose to us? Some say through direct action in the lives of people, or through a direct word of guidance, or through a particular person. While it is possible for God to use many different ways, the Christian belief is that God has chosen to reveal His purpose and express His authority primarily through the person Jesus Christ, and all other ways of revelation must be subject to the revelation or self-disclosure given in Him. But where is the revelation of Jesus Christ to be found? Only in the Bible, because it reveals the purpose of God as this is worked out in the history of Israel and in Jesus Christ and the church. God continues to speak to us through this written record. The Bible, therefore, is the primary source for any understanding of God and is the standard by which other knowledge must be tested. It is the inspired record of the special actions of God in the world, and is the source of truth in understanding His purposes. So Christians accept the Bible as the record of God's special revelation of His purpose and describe it as "The Word of God"; that is, the way by which God's purpose is communicated to us.

This emphasis on the Bible as The Word of God, the record of the divine revelation, does not mean that it is against human reason (anti-rational), or against spiritual experience (anti-mystical). These are good gifts of God, but the Bible has a greater authority which informs our reason and interprets our spiritual experience.

Nor does it mean that there is no knowledge of God outside the Bible. There is also a "general" revelation of God in creation and history. His existence can be clearly seen in the created universe (Romans 1:20). However this general revelation is limited and needs to be enlarged and interpreted by God's special revelation in Israel, and in Jesus Christ and the church, and it is this special revelation which is recorded in scripture.

The claim that the Bible is the primary source for our understanding of God does not contradict the fact that Jesus is the full and complete revelation of God to mankind. To see him is to see the Father (John 14:9). However the important question is: "Where is the true knowledge of Jesus Christ to be found?"

Today there are many bogus Christs being offered to the world, many of which are based on human understanding; for example, Jesus Christ Superstar, Jesus Christ the anti-colonial fighter, Jesus Christ the humanitarian moralist, Jesus Christ the master guru, and so on. An example of this is the New Age teaching which describes Jesus as one of the many evolutionary forerunners of a new earth and a new humanity, or a great example of cosmic consciousness (see Chapter 11 on Alternative Healing Movements).

Because there are so many conflicting interpretations of Jesus, we must ask the question: "Will the real Jesus please stand up"? "Which is the true picture of him?" The Christian answer is that the only truly valid account of Jesus' life and ministry is found in the scriptures; so our understanding and confession of Jesus Christ as Lord and Savior must be according to the scriptures. He is the Living Word, who is made known to us through the pages of the written word. Any other Jesus is inadequate and, in the end, is really an impostor. So, we cannot do away with the need for the Bible, because it is the true record of God's revelation in Jesus Christ. It, therefore, is the source of our understanding of God and is the written Word of God which leads us to the Living Word of Jesus Christ. It is not just a dead story about events which took place in the past, but it is living and active and as sharp as a sword (Hebrews 4: 12), as the Holy Spirit quickens and applies its message to our lives. Insight and understanding into the meaning of scripture is given through the ministry of the Holy Spirit, who guides us into all truth (John 14:26; 16:13-15).[1]

Thus, when the question is asked: "What is the authority for the Christian healing ministry?" the answer is: "This authority is found in the words and actions of Jesus, as these are recorded in the scriptures." The Order of St. Luke affirms that "the New Testament clearly teaches that the healing of mind and body was a very real part of the total ministry of our Lord and that he commissioned his followers to continue this ministry."

The healing ministry is therefore accepted as an integral part of the mission of Jesus and the gospel, which is given to the church. This is well expressed by George Bennett:

> The healing ministry is not just a movement we are trying to push, not just a legitimate concern of the church to be placed alongside many others. Healing is not an optional extra, but is basic and central. It derives its authority from the lips of the Lord himself; it is rooted in the gospel and is an integral part of it.[2]

If the authority for the healing ministry is to be found in the teaching and practice of Jesus Christ, as given in the scriptures, then it is important to understand the following:

- The Old Testament perspectives on healing.

- The New Testament understanding of healing in the ministry of Jesus as recorded in the gospels.

- The healing ministry in the Early Church, as recorded in the Acts of the Apostles and other New Testament writings.

- The relevance and authority of this biblical material for our situation today.

This chapter will deal with the first two points and the following chapter with the last two points.[3]

Old Testament Perspectives on Healing

We have already noted some of the Old Testament words and ideas about health and healing which formed part of the worldview of God's people, as they lived out their lives in the cultural situations depicted in the Old Testament. The people of Israel were surrounded by many nations and peoples, all of whom had their particular ideas about healing, and these ideas and practices often influenced the people of Israel. But there were certain foundation ideas which formed the "world-view" of Israel, and it was on these foundational ideas that their understanding and practice of healing was built.

God is the creator and His creation is good. Harmony exists between God and the creation, but this is broken by the human desire for the knowledge of good and evil. This disobedience is met by both judgment and mercy. It results in expulsion from the presence of God, but also in the promise of a future salvation (Genesis 1-3).

As creator, God is the source of both healing and sickness. He is the personal, active Lord, the source of all power and all the issues of life and death. Because of their strong belief in one God (monotheism), the Hebrews rejected any idea of sickness and suffering deriving from demonic powers of various gods and spirits. God is the source of all: good and evil, sickness and health, life and death (Exodus 4:11; Deuteronomy 32:39; Isaiah 45:7).

The belief in the powers of gods and spirits was common to many people; for example, Egyptians, Babylonians, Persians; and they ascribed sickness to these powers of darkness. Israel was only gradually influenced by these ideas, and they did not greatly affect the foundation ideas of God as creator and the source of both healing and sickness for many years. It was later in Israel's history — especially after the exile from about 400 BC onward — that these ideas from other nations began to have a stronger influence in Israel's understanding. Before then, God was seen as the Lord of all, and therefore there could be no other source of sickness but God alone. If God was the source of sickness, then He must have a good purpose in mind.

These two ideas; that is, God as creator and God as the source of both healing and sickness, provided the foundation for the dominant view of healing in which sickness is interpreted as God's rebuke and punishment for sin which involved the breaking of the ritualistic or moral law. Those who were disobedient to God's law received the consequences in natural disasters and physical disease (Leviticus 26:16, 25; Deuteronomy 28:27-29), while obedience to the laws of God, and honesty and justice in living, brought blessing. Health and wealth bring rewards, and sickness, poverty and misfortune are the divine punishments (Exodus 15:26).

In the Old Testament there are many examples of the strong link between sickness and sin. For example, Pharaoh's household is struck down because Sarah is taken into the palace (Genesis 12:17). The Egyptians' hardness of heart brings physical illness and death of the firstborn (Exodus 9:8-10, 12-29). Miriam is struck with leprosy because she slandered Moses (Numbers 12: 10); also Gahazi suffers the same fate for his greed (2 Kings 5:26, 27). (See also Genesis 19:11; Exodus 4:6, 7; Numbers 14:11, 12; 17:12-13, 25:3-9; 2 Samuel 24:10-15.) This *"disciplinary"* understanding of sickness and sin is also expressed in the many Psalms where sickness, both physical and emotional, are seen to come from God (Psalm 38:1-8, 39:1-5, 88:1-9, 102:1-11; Proverbs 3:7, 8, 11, 12). The main point is clear — to follow wisdom and the law will bring health and long life, but to do otherwise will result in misery, misfortune, sickness and death. An important aspect of the disciplinary understanding of the Old Testament is that sickness and healing are *corporate* as well as *individual* experiences. Israel is a people under a corporate covenant with God, and the individual does not stand alone. When one persons sins, the whole community is affected, and the healing of the individual flows on to the healing of the community.

The basis for this **"disciplinary"** theory came from the rejection of any principle of evil or evil spirits apart from God as the cause of sickness. Because there was no spiritual power independent of

God, then God must have a purpose in using sickness as a discipline to motivate people toward holy living. The teaching of the Old Testament prophets on the righteousness of God strengthens this connection between sickness and sin, and it not only became the dominant thinking among the Jews in Old Testament times, but also carried over into New Testament time. For example, compare the disciples' question to Jesus in John 9:1-4: Jesus saw a man blind from birth. His disciples asked him, `Rabbi, who sinned, this man or his parents, that he was born blind?' Jesus answered, `Neither this man nor his parents sinned, but this happened so that the work of God might be displayed in his life.'" (The disciples' understanding appears in much thinking about sickness and healing, and remains strong in many quarters today). For Israel, then, the dominant belief was that sickness represented a break-down in relationship between God and His people, and it could not be healed until the relationship with God had been restored through repentance, confession, obedience to the requirements of the law, and forgiveness.

However, there was another important strand of teaching which never became the dominant understanding of the Hebrew people. It is expressed in some healing stories; some Psalms; some Isaiah passages; and especially in the book of Job. There are examples where it is clearly recognized that God can and does heal, but where there is no apparent connection between the sickness experienced and sinful wrongdoing. For example, many women who were unable to have children were blessed by God, as He healed their barrenness. There does not appear to be any sin involved in their situations (Genesis 18:10; Judges 13:5, 24; 1 Samuel 1:19, 20; 2 Kings 4:16, 17). Both Elijah and Elisha perform healings, but no sin is attributed to the sick person (1 Kings 17:17-23; 2 Kings 4:18-37, 5:14). In some Psalms God protects from plague and pestilence (Psalm 91), and God heals all diseases (Psalm 103). He is the healer of body, mind and spirit, and also of social and political situations (Psalms 41, 46, 74, 116, 121). Isaiah also refers to the Day of the Lord, the coming Messiah, when the ills of humanity will be healed (Isaiah 35:5-6, 61:1-11). In all these references healing is given by God, but it does not appear to be directly connected to sin, although it can be said that man's disobedience may form a general background in all of these situations.

The greatest challenge to the dominant "disciplinary" theory is the book of Job, which emphasizes that sickness and misfortune may not always come as a result of sin and disobedience. This is the story of a righteous man who fears God and does no evil, but who suffers terribly in relation to his possessions, family, physical health, reputation, friendships, and status in his society. Job suffers physically, yet there is no apparent cause for this in his faith and lifestyle. His friends try to maintain the legalistic "disciplinary" theory of the origin of sickness as due to sin, but this cannot be upheld in this situation. There are also suggestions that alien forces are at work in the world which are opposed to God, and they are partly responsible for many of the trials and difficulties that humans encounter. In spite of all the adversity and the taunts and advice of others, Job maintains his faith in God and in the end, he finds healing in a new and vivid experience of God's power. The book does not give a clear answer to the problem of sickness and suffering, but it does present a different perspective which does not fit into the dominant and accepted understanding of that time.

(It is the broader understanding which Jesus develops in his ministry, even though it runs counter to the official teaching of the religious leaders of his day.)

In summary, the Old Testament sees healing as involving a restored relationship with God and the community. The causes of sickness may be varied, and there is a strong emphasis on the connection between sin and sickness. But there are also other ideas which do not emphasize this connection, and begin to question its validity as a way to explain all sickness and misfortune. Overall, healing is described and experienced as *shalom*, and includes the idea of well-being, completeness, justice, self-discipline and obedience, leading to a true community with others and with God.

Healing in the Ministry of Jesus[4]

When Jesus began his ministry there was a lot of healing being practiced in the world of the first century. There were many healing cults and shrines to which people flocked to gain relief from illness and disease. In Judaism, there were popular healing places where it was believed healing could be experienced at certain times; for example, at the Pool in Jerusalem (John 5:1-14). Jesus therefore did not come into a vacuum situation, as far as healing is concerned. He was one of many healers, and he would be familiar with the ideas and practices of healing at that time.

His uniqueness, therefore, is not that he was the only healer (he was one amongst many), but it was rather in his understanding and practice of healing as revealing the power of the kingdom, and releasing God's creative and loving Spirit to act upon the moral, mental, and physical illnesses of the people around him. As the promised Messiah, Jesus revealed God's essential nature. He was God's special messenger and his healings revealed the true attitude of God toward sickness and all forms of "dis-ease," personal, social, and spiritual.

The healing ministry of Jesus is given an important place in each of the gospels. The general references to healing, including the narrative stories of healing (for example, the healing miracles), occupy approximately one-fifth of the gospel record. This shows that the gospel writers regarded healing as an important part of Jesus' total ministry. However, it is also clear that healing was only one aspect of his ministry, and therefore should not be either over-emphasized or under-emphasized. Matthew 4:23 and 9:35 give a threefold emphasis in his ministry of teaching, preaching, and healing. On some occasions, Jesus emphasized the primary importance of teaching and preaching the good news of the kingdom (for example, Mark 1:38). This emphasis on teaching and preaching is especially strong in Matthew and Mark, so healing must always be seen in relation to these other activities. It is important, but should not be seen as the primary or the only purpose of his coming.

Also, within the healing ministry of Jesus, there was both a "narrow" and a "wider" expression of this ministry. The "narrow" expression is seen in his concern for **the individual** person, in their physical, emotional, and spiritual need. So the paralyzed, blind, diseased, demon-possessed received his attention. A quick reading of the healing incidents could suggest that his ministry was therefore only directed to individual people. Certainly the church over the centuries has interpreted the New Testament in this way, and has therefore focused more on the individual approach, and directed its teaching and ministry toward the spiritual, emotional and physical healing of individual people, whether through prayer, and other spiritual means, or through the practice of medical care.

However, there was also a "wider" dimension in Jesus' ministry. He was concerned to restore health, not just to the individual, but to the **"individual within community"**. That is, Jesus responded to people who were part of wider social structures involving many complex relationships. For example, see Luke 4:18-21 and Luke 7:18-23, where he applies the words of the prophet Isaiah to describe his ministry. Issues relating to poverty, oppression, injustice are affirmed as essential aspects of his mission to transform and renew the whole of human society; these are social rather than strictly individual issues.

This wider concern has often been neglected by the church because it is not immediately apparent in the way Jesus' ministry has been described and interpreted. This is especially so when the healing stories of the gospel are read, interpreted and applied by people from "individually" oriented communities and cultures, especially many Western cultures. Both the "wider" and the "narrower" expression of Jesus' healing work need to be kept together to form a balanced understanding. [3]

The following points summarize some of the main features of Jesus' healing ministry. No detailed study of any of the healing incidents is given, because this would be a separate study in itself.[4]

Jesus healed a great variety of sickness: physical, emotional and psychological.[5] (Refer to Appendix I for outlines of healings, types of diseases healed, and other information as categorized by J. Wilkinson.)

In some situations, *Jesus took the initiative* in seeking out the sick person (Luke 7:14, 13:12, Jesus took the 22:51; John 5:6). At other times the sick person took the initiative (Matthew 9:27; Mark 1:40, 5:6, 5:27, 10:17; Luke 17:13). Sometimes, other people acted on behalf of the sick person (Matthew 8:5; Mark 2:3, 5:23, 7:26, 8:22; John 4:47, 9:2, 11:3). On occasions, it appears that his enemies tried to ensure that a sick person was present, in order to trap Jesus (Luke 6:6, 7, 14:1-3).

Jesus' *motives* for healing were varied and included:

- An expression of compassion (Matthew 14:14, 20:34; Mark 1:41; Luke 7:13).

- A response to a cry for help (Matthew 9:27, 15:22, 17:15; Mark 10:46, 47; Luke 17:13).

- A response to faith (Matthew 8:10, 15:28; Mark 2:5, 9:24, 10:52).

- A fulfillment of the Messianic scriptures (Matthew 8:16, 17; 11:2-6; 12:15-21; Luke 7:18-23). Jesus appeals to the fulfillment of Old Testament scripture to make clear that he is the promised Messiah.

- A sign of his glory, revealing his deity; showing that his presence and power is the presence and power of God (John 4:54, 9:3, 11:4).

All of these motives were present, but the writers of the gospels do not explain them in detail. Overall, it can be said that Jesus healed people because of his love for them. This was clearly shown in his coming to share human life and supremely, in his suffering and death. He healed because of who he is, the Christ, the Son of the Living God, and his healing ministry witnesses to this fact. The Gospel of John states clearly the reason the particular stories are written — that people may believe that Jesus is the Christ, and may have life through his name (John 20:31).

Jesus used several *methods* in his healing, all of which were simple and effective:

- He healed by a word of command; for example, to demon-possessed people he commanded the demon to leave (Mark 1:25, 5:8, 9:25; Luke 4:35). To the physically ill, he commanded the person to take certain actions — "get up," "stretch out your hand," "go and show yourself to the priest" (Mark 2:11, 3:5; Luke 17: 14; John 5:8). To the dead his command came, so that his words could be heard by the crowds, to make it clear that his power was from God (Luke 7:14; John 11:43).

- He also healed by touch; for example, when he touched others (Mark 6:5; Luke 4:40, 22:51), or when others touched him (Mark 3:10, 6:56; Luke 8:44). Sometimes word and touch went together (Matthew 8:3, 9:29; Mark 1:41, 5:41; Luke 8:54, 13:12, 13).

- On three occasions Jesus used saliva as part of the healing process (Mark 7:33, 34; 8:23-25; John 9:6, 7).

- On three occasions he healed at a distance (Matthew 8:13; Mark 7:29; John 4:50).

Whichever method Jesus used, each one awakened something within the sick person, and opened that person to the Spirit of God working in their lives, bringing harmony and healing. The power of God flowed through Jesus' words and actions, and people were made whole. Whatever the method used, his purpose was to bring people to a faith relationship with the living and loving God, so that the power of God would bring restoration and healing to their lives.

Jesus also drew upon the faith of the individual and the faith of those around the sick person (Mark 2:1-5). Faith played an important part in this ministry. He looked for faith, rejoicing when he saw it, and was disappointed when it was not present. The presence of unbelief prevented healing (Mark 6:5, 6). In doing this, Jesus looked for a response, even though it may have been very weak. He himself was full of faith in the power of God, and he used his faith to inspire others to faith. It was as if a healing circle operated, as faith by or for the recipient joined with the faith of Jesus, and this completed the healing circuit, so that the power of God could flow into that person's life. However, on some occasions it seems that Jesus healed people where there was no emphasis on faith at all. Usually however, faith was seen as very important and significant.

Jesus endorsed the Old Testament understanding of God as the healing creator, who showers all people with his providential care, and He called people to become his disciples and to enter God's kingdom of righteousness and peace. The healing Jesus offered addressed the whole person in all their relationships and his words and actions deepened and demonstrated the Old Testament perspectives.

However, there were some significant differences in Jesus' approach, as he showed a new way of thinking about healing.

He was not confined to the "disciplinary" theory of sickness, which was the dominant understanding in the Old Testament. Rather, he appeared to follow the teaching which did not emphasize the connection between sickness and sin, and which gave a much greater emphasis to the power of God working in people's lives, quite apart from the rigorous requirements of obedience to the law. Jesus did accept the fact that there was often a connection between human failure/sin and sickness, and on at least two occasions he seemed to equate sickness with sin, presumably some moral or religious failure (Mark 2:5; John 5:14). To sin is to turn away from God's way and refuse His forgiveness and wholeness. And this opens people to fear, hate, meaninglessness, despair, and other destructive emotions, which can lead to a variety of mental and physical illnesses. So there can be a very direct connection between sin and sickness.

However, Jesus did not accept that *all* sickness and suffering has its origin in human sin and failure. He rejected the current thinking of his time, which saw all sickness as a result of sin and, therefore, God's punishment for disobedience to the divine law. For example in Luke 13:2-5, Jesus spoke of two human tragedies: of people killed by the Roman authorities, and others who were crushed under a falling tower. He concluded that those who suffered in these ways were no more sinful than others. Also in John 9:3 the same response is given in relation to physical blindness.

But if sin was not the sole reason for these tragedies, then what is the reason? Jesus dearly believed that a primary cause of sickness was a force of evil, hostile to God and His purposes, and that people could come under the control of this power which exerted a destructive influence over their lives — morally, physically, and psychologically. He described this as the power of Satan, and all the evil spiritual forces. The powers of the kingdom of darkness are opposed to the kingdom of light. On several occasions, he rebuked the evil forces which were binding people emotionally and physically, and he made a direct connection between the power of Satan and sickness (Mark 1:25, 5:8, 9:25; Luke 13:16). His coming and his healings were the beginning of the destruction of this power and the establishment of the kingdom of light (Matthew 12:22-29; Luke 10:17-20, 11:14-23). The power of evil could only be overcome by the greater power of the Holy Spirit, unleashed in the person of Jesus himself. (Note that the writer to the Hebrews sees this battle against the devil as the primary purpose of Jesus' coming, and the death and resurrection of Jesus as the pivotal battle in the conflict between good and evil (Hebrews 2:14-18). Other writers see Jesus' death as the focal point of the battle against the powers of evil, including sickness, and it is in his death that Jesus bears human sin and sickness and brings healing and salvation (for example, Matthew 8:17).[6]

So Jesus did not subscribe to the accepted idea that God always put sickness on people because of sin. He did not seem to enquire whether people had repented before he healed them, although he did point out the necessity for responsible living after healing (John 5:14). In his ministry Jesus expressed God's compassion toward people who were caught up in both sin and sickness, and he healed both. One writer sums up the attitude of Jesus:

> There was no hint of sitting back to wait for suffering to teach human beings their lesson, and bring them back to relation with God. Jesus knew that healing could accomplish God's will in people far better. God through Christ is interested in whole, redeemed men and women, not in using them to satisfy divine anger. This is one of the fundamental conceptions of Jesus and vital Christianity. Jesus underwent crucifixion and resurrection for human beings, before people thought of accepting God's way of love.[7]

Jesus commissioned his disciples to be involved in the healing ministry and to model their ministry on his. So the disciples were sent to preach the kingdom, to heal the sick, and so on (Matthew 10:7, 8; Luke 9:2, 10:9). However, in his final commissions after the resurrection, there is no mention of healing and this has led to the idea that healing was not meant to be part of the life of the church, but was intended only for the time of Jesus' earthly ministry. However, this cannot be accepted.

- In Matthew 28:18-20, Jesus speaks with authority, and commissions the disciples to go and make disciples . . . and to teach them "to observe all that I have commanded you." Jesus had already commanded them to heal the sick, so we can assume that this was part of the teaching they were to pass on to all future generations of believers.

- Mark 16:9-20, although often treated as a disputed passage, also includes the command to go into all the world to preach the gospel, and to continue the ministry of signs and wonders, which includes the laying on of hands on the sick, and healing.

- Luke 24:44-49 and Acts 1:6-8 link the power of the Holy Spirit with the future ministry of the apostles. They obviously understood that this included healing, as many healing incidents occur in the Acts of the Apostles, apparently as part of the normal witness to the gospel.

- John 20:21-23: Jesus sends the disciples as the Father had sent him. In doing this, he is affirming that his ministry, which included healing and deliverance, is to continue through them.

In all of these commissions, it is implied that the healing ministry was meant to be an essential, continuing part of the church's ministry. And if the church has been commissioned to continue the ministry of healing in the name of Jesus Christ, and to proclaim Him as the contemporary healer, it is essential that the church focuses on the ministry of Jesus as the norm, touchstone, standard for its understanding and practice. This means that the Old Testament perspectives must be read and interpreted "through the eyes of Jesus." Just as Jesus refines, focuses, and deepens other Old Testament ideas, so he deepens and fulfills, that is, brings out the deeper meaning of healing. Jesus is the key to understanding both the purpose and scope of healing, and any interpretation and teaching of the Old Testament must be subject to his teaching and practice. So the Old Testament perspectives are accepted and used, provided "it is Jesus who reads it to us."

In summing up, the healing ministry of Jesus can be seen as varied and dynamic, including the following emphases:

- The source of healing is in the nature of God, and is an expression of God's love.

- Healing of sickness may involve issues of disobedience and sin — but this does not apply in all situations.

- Healing comes through the activity of the Holy Spirit moving into the lives of people.

- Healing involves warfare with evil spiritual forces.

- Healing relates to salvation and wholeness, and involves both individual and social health.

- Healing is not to be found in any form of ritual or magic, but it is to be found in Jesus alone.

- Healing is an expression of the kingdom which has come in Jesus, and is a present reality in the world. It is a sign that God's power has entered into the world, and people can experience the presence and power of God in their lives, bringing healing and restoration. However, it is also apparent the full blessings of the kingdom are not yet present, and will only be fully revealed at the end time. This means that some healing is to be experienced as a kingdom blessing here and now, but complete healing will not be possible until the kingdom is fully established.

Sharing and Discussion

1. How strong is the idea that sickness is the consequence of and punishment for sin and wrong-doing, in people's thinking today? Can you give examples where you see this idea operating? What are the strong and weak points of this idea?

2. Why is it important for our ideas about the healing ministry to be based on the biblical teaching? Discuss some of the popular contemporary ideas which are different from the biblical understanding.

3. Morton Kelsey emphasizes an important point in the following statement:

> The whole body of scripture needs to be evaluated in the light of Jesus' teachings and actions . . . Jesus' teachings in the New Testament give Christians the basis for their interpretation of healing in the Old Testament.[8]

Do you think this is a valid way to interpret the scripture; that is, "through the eyes of Jesus"? What does this mean for the way we use the Old Testament, particularly the way some people take texts out of the Old Testament without any reference to the original background situation and meaning, or to the teachings of Jesus, and apply them directly to the healing ministry today?

4. Choose two or three of the healing incidents in Jesus' ministry and discuss how these particular experiences of healing would affect both the individual and the community; the physical, emotional, psychological and social aspects. You will need to investigate the social situation of the time, including the prevalent beliefs about sickness and disease. Three particular incidents will repay careful examination (Mark 1:40-45, 5:21-34; John 5:1-9). See suggested helpful reading in Endnote 9.

5. Bishop Morris Maddocks defines the healing ministry as "Jesus meeting people at the point of their deepest needs." From the New Testament, give four or five examples where Jesus met people in this way. How did Jesus help the person either to cope with, or overcome, their particular need?

6. In the hymn "At even, when the sun was set" (Australian Hymn Book 169), one verse says:

Thy touch has still its ancient power;
No word from thee can fruitless fall.

Is this still true? How does Jesus touch people today, to bring healing and hope? Does he still meet people at the point of their need? Give some examples where you have seen this happening in people's lives.

7. Jesus spoke of healing as one of the signs of the kingdom breaking into people's lives. Can we think of modern healing in this way, when we also use medical and other resources to bring about healing? Are these also "signs" of the kingdom?

8. How should we think about the methods Jesus used in his healing ministry? Are they applicable for use by his followers today, or are they no longer relevant to the modern technological situation?

9. What motive(s) should Christians have to be involved in the healing ministry? Are there some doubtful motives which may entice and attract people to become involved in this ministry?

10. Christians have different viewpoints to the idea that "healing is in the atonement," and that Jesus death offers healing from sickness, in the same way as his death offers freedom and salvation from sin. Study some of the suggested references (see endnote 6), and discuss this issue.

References for Further Reading

Bennett, G., *Commissioned to Heal,* Divine Healing Mission, London, undated.

Cowie, I., *Jesus Healing Work and Ours.* Wild Goose. Glasgow, 2000.

Epperley, B., *God's Touch,* Westminster John Knox Press, Louisville, Ky. 2001.

Harper, M., *The Healings of Jesus,* Hodder & Stoughton, London, 1986.

Kelsey, M., *Psychology, Medicine & Christian Healing,* HarperCollins, New York, 1988.

Pilch, J., *Healing in the New Testament.* Augsburg Fortress, Minneapolis, 2000.

Wilkinson, J., *Health and Healing,* Handsel Press, Edinburgh, 1980.

Wilkinson J., *The Bible and Healing,* Handsel Press, Edinburgh; Eerdmans, Grand Rapids, Michigan, 1998.

3
THE AUTHORITY AND COMMISSION TO HEAL PART II — THE EARLY CHURCH AND CONTEMPORARY APPLICATIONS

Having seen the very important place which healing had in God's dealings with Israel in the Old Testament, and how healing was central to the ministry of Jesus, and noted his command to his disciples to continue this ministry, two questions must be answered:

1. Was the healing ministry carried into the life of the church, or did it gradually fade out? Was it a special ministry, which was only meant for the breaking in of the kingdom and the establishment of the church, or was it to continue as an essential part of the church's ministry through history?

2. Can the healing ministry today claim to be a continuing part of that ministry begun by Jesus, or are the healing gifts and ministries no longer part of the church's resources? Does the healing of sickness belong to the health professionals only?

This chapter aims to:

- Review the healing ministry in the early church;

- Understand the relevance of the biblical teaching for the continuation of the healing ministry today.

Healing in the Early Church

The Acts of the Apostles, written by Luke, is the record of how the church developed after the resurrection of Jesus Christ. The other New Testament books are either letters or messages sent to the various local or regional churches, which had been established. The disciples of Jesus in the gospels are now the apostles in the Acts, sent out by Jesus to continue his ministry and empowered by the Holy Spirit at Pentecost. They have received the same "dunamis" or power, which is seen in Jesus' power and authority to heal in the gospels. In the Acts of the Apostles, Luke does not emphasize the healing ministry, but assumes it to be an essential part of the apostolic proclamation and action. Luke simply records the healing events, without explaining or proving their reality. These events are signs and wonders by the Holy Spirit, which point to the new reality of the kingdom, following the life, death, resurrection and ascension of Jesus Christ. This acceptance of healing is significant, as Luke himself was professionally trained as a doctor, and he therefore writes from this perspective.

The healings in Acts include physical healings of individuals, the exorcism of demons, the raising of people from the dead and the healing of several groups of people. There are also several references to signs and wonders, which would include healing. (Refer to Appendix 2.)[1]

The methods used by the apostles are similar to those used by Jesus. For example, by word (Acts 9:34, 14:10, 16:18); by touch (Acts 5:12, 14:3, 19:11, 28:8); by a combination of word and touch (Acts 3:1-10, 9:17-19). There were also other unusual methods used. For example, a type of resuscitation (Acts 20:9-12), the effect of Peter's shadow (Acts 5:15) and the use of clothes from Paul (Acts 19:12). But whatever the method used, healing is effected through the name and the power of Jesus Christ, and not through any power of the apostles (Acts 3:6, 3:12-16, 9:34).

It is clear that the healing power of the Holy Spirit, expressed through the apostles, was an important means of witness and evangelization. It is also clear that ordinary people like the apostles, who were often regarded as common and uneducated in terms of religious law and knowledge, were filled with a power greater than any natural power, which enabled them to deal with the physical and mental illness of sick people (Acts 4:13,14).

As the church developed, there is no indication that the healing ministry diminished in importance. It is true that there are fewer specific references to healing in the New Testament letters, but this can be explained by the fact that most of the letters were written to deal with specific issues and situations. So, only subjects which were relevant to those situations were discussed. Indeed, the fact that healing is not mentioned probably means that it was not a problem issue, or it was taken for granted. (See later discussion on this point.)

In his earliest letters to three different churches, Galatians, Romans and Corinthians, Paul refers to miracles, signs and wonders as valid proof of the presence and power of the Holy Spirit: (Galatians 3:5; Romans 15:18, 19; 2 Corinthians 12:12). Paul appeals to these acts as the authentic signs of the true apostle. Although healing is not specifically mentioned, it can be assumed that it would be included. This is because Paul uses the same Greek words to describe these signs and wonders as are used in the gospels to refer to the miracles of Jesus. These miracles often included healing, and it is significant that the same word is used to refer to the healing miracles through the apostles.

Paul was himself involved in many examples of healing, so he did not have to emphasize something which was so obvious. He also taught that people were under the influence of various forces of evil, of demons, idols, the flesh, law, sin, death, sovereignties and powers, and so on. One of the reasons for the coming of Jesus was to rescue people from this domination, and to set them free from evil forces and from the dis-ease, moral, social, mental and physical, that came from these evil powers (for example, Ephesians 6:10-12).

However, there are some passages in Paul's writings which are often used to dispute the claim that healing should be a continuing part of Christian ministry. These refer to the sickness of Paul's friends, and also to Paul's "thorn in the flesh."[2]

Philippians 2:25-28 refers to the sickness of Epaphroditus, who was so sick that he almost died. 2 Timothy 4:20 refers to Trophimus, who was sick. The question is asked, "If Paul believed in healing, why were Epaphroditus and Trophimus not healed?" However, there is no contradiction here. No one suggests that Christians never fail, nor that Christians never get sick. What the New Testament teaches is that they can often be healed, by physical, psychological and spiritual means. There is no way of knowing if Epaphroditus was restored, or whether Trophimus was in the process of getting well. All that is reported is their particular situation at that time. These are arguments from silence, which rest on the assumption that all Christians who are sick are a contradiction of the healing ministry. We simply do not know whether these people were subsequently healed. To deduce that because two people happened to be sick at a particular time this invalidates the healing ministry, is quite unreasonable. Likewise, when Paul advises Timothy to drink wine to relieve his digestive problem (1 Timothy 5:23) this does not contradict the healing ministry. Paul is simply recommending a long-standing remedy, and showing that God can and does provide healing through various means; in this case, accepted medical means. It is simply recognizing another valid way of healing, but does not thereby invalidate healing through spiritual means. With Paul's "thorn in the flesh" (2 Corinthians 12:7-9), it is clear that Paul struggled with this discomfort which he regarded as a messenger of Satan. However, he accepted it as a means to humility, and to keep him focused on God as the source of his strength. But this did not stop

Paul from healing others and commending the healing ministry, and the passage cannot be used as an argument to invalidate such a ministry, nor can it be generalized as a basis for Christian action.[3]

There are two further passages which do seem to indicate some development in the understanding of the healing ministry in the life of the early church. In his letter to the church at Corinth, Paul speaks of healing as a special gift, or *charisma,* of the Holy Spirit (1 Corinthians 12:9, 28-30). Whether this refers to a divinely-given power or skill, quite separate from normal human capacities, or whether it refers to a heightening or strengthening of human capabilities already possessed, is not clear. What is clear is that certain people were recognized as possessing a special charisma in the area of healing, and they were given a place of honor in the church and constituted as a special group of healers. However, there is also the reference in James 5: 13-16, which makes no specific reference to any special gift, but locates the healing ministry as a normal part of the elders' work in each congregation. The sick person is to call for the elders who are to pray over the person, anointing with oil in the name of the Lord and the prayer of faith is to be offered in expectancy and trust. Healing and forgiveness are recognized as the result of the Lord's work in the sick person's life.

Are these two different ways: for example, a special healing gift to an individual, and the elders' role in healing? Are they in opposition to each other, or are they meant to complement each other?

There seems to have been a gradual process of consolidation in the way the church functioned. The Holy Spirit gave gifts to individuals according to His will and purpose (1 Corinthians 12:4). These gifts were a direct infusion of grace for a particular purpose, but all were to be used for the common good (1 Corinthians 12:7). All the gifts, including healing, were given for the one purpose of furthering the kingdom. As the Holy Spirit is a Spirit of order and not disorder, Paul writes to analyze and make some kind of order out of the many spiritual gifts. But there is also a development in which the gifts of healing appear to be vested in the eldership of the church. The gifts are still given to the Body, to be used for the Body, but for the sake of order are to be administered by the eldership. This probably became the normal pattern in the life of the church, and has continued in many churches to the present day. However, this focus on the role of the elders does not mean that the Holy Spirit no longer gives special gifts to certain individuals. The history of the church offers many examples of gifted individuals who have exercised a ministry of healing, either apart from, or alongside, ministry by the elders. It is true that some Christians who claim to possess this special healing gift have exercised it quite apart from the church, and this has resulted in opposition and confusion. But this wrong use of the gift does not invalidate the gift itself.

In the church these two ways seem to operate side by side, with individuals exercising a special gift of healing, alongside or supplementary to the healing ministry of the elders. Some churches refuse to recognize any special healing gift, or any special role of individual healers, and will only accept the healing ministry through the appointed elders. On the other hand, other churches tend to ignore the role of elders and focus almost entirely on the work of specially gifted healers. What seems to be clear is that the Holy Spirit is not bound by church systems or structure. He may choose to use particular people who are open to receive His power, whether they form part of the official leadership of the church or not. And He also uses the more structured form of church leadership. Either way it is the Holy Spirit at work to bring about His purposes.

Relevance of Biblical Material for Today

Having briefly surveyed the biblical material, the original question can be asked again: "Has the church today any authority to be involved in a healing ministry?" This chapter has suggested that the same healing gifts are available to the church today, and therefore the church should be involved in the ministry of healing. However, some Christians, whilst agreeing that God continues to work miracles and to answer prayer for healing by His people, are strongly opposed to the idea that the healing gifts given to certain people in the New Testament church (as in 1 Corinthians 12:9, 28-30) are still applicable to the church today. They argue that these particular gifts of healing are no longer given, for the following reasons.[4]

- Their purpose is no longer relevant. Why were these gifts originally given? It is clear from the New Testament that the purpose for the gift of healing and other miraculous gifts was to accompany new, special revelation; authenticating that revelation and vindicating God's servants through whom He was speaking: That is, the healings of Jesus were never done for their own sake, but always to point to a deeper truth that Jesus was the Son of God, with power to forgive sins and to vindicate his status as Messiah (Matthew 9:2-6). In the same way, the gift of healing was not given to the apostles simply to heal but to accompany and authenticate the new revelation of Jesus Christ as the eternal Son of God. They were meant as signs to validate and clarify who Jesus is. They were a special revelation for a special purpose (Hebrews 2:3a). That special revelation of Jesus as the Son of God is now contained for us in the scriptures and there is therefore no longer any need for such special gifts, because their purpose (to reveal Jesus as Son of God) has been accomplished. The biblical record is now sufficient to point people to him.

- These healing gifts were only given to the apostles and others who worked closely with them (Acts 2:42-43, 5:12, 6:8, 8:5-6, 14:3). The apostles were a unique group of individuals, because they were personally called by Jesus and received their commission from him (John 6:70, 13:18, 15:16; Galatians 1:1, 2). Signs and wonders were the unique mark of an apostle (2 Corinthians 12: 12) given to authenticate them as "the men through whom

God was speaking infallibly with new revelations." They were the signs suitable to the inauguration of the church, as at a spectacular premiere, and were not meant to be passed on. Only the apostolic band; that is, the apostles and their right-hand men had the gifts of miraculous healing, and these gifts finished with this group. Today there are no such apostles, so the gifts given to them are no longer applicable.

- In the New Testament, miraculous healings fade out after the apostles. Following the writing of the New Testament scriptures, there was no further special revelation, so the miraculous healings were not needed. In the early period of the church's life from 33 AD to 60 AD, there were many instances of healing (as in the Acts), but after 60 AD these special gifts are not mentioned, which implies that they were no longer available. For example, Paul could not heal Timothy of his problem and prescribed a purely medicinal cure (1 Timothy 5:23); also he had to leave Trophimus sick (2 Timothy 4:20).

- Miraculous healings are spoken of in the past tense in the New Testament; for example, Hebrews 2:3, 4, implying that when they confirmed the new revelation of the gospel these gifts were no longer needed.

- In later New Testament writings, it is the gift of teaching which is emphasized, and not the gift of healing. This gift is mentioned in 1 Corinthians 12, written about 56 AD, and in Romans 12, written about 57 AD. But by the time of the Letter to the Ephesians, 60-67 AD, there is no mention of such gifts, but the emphasis is on the preaching of the gospel rather than any healing signs and wonders. Other writers support this idea that the epistles are almost devoid of any reference to physical healing as part of the ministry of the church life in its settled state. We find many references to the power of God evidenced in the actual preaching of the gospel, and therefore, there can be little doubt where the priority of ministry is to be found.

It is clear that the power of the Spirit is to be seen primarily in the effect of the message proclaimed with conviction . . . the New Testament writings do not see the early Christian community as having a healing ministry. Apart from the reference in James and in an almost incidental reference to healing in 1 Corinthians 12, there is virtual silence on the theme of physical healing in the early Christian community, beyond the Acts of the Apostles . . . It would be very difficult to deduce that this physical healing ministry was a primary task of the church, when there is such a massive silence on the subject.[5]

- In James 5: 14-15, the sick person is to call for the elders of the church, and not for any miraculous healer. The elders are not described as having any special gift, but they are the ones who are to pray for the sick. Healing comes by prayer, not as the result of some miraculous gift. The apostolic gift of healing was rare, and was given only to the original apostolic band. Today, there are no such apostles and the church therefore uses James 5:14-15 as the guideline for prayer, rather than any dependence on special miraculous gifts.

This position strongly contends that any special gifts of healing were limited to the time of the apostles, and that the New Testament emphasis is on evangelism, not healing. What is essential for the church today is to make evangelism a priority, and not become sidetracked by an over-emphasis on, and search for, special healing gifts.

There is no evidence of any kind of healing missions, or groups of people, traveling around with a kind of healing circus in the New Testament. There is evidence of traveling evangelists moving into pioneer areas, and Paul saw this as one of his greatest ministries (Romans 15:17-20). This follows from the clear New Testament pattern that evangelism must be the priority. The gospel of eternal life is needed by all, whereas healing, in its narrowest physical sense, is not that universal a need.[6]

Are these arguments valid? There is value in the objection against the over-emphasis on special gifts for self-appointed leaders. This over-emphasis can lead to a focus on specially gifted individuals, whereas the emphasis should be on the role of the church as a whole, especially the elders, as in James 5. There is also some validity in emphasizing that the purpose of the healing gifts was to authenticate the new revelation in Jesus. But authentication of the new revelation in Jesus cannot be regarded as the only purpose of the healing gifts. In the ministry of Jesus, healing gifts were also a sign of his compassion, and a sign that the kingdom of God had broken into human life and society (Luke 7:18-23). As a sign of the kingdom these signs continue, and there is no indication that the gifts have been withdrawn. The completion of the scriptures as the final source of authority remains valid, but there need be no clash between the acceptance of the scriptures and the continuation of these gifts. In addition, many writers dispute the claim that the apostles have no successors. It is true that the original apostles were unique, but this does not mean that the apostolic commands finished with them. For example, does Matthew 28:18-20 apply only to the apostles? Some in the church have argued this, especially at the time of the Reformation and through the eighteenth and nineteenth centuries. However, most scholars agree that the apostolic command to world mission remains applicable to the church today. Presumably the gifts necessary to carry out that command have not been withdrawn. Why, then, should the gifts of healing be withdrawn?

Also, it is always dangerous to argue from silence, and the lack of references to healing in the New Testament letters may simply mean that the subject was not an issue, and therefore did not need to be mentioned. There is little or no reference to many aspects of faith in the New Testament letters; for example, God as creator, the Lord's Supper, and so on. But it is not suggested that these beliefs were no longer important. In the valid attempt to show the dangers of miraculous healers claiming special gifts and thus ignoring the role of the church in any healing ministry (as has been seen in many examples in charismatic renewal in recent years), those who support these arguments tend to overstate their particular viewpoint. They imply that any ministry today can only be patterned on that of Jesus and the early church if it receives explicit mention in the Commission of Jesus, or explicit statements in the rest of the New Testament. But there are many aspects of church life and ministry today about which there is no explicit mention. One writer who responds to this argument is David Huggett, who writes as follows:

> The implicit requirement that ministry today may be patterned on that of Jesus and the gospels only if it receives explicit mention in the post-resurrection commission of Jesus, is altogether too narrow a bottleneck. Our justification for taking Jesus' ministry of healing, miracles, signs and wonders as a pattern stands chiefly on the direct teaching of Jesus on this point. It will be backed up in the way he taught, trained and commanded his disciples on this point; how he directed them to pass this ministry on to others. It will be further undergirded by the record of Acts and the teachings of the Epistles, concerning these gifts and ministries in the church. Further support would be lent by the example and experience of the church down the ages, and the contemporary witness of the church throughout the world . . . The Epistles clearly teach people to expect these gifts and ministries of healing and miracles. In some eight passages concerning gifts and ministries, at least twenty are spoken of. Many are only mentioned in one passage; healing and miracles, however, are mentioned in three passages, and only three gifts of ministries receive greater mention than them in these passages.

> Clearly, the expectation and teaching of the early church was that it would continue to receive these ministries and gifts. The

story unfolded by church history shows a continual thread, but with shifting intensity and weakness, which saddens the student. The same waxing and waning is also sadly present in the record of evangelism and missionary concern over the centuries. Graciously, God has brought us back to an awareness of the centrality of evangelism and mission, so also now, to the importance and centrality of healing and miracles.[7]

In evaluating these different perspectives, it is clear that there are differing opinions among Christians as to the continuation of gifts within the church. This has always been a debatable issue, but there are very strong arguments for affirming that the church today has a continuing authority to be involved in the healing ministry. These can be summarized as:

• The contemporary church remains under the commission of Jesus, given to the disciples and apostles. Even though the original commissions may have been local in application, they continue to speak to the church today, in the same way as the commissions to teach and evangelize continue to speak to the church. There is no indication that the command to heal was for a limited time only, and there is also no indication that this command has been withdrawn.

• Jesus promised that his disciples would do the same, and even greater works, than he had done when he was with them John 14:12). It is generally agreed that this would include the works of preaching and teaching, but there is no valid reason why these greater works should not also include healing as well.

• The scope of the gospel is the same today as in apostolic times. Healing of the sick was an accepted part of the Good News included in the healing and salvation of the whole person — body, mind and spirit. All are important to God and share in true wholeness (1 Thessalonians 5:23).

- The main method in the church's ministry of healing is prayer, and that is still available in the church today. John 14:13 contains the promise of Jesus to the church, and as has already been noted, James 5:13-16, remains an essential part of the church's life. Healing occurred in the apostolic church in response to the prayer of faith, and there is no reason why this should not continue to happen.

- Where there seem to be special healing gifts given to particular people (there is much contemporary evidence to suggest that these gifts are still given), it is essential that they be recognized by the church and used to strengthen the ministry of the church. They are not to be used in such a way that gifted people arrogate power to themselves.

- The in-breaking of the power of the Holy Spirit is still the same, and all healing is achieved through His work in people's lives, as they are open to the healing which is available in the name of Jesus Christ.

Throughout the long history of the church, the healing ministry has been present; at times very strong, at other times very weak, but there has been evidence of this ministry present in every age. (Refer to Chapter 4). The church today stands in a long tradition when it accepts that it must fulfill the commission of Christ to preach the gospel and to heal the sick. Two statements from the Lambeth Conferences of the Anglican Church sum up the question of the authority for the church to be involved in this ministry. Firstly, the Lambeth Conference of 1920 affirmed the following:

> Within the church . . . systems of healing, based on the redemptive work of our Lord . . . all spring from a belief in the fundamental principle that the power to exercise spiritual healing is taught by Christ to be the heritage of all Christian people who are living in fellowship with God, and is part of the ministry of Christ through his Body, the church.[8]

This was reaffirmed in 1958, and again in 1978:

> This Conference praises God for the renewal of the ministry
> of healing within the church in recent times, and reaffirms:
>
> • That the healing of the sick in his name is as much part
> of the proclamation of the kingdom as the preaching of the
> Good News of Jesus Christ.
>
> • That to neglect this aspect of ministry is to diminish our
> part in Christ's total redemptive activity.[9]

The healing ministry is now widely accepted and practiced as an
essential aspect of the ministry of the church. It is not confined
to any one church or tradition, but is truly a global ministry of the
whole church, a truly ecumenical expression of the gospel. Most
branches of the church have statements on healing, and appropriate structures and training to enable this ministry to be effectively
practiced.[10]

Sharing and Discussion

1. Why should the church be involved in the healing ministry today? Do some churches and individual people get involved in this
ministry for the wrong reasons?

2. Is the healing ministry meant to be part of the evangelistic witness of the church; to reach non-Christians outside the church, or
is it meant to be a ministry which is directed primarily, or only, to
those within the church fellowship?

3. Look up material on Paul's "thorn in the flesh" (2 Corinthians
12:7-10) and discuss the various interpretations given. (a) Which
do you think is the most valid interpretation? (See discussions
in Glennon, Goldingay and Maddocks.) (b) Is it still true that
God's power is made perfect in weakness and that God's grace

is sufficient, as in 2 Corinthians 12:9, 10? Can you give examples where this has been a reality, either in your own life or in the experience of others?

4. Read the six reasons why it is believed that the healing gifts have ceased. Imagine that one of your friends has written to you, giving these same reasons why they should not get involved in any healing ministry, and asking for your opinion as to whether these reasons are valid. Write a letter to your friend giving your response.

5. What does your church believe and teach about the gift(s) of healing? Are they seen as an essential part of the witness of the church?

6. Does your church take James 5:13-16 seriously and attempt to put it into practice? Discuss ways in which these verses could become more significant for the life of your church.

7. What is the official attitude of your church or denomination to the healing ministry? Are there any statements or affirmations by the church like the Lambeth Conference statement? How are these statements communicated to each worshipping congregation to enable members of the church to understand and become involved in this ministry?

8. If your church is involved in a healing ministry, what sort of training is offered for members to become involved in this ministry?

References for Further Reading

Goldingay, J. (Ed.), *Signs Wonders and Healing,* IVP, Leicester, England, 1989. An excellent source of material to clarify the different interpretations of the New Testament, and its meaning for today.

Glennon, J., *Your Healing is Within You,* Hodder & Stoughton, London, 1978.

Kelsey, M., *Psychology, Medicine and Christian Healing*, HarperCollins, N.Y., 1988.

Maddocks, M., *The Christian Healing Ministry*, SPCK, London, 1990.

Wilkinson, J., *Health and Healing*, Handsel Press, Edinburgh, 1980.

Wilkinson, J., *The Bible and Healing*, Handsel Press, Edinburgh, and Eerdmans, Grand Rapids, Michigan, 1998.

4
DIFFERENT APPROACHES TO HEALING THE SICK: HISTORICAL DEVELOPMENTS AND CONTEMPORARY PERSPECTIVES

Today there is a renewed interest in the healing ministry and a growing concern for it to be taken seriously, and restored to the life of the church, rather than being a fringe interest. There is also a general acceptance of healing as wholeness, although there are some differences as to what this actually means.

However, when it comes to the content and practice of any healing ministry, there are wide differences in approach and understanding. These differences often cause confusion and misunderstanding among those who are involved or interested in the healing ministry. Many Christians feel comfortable with one particular emphasis and become confused by different approaches, each of which usually claims to be based on particular interpretations of the Bible.

One of the aims of the Order of St. Luke is to help people to understand some of these different approaches to the healing ministry, and to encourage discussion among those who are actively involved in health and healing, so that they will appreciate the work of others who may approach the work of healing quite differently from themselves. So the question which we ask is this: "If healing the sick is a valid ministry for the church today, which is the most effective model for this ministry?" Is it to develop a healing ministry which uses the ministry of Jesus and the early church as a model, with little or no reference to modern medical and psychological understanding and skills? Or is it to develop a ministry largely based on the insight and skills of counseling and psychotherapy and medical skill, which are seen as God's good gifts to people today? Or is the best way a combination of both of these approaches?

John is a highly trained medical doctor who has a keen interest in the healing ministry. He believes that God has given gifts of scientific knowledge and medical skill to help in the struggle against sickness and disease. John has also been trained in counseling, which enables him to understand and help people with their personal problems. John is a sincere Christian who tries to see where and how God fits into his busy medical practice/health world. John is aware that many doctors and health workers have little or no understanding of God and Christian healing, and do not see the relevance of faith in God for their work of caring for people. John's colleagues do not talk much about healing but rather about caring, or curing, or helping people to recover. Although he is a keen Christian, John has strong reservations about some of his Christian friends who seem to ignore what medical science has to offer, and who sincerely believe they are able to heal people by following the methods of Jesus and the apostles without any recourse to modern medical care. John thinks that accepting the Bible as the source of authority for their involvement in the healing ministry is rather naive. He is convinced that where people ignore the insights of doctors and counselors, and rely solely on the supernatural power of God to bring healing, such people and ideas are wrong and need to be exposed and corrected.

John's friend, *Fred*, has also developed a counseling ministry, but he views counseling in a completely different way. Fred readily acknowledges the insights and treatment available through medical science, but is very critical of the fact that many health workers completely ignore the spiritual dimensions of healing. This has been a change in Fred's perspective. Fred was trained in the social sciences, and as a student he agreed completely with what he describes as their basically humanistic approach. However, after a deep experience of the love of God in his life, and receiving the gift of the Holy Spirit, Fred's understanding and attitude have changed. Whereas earlier he saw counseling and the social sciences as the key to healing people's lives, he now strongly believes that healing can also occur through prayer and the laying on of hands; and that God gives healing in response to prayer and faith in God's promises, often quite apart from a reliance upon any of the social science skills. Fred now believes that a model for healing is found in the ministry of Jesus and the early church, and that often there is little or no need to seek medical help. When necessary, such help is valuable, but should never be allowed to replace the promise of healing through prayer and the gifts of the Spirit, for these are given to the church to heal as Jesus healed. Fred feels that, because of a refusal to give any place to the work of the Holy Spirit in healing sick people, the medical and counseling professions are often an impediment to real healing.

- How do you respond to these different approaches by John and Fred? Is one right, and the other wrong, or do both offer important insights?

This chapter aims to:

Clarify different approaches to the work of healing by:

- Giving a brief overview of how the healing ministry has developed in the life of the church;

- Clarifying the emphases in three main approaches or models of healing;

- Suggesting how these models supplement each other in the total ministry of healing.

There are many different approaches to the process of healing. To clarify the issues, *three main models* are suggested. (Note that any attempt to limit the different approaches risks the problem of over-generalization. Remember that the aim is clarification, rather than giving an exact description of each approach). The main approaches (with variations in each), can be described as:

- A spiritual-charismatic-sacramental approach, which is based mainly on the ministry of Jesus and the early church, as being the model for ministry today;

- A medical-counseling-psychotherapeutic approach, which draws heavily on modern psychological therapy and medical models for its methods;

- A middle-of-the-road approach, which draws on both of the others, and tries to relate them to each other, as being complementary and not in opposition to each other.

Each of these approaches draws from the Bible, and the history of the healing ministry in the church, to support its position; but gives different emphases and interpretations as to how to understand God's work in healing. To understand these different approaches, it is helpful to see how the healing ministry has developed in the long history of the church, from the time of Jesus until now. This ministry is not a new thing, but has always been present in the church in some measure; sometimes strong, at other times weak. However, there have always been people involved in healing, whatever the official attitude of the church has been. Even when the church officially ignored healing, it was still present and there has never been a time when some form of healing has not been practiced.

Within a single chapter it is not possible to provide a detailed history of healing ministry in the life of the church. It is possible only to describe the main trends, without much detail. The first section below gives a brief overview of the progress of the healing ministry from the early church to the present; and the second section discusses some contemporary approaches to this ministry.

Historical Overview of Healing Ministry

In previous chapters, we have seen that healing is related to the purposes of God. In both Old and New Testaments, we have a reliable and authoritative record of God's saving actions for His people and the world.

The Old Testament emphasis on the whole person in relation to God, others, and the creation itself, is worked out in the understanding of health as "shalom." But "shalom" has been infected by human disobedience, and disharmony has resulted. Health is seen as a blessing from God, with illness often seen as divine punishment, or chastisement for wrong doing. The truly healthy person is in a right relationship with God, which affects all other relationships. Health or "shalom" is broader than the individual and extends to family, social, community, and national relationships. In the book of Job, there is a development of the idea that illness and affliction may not always be seen as divine punishment, rather it can result from an evil source (for example, Satan), which ultimately derives its power from God. So illness and affliction may be quite separate from human goodness and virtue, and may not necessarily reflect a broken relationship with God, but may be part of His deeper purpose to bring spiritual growth and deeper commitment to Him, as well as a deeper understanding of the vastness and mystery of His will.

The New Testament portrays Jesus' concern with healing the physical, moral and mental sickness of people, and restoring them to a true relationship with God. Approximately one fifth of the gospels are focused on his healing ministry, and the Acts of the Apostles show how the disciples carried on this ministry as the church was established. The remainder of the New Testament does not give much emphasis to the healing ministry (apart from 1 Corinthians 12 and James 5), but this is not surprising because the work of healing was an accepted part of the gospel, and there was no need to continually emphasize the obvious. The central emphasis is that healing is a sign or indication that the kingdom of God has burst into the world, and is now present in human society. The gospel is focused on Jesus Christ who brings the blessing of God's presence to human lives. One aspect of this divine presence is the restoration of bodily wholeness, emotional and mental well-being, and harmony with God and others. Sickness and disease are a bondage to evil forces, and a part of the evil devices of Satan, who seeks to thwart God's healing purposes. The power of evil is broken in the life, death and resurrection of Jesus Christ, and the blessings of the new age of the kingdom can now be experienced in human lives. These blessings are experienced as people are open to the healing presence of the Spirit, and are often accompanied by the need for forgiveness, repentance, a change of attitude, and faith.

Jesus commissioned his disciples and their successors to continue this ministry, and church history provides many examples of how the commission was carried out. In the church's long history, there are six main periods with significant developments affecting the ideas and practice of the healing ministry.[1]

Up to 300 AD - The early church
300-600 AD - The Church in the Roman Empire
600-1500 AD - The Church in the Middle Ages
1500-1600 AD - The Church in the Protestant Reformation
1600-1900 AD - The Church in Post-Reformation/Modern period
Since 1900 AD - The Church in the Modern/Contemporary period

Up to 300 AD

During this time, the ministry of healing was an important part of the worship and mission of the church. The church affirmed the goodness of the human body, and continued to see people as a unity of body, mind and spirit. This was in opposition to the Greek thinkers (called Gnostics) who saw the human body as sinful and therefore subordinated it to the soul. The healing ministry as practiced in the New Testament church continued without much change. Healing was linked to the victory of Christ over Satan and death. During this time the church suffered persecution from the Roman authorities, but this strengthened rather than weakened the church in its mission.

> For nearly three centuries this healing was an indispensable ingredient of Christian life. The same strengthening force was at work, not only in dealing with physical and mental disease, but in meeting persecution. A truly supernatural power was given to these men and women . . . thus (there was) continuous evidence of a power able to strengthen them beyond normal expectations and of the Christian's relation to that source of power.[2]

300 to 600 AD

After the conversion of the Roman Emperor Constantine in 313 AD, the church entered a new era. Instead of being an outlawed faith, Christianity became accepted and was soon recognized as the official religion of the empire. With the ending of persecution, many people flocked into the church, and the level of spiritual understanding and commitment declined. To counter this, some Christians separated from the church to form separate communities where they could more effectively live out a true devotion to God. These communities were the beginning of what is known as the Monastic Movement. The attitude toward healing also began to change, especially between what is called the Eastern and Western sections of the church. The Eastern section was the church based around the eastern part of the empire, in the area of modern Turkey, Yugoslavia, and Greece; whereas the Western section was based around the modern area of Italy, France and the northern European countries. In the Eastern section of the church, the healing ministry continued strong, but there were some important changes in the Western church. The Western church gradually lost its spiritual vitality, became formal and nominal in its faith, and was affected by the decay and eventual collapse of the Roman Empire. The growing violence, confusion and despair led to an emphasis on the wrath and judgment of God on this decaying society, and a moving away from the understanding of God as a loving Father.

There was also an important change in the attitude toward the human body. It came to be seen as less important than the spirit, and this present life as less important than the life to come.

The care of the soul became more important than the care of the body. Sickness was regarded as the result of sin, and was to be accepted as God's discipline and chastisement. It was a sign of the sickness of the soul, and this soul-sickness must be healed. Healing began to be interpreted as healing the soul in preparation for heaven. The healing miracles of Jesus were interpreted in a symbolic way, as healing from the sickness of sin. Thus, sickness was changed from being an evil to be overcome, to being a "hidden blessing," through which God would discipline His people. The sick were taught to see themselves as true children of God, because God disciplines and chastises those whom He truly loves (Hebrews 12:7-10). The emphasis in healing related very strongly to the Old Testament view which saw a direct link between sickness and sin, and there was a corresponding movement away from the emphasis found in the ministry of Jesus and the early church. Kelsey describes the situation in the Western church about 600 AD:

Western thinking about healing had come full circle. Sickness was no longer understood as the malicious work of demons, or the evil one, to be countered in every instance. Instead, it was a mark of God's correction, sometimes inflicted by the negative powers with divine approval, to bring moral renewal.

There was no question about God's power to heal, or ability to intervene, but only of God's will to heal. Only the righteous were likely to find healing. We find in Pope Gregory's attitude the theme that grew more and more prevalent in the West. Here, the Old Testament view of sickness largely displaced that of Jesus, the apostles and the early church, both East and West.[3]

600-1500 AD

Even though healings were present in the Western church, this change of emphasis continued as the main understanding of healing for the next 1000 years. By the ninth century, the practice of anointing for healing (as in James 5:13-15) was changed to preparing people for death, and became the practice of extreme unction. Even though there were still healing centers and some healing orders in the church, healing was no longer an essential part of the life and mission of the church. Sickness was accepted as a divine discipline and forgiveness of sins became more important than healing.

The welfare of the spirit became more important than healing the body. The healing miracles of Jesus were interpreted to prove that he was the universal and spiritual Savior, who worked miracles on the soul, because the soul is more important than the body. One of the leading teachers of the church in that time exemplifies this understanding: "By how much soul is of more account than the body, by so much is the forgiving of sins a greater work than healing the body."[4]

The church thus came to regard the "lower" needs of the body as being in conflict with the "higher" needs of the Spirit. Also, in order to curtail some of the activities of groups who were actually involved in caring for the sick, the church attempted to control visitation of the sick and the practice of medicine. By the thirteenth century, a Christian doctor could not treat a sick person until a priest had visited that person to give spiritual direction, in case the spiritual value of the sickness should be lost. Any doctor who ignored this rule was disciplined by the church. After the Black Death plague struck Europe in the fourteenth century, millions of people died, sometimes as many as four hundred people each day. One Christian emperor described this as a "chastisement from heaven," and another writer referred to it as "these pestilences were for pure sin." As late as the mid-sixteenth century, Roman Catholic doctors had to agree that they would only visit patients who had confessed their sins and had a signed statement which showed this. If they continued to treat patients who had not confessed, the doctor could be barred from practicing medicine. The result was that the practice of medicine itself began to look with suspicion on the church, and also started to develop its own view of the human body as strictly material. It is obvious that these ideas concerning healing and sickness bore little or no connection to the biblical idea of wholeness, and to the teachings of Jesus.

1500-1600 AD

The Protestant Reformation began in 1517, as Martin Luther rebelled against the teaching of the Roman church. The Protestant reformers rejected much of the church's teaching about salvation and also much of the liturgy and rituals of the church. But they did not change the basic emphasis on the welfare of the soul. They agreed that illness was a punishment from God. They did urge compassion toward the sick, however, and encouraged prayer and support for the sick. Their basic understanding was that sickness was an opportunity to reaffirm God's mercy and grace, by receiving the forgiveness of sin. If the sick person died, then death became a merciful release from the sin and evil of the world, and the time to receive the full blessing of God.

What about the healing miracles of Jesus? The miracles were to prove that Jesus Christ was the true Savior, but the church could now do "greater works than these" (John 14:12), by teaching, converting and saving people "spiritually." The true miracle was the spiritual healing of the soul by God's grace, to be received by faith. Physical and emotional illness could, therefore, contribute to spiritual growth, whether or not any healing occurred. In fact, the true healing was spiritual and not physical. The important thing was the healing of the soul through forgiveness. It was believed that the day of miracles was past, and so was the gift of healing, which had been given to the church.

Two statements from Martin Luther and John Calvin explain the Protestant view of healing miracles. Firstly, from Martin Luther:

> Now that the apostles have preached the Word and have given their writings, and nothing more than what they have written remains to be revealed, no new and special revelation for miracles is necessary.[5]

Secondly, from Calvin, speaking about the anointing of the sick:

> The gift of healing disappeared with the other miraculous powers which the Lord was pleased to give for a time, that it might render the new preaching of the gospel for ever wonderful. Therefore, even were we to grant that anointing was a sacrament of those powers which were administered by the hands of the apostles, it pertains not to us, to whom no such powers have been committed.[6]

The Reformers believed that healing gifts were given to the early church, but were meant for that particular time and were relevant only to that time. However, this did not mean that there was no ministry of healing to the sick. The Reformers believed that God could heal. As the Sovereign Lord, He could do all things. But the important question was: "What is His method, now?" "Should special healing gifts be sought?" The answer given was, "No!" We should not seek after healing miracles, but only seek for that which brings glory to God. Was there no place for healing then? "Yes!"

But not through healing miracles, special gifts, or any special spiritual means; rather, through those whose specific task is in the healing professions, and through the faithful prayer of God's people, but apart from any special spiritual gift or spiritual healer. This was an important development in the understanding of healing, which became very strong in those Reformed churches based on the teachings of John Calvin. The teaching can be described in the following way: because God is the Sovereign Lord, He is the source of all good gifts (James 1:17), including the gift of healing. This gift of healing is not a special spiritual endowment, but is ordinarily exercised by those who are engaged in the specific work of caring for the sick; namely, those within the recognized healing professions. It is through these human skills that God's healing is to be experienced. God alone is the healer, but He does this through these special skills. Healing therefore is through the human sciences, which are in themselves the good gift of God. All of life is a gift from God, and is part of His purpose for all people. So, all healing, whether through human skills as in medicine, or through the prayers of God's people, proceeds from God's Spirit. God may still choose to work in a miraculous way apart from these skills, but not normally, for these healing arts are miracles in themselves.

Thus healing remains as one of God's good gifts, but it is to be exercised through the more formal structure of medical practice, clinics, hospitals, and so on. Prayers for healing remain important, and are complementary to those healing skills which have been developed in the healing professions. The authority for this approach comes from an understanding of God as the sovereign creator, whose common love for all people is expressed in His care and providence. He is the giver of every good and perfect gift, and these include the development of human skills in the various professions which seek to bring healing to the sick. What Jesus did in his ministry was to show God's healing in a particular way, as the new sign of the kingdom, and it was to validate the beginning of this new age that special gifts, signs and wonders were given. However, once the kingdom had been inaugurated and the church established, there was no further need for miraculous healing gifts, so they are not to be sought after. What the church has are the good gifts of God, expressed in the many healing skills, and also the Word of God and prayer. There is, therefore, a definite place for healing, but it is not to be based on trying to imitate the methods of Jesus or the early church, but rather on the careful development and use of the natural gifts and skills which God has given to the world. God is still the healer, as He operates through these skills, which are all ultimately given by Him. So the Protestant church strongly emphasized the need for adequate medical care and hospitals, based on this model of healing, and the healing ministry was largely expressed through this medical model, and became an important aspect of Protestant missionary outreach.

1600-1900 AD

One further development which has affected the understanding of healing, was the reversal of the previous emphasis which dominated the thinking of the church for many centuries; that spiritual healing of the soul is more significant than the healing of the body. Beginning in the seventeenth century, greater emphasis was given to the health of the body, and the natural physical processes of living. Rene Descartes, the French philosopher, developed the idea that body and mind are completely separate and belong to different spheres. According to Descartes, there is a material world and a separate spiritual world, with little in common. The created world is the basic structure of reality, and this is primarily material, not spiritual. God is the creator of this material reality, and it runs according to fundamental laws of motion with no involvement by God. It is if God has left the world to run on its own, like a machine. Consequently, God becomes a remote king, who orders things from above, without any direct involvement. In the material world of Descartes, there is no room for miracles or supernatural intervention of any kind.

This created a division between the material and spiritual worlds, the natural and the supernatural. The supernatural world was removed from many people's thinking as remote, and having little or nothing to do with the real world. Spiritual religion was relegated to the supernatural, and was important for that sphere only. So too was any type of healing through specifically spiritual means.

Descartes' world-view became the basis for modern medical practice, where the body is often seen as a well-ordered machine that functions according to certain laws. Illness is the breakdown of this functioning, and healing consists in restoring the proper functions through appropriate intervention. Various bodily functions tended to be isolated to particular parts of the body, and there was little connection between the various parts of the body and its social and physical environment. Emotions, values, mental functions and spiritual factors do not play much part in the process of disease and healing. The person becomes an isolated ego inside the body.

This view has led to amazing developments in medical science, and in recent years, to the establishment of large industries to develop and improve bodily health. Many within this development simply ignored God, and became completely secular in their thinking and work. However, many Christians interpreted this development differently. They saw these developments as evidence of God's providential gifts, and they regarded medical healing as originating in God, whether or not it was performed by believers. As a result of this development, the human person was divided into two parts, physical and spiritual, with the physical to be cared for by the medical profession, and the spiritual to be cared for by the church.

1900 to the present

In recent years, especially in the mid- to latter-part of the twentieth century, the division between natural and spiritual has been under attack, and the purely secular approach to healing has been severely questioned and tested. There has been a rediscovery of the Jewish and early Christian views about the unity of body, mind, emotions and spirit in each individual, and a rediscovery of the importance of social and environmental factors in the healing process. Healing was again reinterpreted as *shalom,* and a new interest developed in the concept of wholeness, both within the church and in society in general. In recent years, different churches have shared in this development, and healing has become a major topic for discussion and debate. This has been stimulated by a renewed emphasis on spiritual-charismatic-healing ministries and many churches have been established in which the healing ministry is central to their life and mission. Much of this emphasis has come from a renewed study of the healing ministry of Jesus and the early church, and a deeper experience of the healing gifts of the Holy Spirit.

In the second part of the twentieth century, the renewed interest was also expressed in the re-establishment of the healing ministry in many churches, together with the growth of special ministries focusing on signs, wonders, prophecy, deliverance, and so on. It has been recognized that whilst there has always been some healing ministry in the church, healing ministry has often been given a low rating in importance. The institutional ministry of healing has been offered, largely through the medical establishment, and the churches have supported this, and Christians have a wonderful record of service and care in these institutions. But the spiritual-charismatic-sacramental approach to healing has been neglected, and it is this approach which has received renewed emphasis in recent decades.[7]

However, now that the spiritual-charismatic-sacramental approach is receiving more attention, a tension has sometimes developed between an approach which concentrates on God's gifts, expressed in the healing professions, and an approach which emphasizes the special healing gifts, which often operate apart from the established healing professions.

Of course, many who are committed to the healing ministry affirm both of these approaches, and do not see any conflict between them. Whatever approach is taken, God is the healer. All the good gifts of God are to be used; all are spiritual in purpose whether they are expressed through the natural healing skills, or through specific spiritual gifts. God's involvement is true even if it is not recognized by those involved in the healing professions. This tension does exist, however, and it needs further clarification.

Different Approaches in Today's Church[8]

Having noted some of the developments in the healing ministry through the life of the church, we now look in more detail at the major approaches to healing, which are present in the church today. There are many variations and hybrids — we are looking only at the broad picture and are trying to gain some understanding of the complex nature of the contemporary healing ministry.

Spiritual-Charismatic-Sacramental Approach

This approach has been taken throughout church history, especially by those recognized as having special healing gifts seen as channels of God's healing power. The emphasis in the spiritual-charismatic-sacramental approach is usually on physical restoration, and on emotional and spiritual renewal. This may involve a recognized healer within a particular church group or believers who are committed to this ministry. It may involve any, or all, of the following methods: spiritual discernment, anointing, laying on of hands, sacraments (especially the eucharist), prayer, repentance, confession, tongue-speaking, praise, meditation, and exorcism.

Special healing services are often held in the spiritual-charismatic-sacramental approach. These services may involve just one or several periods of time, depending on the depth of the problem and the progress made. This approach may involve forms of prayer counseling and other methods of diagnosis and support. This approach is often described as "charismatic" or "Pentecostal" or "third wave" and is practiced in churches which are part of this movement. However some churches and individuals within the traditional or "established" churches also share this approach.

The spiritual-charismatic-sacramental approach is often difficult to examine in any detailed way, and like any method used, has both successes and failures. The important fact about this approach is that it is entirely dependent on the grace and power of God. Healing is not given as a result of human activity, knowledge or skill; but occurs as the power of God works in the lives of those seeking wholeness and healing. Human agents are not the source of healing, but channels through which God moves and heals by the power of the Holy Spirit.

Medical-Counseling-Psychotherapeutic Approach

This approach shares some of the methods of the spiritual-charismatic-sacramental approach, but also draws heavily on the insights and skills which have come through the development of the sciences of medicine, psychology, psychiatry, psychotherapy, and others. The medical-counseling-psychotherapeutic approach often links these with an awareness of the religious dimensions of life, and seeks to help people to understand their situation and grow in personal awareness and wholeness. Progress is achieved through a process of listening, in which various interpersonal and intrapersonal skills are used. The medical-counseling-psychotherapeutic process seeks to understand what the sickness means to the person, it supports the person's strengths in coping with negative experiences (like anxiety, guilt, shame), and sees the sickness in the context of family and other relationships. This approach aims to bring the person to an experience of healing through the careful use of what are often called religious or spiritual resources, such as prayer, sacrament, scripture and other means. The extent to which such spiritual resources are used depends upon the counselor. Some use such resources extensively, whilst others do not use them at all, preferring to see God at work in the total process of healing, rather than in any specific spiritual resource.

There is a great variety in methodology, but the main focus is on listening to and learning from the patients, following an accepted medical-psychological model by working in close co-operation with other people involved in the total healing team. This approach to healing has been taught frequently in clinical pastoral education programs, and many people entering the ordained ministry receive this training. Whilst this approach does not entirely ignore the spiritual-charismatic-sacramental approach, it does rely heavily on the use of skills derived from the social sciences and health sciences, which are seen as healing gifts from God.

A Mid-way Approach

Mid-way between the "spiritual-charismatic-sacramental" and the "medical-counseling-pastoral" is a third approach which derives insights from both. The "mid-way approach" gives special emphasis to the laying on of hands, anointing with holy oil, and the celebration of the eucharist. This approach is strong in liturgical-sacramental churches, as in the Roman Catholic and Anglican traditions, where liturgy and ritual are important means by which the healing power of God is received. Combined with this strong liturgical-sacramental emphasis is an equally clear insistence both on the empowering role of the Holy Spirit, and on the role of modern medical and social sciences in healing. These are not seen as opposites, but rather different channels in which God is at work in the total healing process. There is close cooperation with the various helping professions, to provide a "wholistic" approach to healing. This mid-way approach is represented in healing groups such as the various Guilds of Health in U.K., the churches' Council for Health and Healing (U.K.), OSL International, and healing homes and centers situated in many countries. In Australia, the mid-way approach is offered in such ministries as St. Andrew's Healing Ministry (Sydney) and St. Paul's Healing Ministry (Melbourne).

Whilst within the "spiritual-charismatic" stream, it differs from the more overtly Pentecostal type approaches, which tend to give more emphasis to specific healing gifts and the believer's authority, and to the role of the faith healer as seen in many acknowledged leaders within the charismatic-Pentecostal and third wave ministries. (Note: There is no attempt to list and classify particular authors and leaders in these various styles of ministry, because those named may recognize and include several approaches in their ministries. See the suggested reading for references to various authors and approaches.)

It is important to recognize that this "mid-way" approach, while it relates to both the "spiritual-charismatic-sacramental" and the "medical-counseling-pastoral" approaches, is not completely contained in either one. Those who live within this "mid-way" stream would probably affirm that they have the best of both worlds!

Is one **approach** more effective than others? Is one more spiritual than the other? This depends on what we mean by "spiritual." This can mean:

- The inner creative energies which exist in every person; such as the human spiritual energies which are part of our human make-up, and which are given to us by God. We can refer to this as S.1.

- The divine activity of the Holy Spirit who brings more than human resources and power into any situation. This can be referred to as S.2.

Whenever we are involved in caring and healing with another person, there is a sense in which this is a spiritual relationship. It may not have a specifically Christian emphasis, but it is "spiritual" because the meeting of human spirits takes place. Many Christians would emphasize that the Holy Spirit is present in each situation, whether His presence is acknowledged or not.

However, other Christians stress the need to be more open to the special divine resources and special healing gifts of the Spirit (as in 1 Corinthians 12:28-30 and the special blessing of the baptism of the Spirit), and would therefore affirm that an intentional dependence on the Holy Spirit is essential for true healing. This can only take place as the Holy Spirit moves into that particular situation. This ministry of the Holy Spirit is essential, quite apart from any healing which may be brought through the use of human skills.

One approach tends to emphasize the spiritual aspects which are present, through a medical-pastoral-psychological-therapeutic approach (such as in S.1.); while the other more explicitly uses the language of faith and the methods of prayer, laying on of hands, anointing and the like, and deliberately seeks the presence and power of the Holy Spirit in the healing process (such as in S.2.)

The difference between these approaches can be traced to a different theological emphasis which underlies each approach. For example, the medical-psychological model tends to stress the fact that God is present within the total healing process: this could be called the immanence of God; while the spiritual-charismatic-sacramental model tends to stress the power and the presence of God beyond the situation, which moves into the situation to bring healing: this could be called the transcendence of God. When one approach stresses these particular understandings of God's presence and excludes other approaches, then a gap can come between a medical-psychological approach and a spiritual-charismatic-sacramental approach. This may help to explain why some people who are comfortable in one approach are opposed to, or find it hard to understand, other approaches. For instance, it may help to explain why many health professionals and some clergy who are trained in the medical-psychological model often feel uncomfortable with the less-structured spiritual-charismatic-sacramental approach; and also why those who work more in the spiritual-charismatic-sacramental approach feel uncomfortable with the more structured medical-psychological approach.

Is one way more effective in bringing God's healing to sick people than the other? The answer is that both ways are effective and need to be seen as complementary rather than in opposition to each other. Both ways can claim sound theological and biblical foundations. The medical-psychological model is based on the revelation of God as creator, provider, caregiver, giver of all good gifts, the author of all healing, whose concern is revealed in Jesus Christ, and who works through human skills which are themselves His gift. The spiritual-charismatic-sacramental approach is based more directly on the practices of Jesus and the early church, and gives a greater emphasis to the supernatural work of the Holy Spirit. There have been variations of both approaches in the history of the church, especially in the last hundred years, and there are strengths and weaknesses in each approach. In evaluating these approaches, it is clear that any specifically Christian understanding of healing must go beyond that which can be found in human resources alone, and be open to the power and grace of God, if healing is to be true wholeness. We are not truly healed if we ignore the reality of God's power and presence, because the basic relationship with God has not been restored.

Denis Duncan pleads for these different models to recognize the value of each approach.

> What is needed is a much greater determination to try to create some sort of mutual understanding of the way others minister in Christ's name and to bring about the integration of healing and counseling as the full expression of the healing ministry in our time. The roots of the separation go deep into theology but, in the end, there must be a coming together of the approaches that are each based on an over-emphasis of one element in our experience of God as immanent and transcendent. I see the process presently at work as integration through the Spirit.[9]

Over the past decades there has been a growing recognition of the validity of different approaches in the healing ministry. A recent report on global health and healing ministries stated:

> Experiences of healing have acquired a growing importance . . . in the historical churches as well as in charismatic-Pentecostal movements and independent churches . . . There has been an increasing interest in intercultural dialogue on the understanding of health and healing and the role of faith, as a result of the recognition of the limits and necessary complements to the western scientific model of medicine.[10]

The report outlines a wide variety of healing perspectives and practices from various cultural situations, including Africa, China, South India, the Philippines, and the Caribbean. Some of the differences relate to varieties of medical and health practices, charismatic emphases, liturgical practices, counseling methods, and theological issues as suggested in this chapter.

There is an urgent need, especially in the western church, to become more aware of the global dimensions of the healing ministry, and the way many churches combine a variety of approaches and theological and biblical perspectives, rather than suggesting (and sometimes insisting) that one particular approach – either the charismatic-Pentecostal-third wave, OR the more traditional medical-health-counseling models — are the truly biblical models, and therefore the only perspectives worthy of attention.[11]

Sharing and Discussion

1. Can you give examples of these different approaches to healing, as you see them in the Order of St. Luke, in the church, or in particular people? With which approach are you most comfortable? Do you see problems or weaknesses in any of the approaches?

2. Interview a Christian medical doctor, who is sympathetic to the healing ministry, and ask him or her to explain his or her approach

to healing. How does he or she relate to the approaches outlined in this chapter?

3. Ask your pastor, priest, or minister to comment on these different approaches and on his or her understanding and practice of healing.

4. How can the Order of St. Luke help to bring these approaches together to make the church's healing ministry more effective?

5. Review the different attitudes to health and healing in the history of the church. Can you see any present attitudes to health and sickness which have their roots in previous centuries?

6. It is generally accepted that the healing ministry declined in the church when it became the official church of the Empire, and its spiritual life and strength declined (after about 300 AD); whereas in the period of persecution (up to 300 AD), there was more spiritual vitality in the church and the healing ministry was much stronger. Is there any connection between the strength of the healing ministry and the vitality of the spiritual life of the church?

7. In a recent book *The Nearly Perfect Crime*, Francis MacNutt talks about "how the church almost killed the healing ministry" during some periods of its history. Is it possible for the contemporary church to kill the healing ministry today (that is, make it lifeless, ignored, and meaningless to many people, both within and beyond the church)? Do you think this is possible? If so, how could this happen? How can the church guard against this possibility?

References for Further Reading

A Time To Heal, Church House Publishing, London, 2000.

Brown, B., *Liturgy, Ritual and Healing.* Unpublished D.Min Thesis, 1991, Chapter 4.

Blue, K., *Authority to Heal*, IVP, Leicester, 1987.

Duncan, D., *Health and Healing — A Ministry to Wholeness.* St Andrews Press, Edinburgh, 1988.

Kelsey, M., *Psychology, Medicine, and Christian Healing*, HarperCollins, N.Y., 1988, Chapters 7-10.

Kydd, R., *Healing Through the Centuries — Models for Understanding*, Hendricksen, Peabody, Mass., 1998

MacNutt, F., *The Nearly Perfect Crime — How the Church Almost Killed the Ministry of Healing*, Chosen Books/Baker. Grand Rapids. Michigan, 2005.

5

SICKNESS, SUFFERING, AND THE WILL OF GOD

Miriam is a member of the church's healing prayer group, and spends several hours each week praying for the sick and needy. Miriam is very friendly, and is greatly loved by her friends and family all of whom are encouraged by her concern for them and her ability to forget about herself while concentrating on helping and praying for others. Some people find her attitudes hard to understand, because Miriam is an invalid. She is unable to move beyond her small room, and is often in pain as a result of the rheumatoid arthritis which has taken control of many of her limbs. When asked how she is able to respond to her situation and to continue to be concerned for others, Miriam replied that she sees her sickness as the way in which God is training her and shaping her character. She believes God uses her sickness and weakness as a means of blessing others. When asked if she would like to be prayed for, that God would heal and restore her so that she could live a normal life, she declined the offer of prayer and responded by explaining how much she had learnt through her sickness and pain: "God has been able to use my weakness in wonderful ways, which would not have been possible if I had been healthy, so I believe that this suffering and sickness is God's good gift and will for me."

Miriam is concerned about her friend, *Rose,* who suffers from a similar problem, but who often gets very depressed, frustrated and angry, because of her lack of mobility and her inability to do basic tasks. Rose responds to Miriam's offer of prayer by saying that she believes God has given her this sickness as her cross to bear, and that it would be quite wrong to ask for healing, even though she would like to be free from the problem. Rose also implies that

God is too busy, and has too much on His plate to be concerned for her; besides there are many others who are far worse off than she is, so Rose is prepared to accept this sickness as her lot in life.

For *Elaine,* both Miriam and Rose present a real challenge to her faith. Elaine believes that sickness is evil, that it is God's will for people to be whole, and that healing is available through faith in the power of Jesus Christ. While she acknowledges that God is able to bring good out of all situations, Elaine believes that both Miriam and Rose would be more effective if they were restored to good health and strength. While she respects their understanding of the situations, Elaine continues to pray for their physical healing and a complete restoration to full health, believing that this is God's will for them and would be an important contribution to their overall wholeness.

Reflect on these situations. Is Elaine's affirmation of God's healing power valid in this situation? What about the responses of Miriam and Rose? Is sickness/suffering ever the will of God? Spend a few moments reflecting on how you would respond to this situation.

The healing ministry raises many deep questions concerning the problems of sickness and suffering, and how these problems relate to the will of God. For example, if God is love, why is there so much suffering in the world? If the world is created good by God, why is there so much sickness? Is sickness part of God's plan? Is suffering God's way of punishing people? Or, is healing and wholeness God's will and purpose for humankind? There are many such questions, and often we do not have complete or satisfying answers to the deepest questions about sickness and suffering. As in many other areas of life, we know enough to *ask* the questions but not enough to *understand* all the answers.

This chapter aims to:

- Clarify the meaning of sickness and how it affects our lives;

- Understand God's will in relation to sickness;

- Understand the developments in the idea of suffering as a positive spiritual blessing; that is, redemptive suffering;

- Discuss the differences between sickness and suffering;

- Discuss the relationship between God's love, and a suffering painful world;

- Consider the use of the phrase "If it be Thy will" in relation to healing prayer.

To open up these issues, the following seven statements will be used as a basis for study and reflection. The validity of these statements would be accepted by many who are involved in the healing ministry, although questioned by others.

1. Sickness is a reality in the world, and it deeply affects our lives and society.

2. God's *normal* will for people is health and wholeness.

3. Sickness is an evil to be overcome by the power of Jesus Christ.

4. Even though sickness may not be part of God's *normal* will, in some situations it can be accepted as a means for both spiritual and moral growth.

5. Although suffering and sickness are often related in our thinking, they are not the same, and in the New Testament an important distinction is made between them.

6. The fact of suffering and sickness causes many people to question God's love.

In clarifying God's will and purpose in relation to suffering and sickness, we need to think carefully about using such phrases as "Thy will be done," and "If it be Thy will" in praying for healing.

The Reality of Sickness and Its Effects[1]

It is important to understand that there are different kinds of sickness relating to different aspects of our lives, and all of them need to be healed if wholeness is to be experienced. Sickness can be physical, emotional, mental, spiritual, and social, and can affect each of these areas. Sometimes sickness will affect several of these areas at the same time. This chapter is particularly concerned with *physical sickness* as one aspect of an overall "dis-harmony" which affects all people. But while attention is given to physical sickness, it must be remembered that this is one part of a larger problem.

- In defining sickness, two aspects need to be kept in mind. One is the aspect of dis-ease which can be defined as some problem with an organism, when some part of the body or mind is not functioning properly. There is also the aspect of illness which can refer to the experience of the person with the disease, involving both attitudes and feelings. So sickness is a particular malfunction of our bodies or minds, involving feelings and attitudes, which either contribute to the severity of the sickness, or can be a means of healing.

- Sickness is a fact of human life, and few people go through life without experiencing it in some way. The reality of sickness cannot be denied, despite some teaching which suggests that pain and sickness are not real but an illusion. The reality of pain and sickness is expressed in the couplet concerning a faith healer:

There was a faith healer from Deal
Who stated that pain was not real.
He sat down on a pin, and let out a peal,
I dislike what I fancy I feel!

We need to clarify our understanding of sickness, and we can only do that if we accept the fact that it is real, and part of our human life.

• Sickness is an expression of our physical, emotional and spiritual limitations. More than just a lack of health, sickness is a vivid indication that we are human beings, and have a body which is designed to die. When we are healthy we often take our physical body for granted, but when we become sick, especially if the sickness is serious, painful, or of a long duration, we are forced to recognize our human limitations. Sickness inhibits our activities, makes life more difficult, and often poses hard questions for us; such as, "Why me?" or "Why has this happened?" and so on. Often this is accompanied by such feelings as anger, discouragement, loneliness, sadness, bitterness, and confusion.

• Sickness occurs through a variety of causes. It may be through a contact with a virus, poor diet, lack of good body-care, an accident or injury, hereditary disability, drugs or poison, physical degeneration, and other factors. Sometimes there seems to be a direct correlation between a person's lifestyle and their sickness. A sinful lifestyle will often produce sickness in people. Smoking, for example, or intoxicants, may literally make people sick. In other cases, there is no direct connection, as Jesus pointed out in the story of the man born blind (John 9:1-3).

• Sickness involves emotional and psychological responses, as well as physical malfunction; that is, the whole person is affected. Some of the psychological stresses accompanying sickness are that *our integrity is threatened,* and we are forced to see ourselves as not always capable, not always independent, not always self-sufficient, and we may have to come to a new understanding of ourselves. Sometimes sickness can produce *separation anxiety,* in that we are separated from our friends, and from our customary routine. This is especially so if hospitalization is part of sickness. Sickness can also create a *fear of losing love and approval,* particularly if the sickness or injury leaves us physically deformed, or dependent on others, or forced to slow down in some way. Sickness can also create a *fear of losing control,* losing physical strength, intellectual alertness, the control of our bodily functions, the ability to regulate our emotions — all of these things impact our self esteem. Sickness can also create within us a sense of *guilt and a fear of punishment.* Many people feel that their sickness is a punishment for previous sins, and this belief (as in the book of Job) lies deep in the thinking of many people. Sickness also brings *a wide variety of emotions.* We fear pain, we fear possible complications, we fear the future. There can also be anger directed at ourselves, at the sickness, at the doctor, and at God. We can feel depression, with no real desire to get better, sometimes leading to the desire to end our lives. And, over all this, there is often uncertainty and confusion in which we just do not know the answer to our sickness.[2]

• Sickness brings different responses from people . . . These responses are meant to protect us, and they can be both positive and negative.[3] For example, there can be the response of *defense* and *denial.* Because sickness is unwelcome, there is a tendency to deny its seriousness and sometimes even its presence. This is especially true if the illness is likely to be terminal. Sometimes people will respond with an attitude of *projection,* where they pin their feelings of anger, fear, responsibility, on to somebody else; and so the doctor, for example, or others in the patient's life, become the cause of the problem. Occasionally, people retreat into *fantasy,* or magical thinking, where they pretend that healing will come quickly, and "it's not really serious." At times people *suppress,* or, with a stiff upper lip, deliberately forget the unpleasant realities and push them out of their minds. For some people, the response may be *withdrawal.* We need to let others help and love us, but often we feel threatened by such dependence on others, and we withdraw into an attitude of self-pity, despair, resignation, or loneliness. People also respond with *manipulation.* They use their sickness to control others, to get sympathy, attention, and favors from others. Occasionally, people *resist* the sickness through strong complaining and protests; or they can be very positive and refuse to accept the sickness, and come out fighting against it. Sometimes, people will respond by *accepting* all the benefits of sickness; such as attention, sympathy, opportunity to do nothing and freedom from responsibility. Some people enjoy this, and they never get better, and may even experience physical symptoms for which there is no organic basis.

Summing up, we can say that sickness is a sign that we are part of a fallen world. As individuals, and as a world, we are out of harmony, fractured, and broken. Sickness is an indication of this, both in our personal and corporate lives.

God's Will and Purpose for Us is Health

The healing ministry is built on the belief that it is God's will that people be healed and be made whole; that sickness is contrary to His will and purpose, and that His normal will is that people will be healed, unless there is some countervailing reason. This belief rests on the biblical revelation that a fundamental characteristic of God's creation is that it is *good* (Genesis 1:31). God loves what He has made, and He longs for it to be perfect. God loves without distinction and without limit. In Jesus, God is revealed as an all-loving Father, who does not will evil, but rather seeks the good of all people (Matthew 5:45). The will of God is the well-being of all people, and this well-being can be defined in terms of right relationships. There is a right relationship with God, expressed in our obedience to Him, and a response to Him, in love and worship. There is a relationship to our neighbor, expressed in love and service. There is a relationship to our environment, expressed in concern and stewardship. There is a relationship with ourselves, which accepts all aspects of our being as given by God, and therefore to be treated with respect and love.

But this good purpose of God has been thwarted by the evil

which exists in the world. We are part of a broken world, and we share in that brokenness by our own responses, our own desires, and our own brokenness, which the Bible describes as sin. The Bible speaks of human disobedience bringing a fall from God's grace, and it is through this disobedience that disorder has been brought to God's world (Genesis 3; Romans 3:11-20; Ephesians 2:1-4). Within the world, we see powers of evil which work against God's will and are able, to some extent, to limit and hinder His purposes.

The human predicament has been described as God calling His human children to form a very large circle in order to play His game. Everyone is to stand with hands linked together facing toward the light in the center, which is God, and therefore seeing each other all around the circle in the light of that central love, which shines on each one and gives beauty to them. But instead of that, each of us has turned our backs on God, and also upon the circle of our fellow men and women. We face the other way, so that we can see neither the light at the center, nor the faces of our brothers and sisters. Part of this disharmony is revealed in sickness, which is one of the consequences of this thwarting of God's purpose. The healing ministry affirms that in Jesus Christ, God's purpose of healing and wholeness is restored, and in Jesus is released the power which both saves us from our brokenness and alienation, and also heals the sickness which is part of that alienation.

Sickness Overcome through Jesus Christ

In the Old Testament, there is much evidence that God is anxious to heal (for example, Exodus 15:26, 23:25; Psalm 103:3, 107:17-22; Isaiah 53:5; Jeremiah 30:12-17). Sickness is regarded as a punishment for disobedience (Deuteronomy 28:15, 27-29).

In the New Testament, we find Jesus confronting and healing sickness. He described his ministry as doing the works of God, who had sent him (John 4:34, 5:19-21, 6:38, 9:4, 14:10). Jesus cited his works of healing as an indication that he is the Messiah (Luke 7:18-23). In some instances, Jesus regarded sickness as coming from Satan (Luke 13:16). He attributes to Satan the crippling disease that had bound the woman for eighteen years. Throughout the New Testament there is no acceptance of sickness as being part of God's purpose, but there is a confrontation against sickness. Jesus sends out his disciples to heal the sick (Luke 9:1-2, 10:9) because sickness is an evil, to be fought against and overcome.

Both in Jesus' ministry, and the ministry of the early church, there is strong emphasis on healing, because sickness is seen as something which is against God's will and purpose. As the church developed, and became more structured, James 5:13-16 taught how Christians were to respond to sickness. Christians were not to see sickness as part of God's good gifts, but they were to pray against it. Christians were to call for the elders of the church, who would pray and anoint, so that the sickness would be overcome.

Again, as the church developed in history, and as medical science has developed, there has been a constant recognition that sickness is against God's purpose, and is something which reduces our true humanity. If sickness is seen as part of God's will, then Jesus and the apostles, the church in history, and today, doctors, nurses, priests, and all those who work and pray for the sick, including all health care workers, are actively working against the character of God and the will of God. For all of these reasons, sickness can rightly be seen as an evil, as part of the fallen world; to be overcome through the power of Christ; through various medical means; through prayer; but with the realization that this overcoming is only partial, and sickness will not be completely overcome until the kingdom is fully established, when there will be no more tears, or crying, or sickness (Revelation 21:1-4).

It is important therefore, to see that *God's will is to heal,* and to bring complete freedom from sickness, sin, and all the consequences of the Fall. God's primary will is health for His children, so His will is to heal sickness through medicine, prayer, or a combination of means, because sickness is a curse upon our fallen world. Far from being a blessing, sickness is ultimately caused by the forces of evil. Part of the problem will be cured in this life, through the redemption which has been won by Christ on the cross. But the complete answer to sickness will only occur when the kingdom is fully established at the end of time. The healing ministry is based on the belief that substantial healing is available in this life, and this should be seen as God's will and purpose for people, unless there appear to be strong reasons against it. However, there is another way to think about sickness.

Sickness Used by God for Our Growth

Many people who have experienced sickness have interpreted it as an experience which has brought painful benefits to their lives, in their spiritual growth and character development.

Sickness is linked with suffering and accepted as a blessing, and an important aspect of God's refining, character-making purpose. So, while it may be claimed that sickness is not part of God's normal will for us, it can be accepted as a *discipline*, given by God to enable spiritual and moral growth. Sickness, therefore, has a redemptive quality and is an important means which God uses to fulfill His deeper purpose in people's lives.

How did this thinking develop, and is it valid?[4]

Many writers believe that a significant change in the Christian understanding of sickness and healing developed as many church leaders moved gradually from a whole-hearted belief in healing (still strong in the second and third century) to the idea that the body's suffering is preferable for the sake of the soul. With this shift in emphasis, there came a lessening of the church's belief in Christ's healing power. One of the main factors in this development was that some aspects of pagan thought, often described as

"Gnostic" thinking, began to influence Christian thought. One idea was that the human body was like a prison, confining the spirit and hindering true spiritual growth.

Therefore, in the early centuries it came to be thought the human body is not to be trusted, but restricted, controlled, and metaphorically "put to death" through various mortifications and penances. In the battle of the flesh warring against the spirit, the physical body came to be seen as an enemy, to be subdued through punishment, rather than as a wounded friend that needs to be healed. So, traditional Christian spirituality began to emphasize mortification and distrust of the body. This was linked to the belief that sickness was a God-given way to subdue the body; a way of being drawn nearer to God, so that the soul would be purified and conform more perfectly to God's will. Therefore, sickness came to be seen as a *disciplinary* **gift** from God, to be used as a spur toward growth in holiness and sanctification. Prayer for healing began to weaken, because people believed that God wanted them to endure sickness and suffering as a way of preparing the soul for its true passage. In this view, only the human spirit is truly worthy of prayer. Any prayer to heal the broken human body was considered of questionable spiritual benefit. This was a very weak understanding of God's desire to heal our suffering bodies, and this resulted in a strong prejudice against physical healing. If sickness was God's will, then there should be no inclination to ask for release, because sickness was given by God for people's true welfare.

This way of thinking was strengthened by the idea that those whom God loves have to suffer most, as part of their true commitment to Him. In the times of persecution, Christians were called to suffer for their faith as a sign of their loyalty to Christ. The church began to value suffering because persecution helped to both purify and multiply the membership of the church. Those who were half-hearted fell away. By 300 AD a cult of martyrdom had developed, where suffering and especially dying for the faith brought a higher status to the sufferer.

But after persecution declined when the Roman emperor Constantine became a Christian (313 AD), many in the church accepted a lower level of commitment, and there was a sharp decline in spiritual standards. To overcome this drift many began to develop systems of asceticism (self-denial), which were ways of achieving holiness through the denial of normal physical desires. Self-persecution was achieved through living as hermits in the desert, for example, or in separated and isolated communities dedicated to holy living. Often the deprivations included exposure to the elements, sleep deprivation, fasting, self-mutilation, neglect of basic health functions, and other ways to "subdue" the body and "suffer for the sake of true holiness". Sickness was seen as a valuable ally in this quest, and it became linked as a positive blessing to the sufferings of the "true confessors".

Sickness also came to be linked with the idea of "carrying the cross" — an essential mark of the true follower of Jesus Christ (Mark 8:34). The idea was that if you carried your cross of sickness nobly in this life, then you were assured of greater rewards in the life to come.

This popular spirituality taught the importance of suffering, penance and confession, because it offered several important benefits. These disciplines were thought to purge the person of self-seeking and sin (especially the cardinal or deadly sins of lust, gluttony, greed, sloth, wrath, envy, and pride); and helped people to advance in their unselfish love for God and their neighbor (through the cardinal or "Catholic" virtues of chastity, temperance, charity, diligence, forbearance, kindness, and humility). Sickness was thought to enable one to share in the sufferings of Jesus (Colossians 1:24), so personal suffering and its glad acceptance, would fill up what was lacking in the sufferings of Christ for the salvation of the world. Thus the acceptance of suffering and sickness would be a way to imitate Christ; to accept these things as part of his will; and to see them, not as evil, but as a sign of God's love and a way to share more deeply in his crucified life. Therefore it would be wrong to ask for relief from pain or sickness, because any healing would take away an opportunity to imitate Jesus and help redeem the world. A further support for this understanding was the acceptance of the idea that sickness was a punishment for sin. Based on the Old Testament, and given prominence in the teaching of Job's friends, this made a very strong connection between sickness and wrong-doing. This connection was strong in the thinking of the disciples (see John 9:1-3), and it remains important for many people's understanding today. If sickness is seen as a punishment for sin, then we cannot ask for healing from it, but must respond to God in true repentance and accept the just punishment. This idea has been reinforced through the words of the liturgy in the service for the visitation of the sick (dating from the sixteenth century, and only changed in the early twentieth century):

> . . . Wherefore, whatever your sickness is, know you certainly it is God's visitation . . . to try your patience, for the example of others . . . that your faith may be found laudable, glorious, and honorable . . . or else it be sent to you to correct and amend in you, whatever doth offend the eyes of your heavenly Father . . . if you truly repent and bear your sickness patiently, and render unto Him humble thanks for His Fatherly visitation . . . it shall turn to your profit and help you forward in the right way that leadeth to everlasting life . . . [5]

This feeling is evident in the thinking of many people when, following some misfortune or some sickness, they ask the question: "What have I done to deserve this?" thereby making a very strong connection between wrong-doing and sickness.

When these various ideas are brought together, they often result in an attitude of stoicism, where hardship, sickness and suffering is accepted, not just as the normal lot of people, but as part of God's good will and purpose; and therefore not to be changed by any desire for healing. Weak resignation seems to be supported by passages of scripture which emphasize the punishment of sin; the need to share in the sufferings of Christ; the carrying of the cross, interpreted in terms of sickness and suffering; and the example of Jesus, who learned obedience through the things that he suffered (Hebrews 5:7). So sickness is not seen as an evil, but rather a blessing sent by God for some higher purpose. This often produces a conflict in the thinking of many people. On the one hand, when sickness occurs, they eagerly accept the benefits of medical science, in attempting to fight against sickness and overcome it. Yet on the other hand, they believe that not only does God allow it but it is an important part of His purpose, and that you should not pray for the sickness to be relieved.

So, many people are in two minds about sickness. On the one hand they see it is part of God's will and purpose, yet, on the other hand, many in the church and health services are trying to eradicate and overcome it, and their actions are also seen as part of God's will and purpose. But if sickness is part of God's will and a blessing, then are all those who seek to work for the healing of sickness really working against the will of God? This often results in an absurd dichotomy within people's thinking about sickness.

Of course, it is possible to dismiss the idea of sickness being a blessing as outdated and irrelevant. However, there are some important elements of truth within this understanding which need to be accepted. This raises the question of the relationship between suffering and sickness. Are the two synonymous? If sickness is really evil (the concept at the basis of the healing ministry), can there be any purpose to it?

Suffering and Sickness Not the Same

Many writers on the healing ministry make an important distinction between suffering and sickness.[6]

In the teaching of Jesus, sickness is seen as an evil to be overcome, but suffering is to be accepted. However it is not the suffering associated with sickness that is to be endured, but the suffering which results from persecution. On the one hand, Jesus tells his followers that they must bear their cross; yet, on the other hand, whenever he meets sick people, he reaches out and cures them. Jesus thus makes a distinction between two types of suffering. The cross that Jesus carried was the cross of persecution, the kind of suffering that is imposed from "outside" because of the wickedness of evil people. Jesus suffered deeply within himself, but the source of his anguish and suffering was outside himself. Precisely because of who he was and what he did, Jesus drew down upon himself persecution, anger, insults and torture from his enemies, who were infuriated at his life and teaching. But nowhere do the gospels suggest that Jesus was physically sick. Although this cannot be proved, there has been a long Christian tradition that has suggested that Jesus did not suffer from leprosy, epilepsy, schizophrenia, or any other disease or emotional disturbance. We sense that these sicknesses result from a breakdown of our inner being, and are not in accord with God's purpose for us. In Jesus, we see one who was emotionally and physically balanced and healthy.[7]

In his words and actions, Jesus distinguishes between sickness which attacks our life and wholeness from within, and persecution which attacks from outside. He warns his disciples that they will be persecuted; they will be dragged before leaders and authorities; they will be thrown out of synagogues; their enemies will be their own relatives; and that they are to rejoice when all manner of evil is spoken against them (Matthew 5:10-12, 10:16-22). This is the suffering which results from persecution, and it can be expected as a normal part of true discipleship. However in relation to sickness and demonic possession, the gospels never depict Jesus as telling sick people to rejoice and be patient, because their disease is helpful or redemptive — rather, he heals the sick. He does not encourage people to accept their sickness as part of the will of God. He taught his disciples to take an uncompromising stand against sickness; and he commissioned them to preach, to heal the sick, to drive out evil spirits — thus making a clear distinction between the suffering resulting from persecution, which was to be accepted, and the suffering resulting from sickness, which was to be healed.

The Apostle Paul also declares his intention of wanting to know the fellowship of sharing in Christ's sufferings, becoming like him in his death (Philippians 3:10). But this did not refer to sickness, because in his ministry Paul opposed sickness, and he and the other apostles healed people from their sickness (Acts 3:1-10, 9:32-43, 19:11, 28:8-9). Paul emphasized the need to suffer with Christ, but he does not encourage the sick person to see his or her illness as willed by God. He acknowledges the sickness of Trophimus, Epaphroditus, and Timothy, as a reality in their lives, but he does not exalt their conditions as evidence of God's good will and purpose for them (2 Timothy 4:20; Philippians 2:25-30; 1 Timothy 5:23). He was ready to boast of his sufferings for Christ and his weakness, but it is not clear whether this involved sickness. He boasted about suffering which came from persecution, imprisonment, flogging, exposure to death, whipping and shipwreck (2 Corinthians 11:23-29).

There is debate among Christian writers as to the exact meaning of Paul's use of suffering and sickness. Some argue that sickness was included as part of his general suffering, while others argue against this. Both arguments rest on the use and meaning of particular Greek words. A further issue is the identification of Paul's "thorn in the flesh" (2 Corinthians 12:7). Some argue that the thorn was a physical sickness or affliction, given to Paul to accomplish some higher spiritual purpose. If this is so, it supports the idea of sickness being redemptive in purpose; that is, a painful but necessary blessing. However, others suggest that the "thorn" refers to human persecution and harassment, and not to sickness. And even if it could be proved conclusively that it was a physical sickness, Paul did not readily accept it and repeatedly asked for its removal. He accepted it only after a bitter spiritual battle, and only after the Lord specifically told him to do so.[8]

It is possible to present arguments which support either

interpretation; namely, sickness as part of suffering, or seeing these as quite distinctive. The problem is that the English word "suffer" has a wide meaning which may include sickness, whereas the New Testament words are distinct and different. This is shown in James 5:13-14, where suffering and sickness are treated as different issues, and responses to them are also different. Whatever we may decide about Paul's "thorn in the flesh," there is sufficient evidence to accept the distinction between sickness and suffering. Certainly in the teaching and practice of Jesus, suffering and sickness are not the same. Whilst suffering is inevitable for the true disciple, sickness is to be confronted and the sick healed. The teaching and practice of Jesus should be the norm in evaluating all responses to this issue.

So a valid conclusion is that suffering can be seen as part of God's purpose to deepen our faith and trust. It is intended to be a redemptive experience, by which we learn the "obedience of not trusting in ourselves" but in God (2 Corinthians 1:8-9). Suffering is an essential aspect of being a Christian. But being sick is not essential to discipleship, because sickness is an evil to be confronted and overcome.

However, it is possible to affirm that sickness, although not good in itself, can be used by God to bring about a deeper purpose for the sake of the kingdom, or for God's special purpose. In the life of the church there has been a long tradition which regards sickness as a form of suffering which can be accepted and used for a higher purpose. Suffering through sickness in itself is neutral. Suffering through sickness may open new doors and windows into a deeper understanding of ourselves and God, or it can shut us in upon ourselves, and produce distorted lives and destructive relationships. Healing and a deeper purpose come when sickness is met with the response of faith, hope and love. For the suffering caused by sickness to be creative and redemptive, there must be a readiness to accept the situation, rather than react in anger against it, an ability to participate in this suffering, leading to a higher quality of life, and an appreciation of the spiritual elements within that suffering. There are many examples of people who have experienced sickness and have found God to be with them, and that experience of suffering through sickness has become a journey into new life. Many of those who visit the sick have found that they are drawn closer to God through the sick person's faith and acceptance; that is, through the very attitudes which their sickness has formed in them. Throughout the centuries, many have interpreted sickness in this light, and they have used it as a way to achieve a greater reliance on God, a greater purification in their life, and a means of sharing in the pain of the world. So in this sense, the suffering caused through sickness has been seen as redemptive and as a blessing.[9]

So there can be some ambivalence of interpretation about the relation of suffering to sickness. On the one hand, sickness is seen as an evil to be overcome; on the other hand, in certain situations, sickness can be seen as a way that God uses to bring about a deeper purpose for the sake of the kingdom. Many involved in the healing ministry have different perspectives on this issue. What is clear, however, is the command to heal the sick, and the need to be actively involved in this ministry. Whether God chooses to use sickness for a particular purpose does not absolve the church from involvement in the ministry of healing.

However, this ambivalence can create a dilemma. When a person becomes sick, then some will offer that person consolation, suggesting that God has chosen this sickness as a means of imparting some spiritual benefit. Others refuse to ask for healing, because they believe it is God's will for them to suffer — even though they may hate Him for sending the sickness. Then there are some who regard their sufferings as sent by God, as a means of producing spiritual progress and growth. They are able to trust God absolutely, and are convinced that God has allowed this to come for their spiritual welfare. Thus they are able to accept their suffering and sickness without doubting God's love. They overcome the problem of sickness by using it as a way of accomplishing spiritual progress. This is a redemptive response to something which in itself is evil.

So, while the healing ministry may accept the fact that sickness is not to be aligned with suffering as part of our normal Christian commitment, there can be an acceptance of sickness as being part of God's special purpose. However, this acceptance of sickness does not change the basic understanding that health is God's primary will for all His children. This should be regarded as the "normal" understanding of God's will and purpose in relation to sickness and suffering.

However, whilst accepting that healing is God's primary will, the reality and depth of suffering and sickness creates a further difficulty for many people.

"If God is Love, Why Do We Suffer?"

In trying to understand this problem, we must acknowledge that the question of suffering has always exercised the minds of thoughtful people. Healing is intimately connected with suffering, and Christians are not exempt from the world's suffering. The idea is false that by joining the Christian fellowship people will be protected against the hazards, the pains, and the sufferings of life. We need to acknowledge that suffering comes from various sources and is of many different kinds. Suffering may be caused by natural disasters, such as earthquakes, hurricanes, and floods; or by accidents, wars, famine, and political oppression; or from conflict between people; or from disease, sickness, emotional distress, or spiritual torment. Suffering may come as a result of human action, and be directly connected with sin. Sometimes there appears to be no sense or justice in suffering; there appears to be no explanation, and suffering may seem quite arbitrary and pointless. Some suffering seems to be deserved, while much of it seems undeserved. But the real questions in relation to suffering, are: "Where is God in all this?" "Where is God, the good creator, whose purpose is one of love and concern?" "Where is God in our suffering?" As one writer asks: "Where is God, when it hurts?"[10]

The Christian answer has *not* been to try and fully explain the causes of evil and suffering, but to recognize God as being on the side of health and healing, and involved in all the efforts to reduce the suffering which is due to human accident, disease, sin, or some other cause. The Christian believes that, although dreadful things happen, it is still God's world and therefore everything within it is somehow contained within His sovereign purposes. This is often difficult to accept and understand. It has caused people much anguish, and kept some from faith and commitment. It has been well said that suffering is not so much a problem to be solved, but a mystery to be accepted in faith. And yet, we need to keep exploring for some kind of understanding. If God is God, the Sovereign Lord, then where does suffering fit into His plan and purpose? On the one hand, it is clear that God permits suffering. On the other hand, it is equally clear that His concern is for health and well-being. It is usually not helpful to people who are suffering to be told by others that this is the will of God for them. The real comfort for people in such circumstances is the knowledge that God is present in the situation and sharing in their sorrow. This is the specifically Christian understanding of suffering, that, when people suffer, *God suffers with them*. The prophet Isaiah speaks of God being afflicted when His people are afflicted, and speaks of the suffering servant: "He has borne our grief and carried our sorrows" (Isaiah 53:4-7). In the life and ministry of Jesus Christ, God shares in the experience of suffering in a direct and personal way, and it is this involvement of God in our lives which helps to make some sense of suffering, even though it is not fully understood. Jesus did not offer explanations of suffering which made light of human alienation and anguish. Rather, he took these seriously and something about them by bearing the ultimate cost in himself.

The Christian belief is that in the cross, we see the love of God manifested in Jesus for the salvation of the world (2 Corinthians 5:19). This suffering is the outcome of the conflict with evil, and the innocent one bears the pain of the encounter. In that great conflict, evil is defeated and suffering is transformed.

So the cry, "He was wounded for our transgressions, he was bruised for our iniquities, and with his stripes we are healed" brings a note of hope; that Christ has been, and is still involved in the struggle with every form of evil. Through Christ, God has conquered evil and suffering. God is not immune from the suffering of the world, but He is with us in suffering; sharing in the pain of a broken world, and in a strange way, absorbing that suffering in Himself, and transforming it into the victory of the cross and resurrection. God is, therefore, not so much the One who sends suffering, but the One who, for some reason in His own purposes, permits it, and then bears the consequences Himself. In Jesus, we see God as the wounded healer, by whose stripes we are healed (1 Peter 2:24).

Ultimately there is no human explanation of the mystery of suffering. We can affirm that the powers of evil are working against God's will; we can affirm God's participation in this suffering; we can affirm the ultimate and complete victory over evil; but we also have to recognize that this is a slow and gradual process, and whilst we may experience something of the victory, it is not yet complete. There is a loving creator and a suffering and sinful creation. There is an almightiness of love and power which conquers by the power of love, for God's purpose is love. In practical terms this means that we can be helped to bear suffering and loss in the knowledge that the one who bore our grief and carried our sorrows is with us. We can say, with Paul, that nothing can ever happen — tribulation, distress, or persecution — to separate us from the love of God in Jesus Christ (Romans 8:37-39). In our involvement in the healing ministry then, the primary emphasis should be upon the love of God, which identifies with human suffering, as the way by which we can accept suffering and find some meaning in it.

How Do We Pray in Relation to God's Will?

In seeking to understand God's will and purpose in relation to suffering and sickness, we need to think of the use of such phrases as "The will of God," "If it be Thy will," and "Thy will be done."

Sometimes the phrase "the will of God" is used in such a way that actions are ascribed to God that we would never ascribe to another human person, and all kinds of terrible actions, accidents and sicknesses are simply said to be God's will. So God is portrayed as acting in ways which would not be tolerated in human behavior. Evil is attributed to God, simply because we cannot understand where it has come from. However, we should not think of God's will apart from His character, His purpose, and His love. To ascribe evil and inhuman conduct to God, makes a falsehood out of the life and teaching of Jesus, who never ascribed to God, pain, disease, disability, or any other evil. Jesus ascribed these things to the enemy of God's purpose (Satan). Thus, whenever we use the phrase "the will of God," we must interpret it in the light of Jesus' revelation of God. In Jesus, we truly see what God is like (John 14:9), as One who Himself shares in the pain and suffering of the world. God's perfect or highest will for us is for our good. When it appears otherwise and we are confronted with evil, then this must be acknowledged as an enemy doing this. (Compare Matthew 13:24-29). Evil is permitted by God but it is not His ultimate purpose.

Often, in praying for people, the phrase "If it be Your will" is used. This is derived from the words of Jesus in the Garden of Gethsemane who, when confronted with the awfulness of the cross, prayed that the cup may pass from him: "But nevertheless not my will, but yours, be done" (Matthew 26:39). Jesus' prayer was an acceptance of the Father's will and purpose, of His sovereignty and authority, and also an indication of Jesus' commitment to that authority. Often, in praying for people, the desire is to commend that person to God and to seek God's healing in their life, but not to demand from God that healing must be given.

There is a healthy sense in which God is allowed to be God, and there is no desire to impose our demands on Him. God's will is to be done. This may be for healing of the person concerned, or it may not be. So rather than try and appear to force God and demand healing, the phrase, "If it be Your will" is used. This is not seen as in any way doubting God, rather it is a faith which is prepared to leave the ultimate issues with God. It is a faith which does not depend on getting a favorable result, but is prepared to accept God's purpose and outcome, whether it be in sickness, or health, in life, or death. However, whilst this is good in that it does not seek to dictate to God, it may also create confusion in two ways. Firstly, it may suggest that God does not wish to heal or help in any way at all. This is what some will conclude when that phrase is used. Secondly, it assumes that God's will is completely unknowable. However J. Glennon affirms that God's will is revealed in the many promises in scripture, and these need to be taken seriously and appropriated.

> It is frequently said that we do not know the will of God, and therefore we cannot pray with understanding faith that God will answer in the affirmative. So we have to conclude our prayer with the proviso, "If it be Thy will."

> That we have to pray according to God's will, if our prayers are to be answered, is not in question. Nor is the fact that there are times when we do not know God's will. But there are many matters on which we can know God's will, because it is revealed in the Bible. His will for us is contained in His precious and very great promises (2 Peter 1:4), and we search the scriptures to see what these promises are. Once we determine what they are, we can appropriate them by the power of faith. Often the phrase, "not my will but Thine be done," is used to create a false dichotomy. It is agreed that we must pray according to God's will, but His will is revealed to us in His promises; that is, His promises reveal His will. So as we accept His promises by faith, we are praying according to His will.

The view that there may be magnificent promises in the scriptures to do with prayer, but that it may not be God's will for us to have them in reality, is a contradiction in terms, for it runs contrary to the basic concept of a promise-making and promise-keeping God. Our whole relationship with God is built on the magnificent promises in the scriptures. Without them we have no assurance of God's blessing, or salvation, or anything else. We are partakers of this promise in Christ Jesus through the gospel, and all the promises of God find their "Yes" in him, that is, in Christ. If God's will and provision are conveyed to us in the promises, then we are to appropriate them by faith.[11]

This affirmation does not remove all the difficulties, but does call for a greater openness to the power of God in our lives, and a greater readiness to take God at His word. As well as acknowledging that God's will and purpose may be different from our own perception and desires, we must be ready to move forward in faith. A practical way forward is to accept that God's "normal" will is for healing, and to proceed on this assumption, unless there is a clear indication to the contrary; such indications coming through some discernment or understanding which God gives in the situation. Unless some clear indication is given to the contrary, then we should assume that God's will and purpose is for healing, and continue to pray accordingly. However, we must always keep in mind that healing may not necessarily mean physical healing. We have already seen that healing means wholeness, which may or may not involve physical healing. Healing is more than cure, so that we can pray to God to bring the healing which is His purpose for that particular person. It may be physical restoration, or in some situations, it may be the acceptance of death as the ultimate healing. It could be healing in the sense of wholeness, through the acceptance of that sickness as a means of drawing closer to God. We hold in tension the promises of healing and the possibility of a different type of healing than we desire.

We therefore can affirm the promises of God for healing, without demanding exactly what He must do. His purposes may align with our desire for ourselves, or others, but are always greater than our desires. We have to rest and trust in God that He will do what is best in each situation. Therefore, when we are in a dilemma as to how to pray, we can continue to ask for healing in that person's life in the way that God purposes, and leave the results to Him. Because of the negative ideas which may accompany the use of the words, "If it be Your will," many prefer not to use this phrase, but use another form of words, such as, "Lord, heal this person and make him/her whole in the way that you would have him/her be," or "Lord, heal this person according to your loving purposes for him or her." It may be objected that this is only another form of words which really says exactly the same as the phrase "If it be Your will." That may be true. However, the use of a different form of words takes away the problem that the phrase, "If it be Your will" has in many people's minds. It acknowledges God's freedom and authority to act according to His purposes, but it also allows us to rest in the confidence and trust that He will do what is best for the person.

In summarizing this chapter, it is acknowledged that sickness and suffering is a difficult area to understand, and not all the questions can be satisfactorily answered. However, we can strongly and confidently affirm that the healing ministry is based on the fact that God's will is for health and healing, and that sickness is to be opposed and confronted, unless a deeper purpose can be seen in that sickness.

Sharing and Discussion

1. Think about your own experience of sickness. What feelings were involved for you? How did you cope with these feelings? How did others either help or hinder your coping with them? What have your learned from your experience?

2. Is sickness an evil to be fought against, or is it a discipline to

promote spiritual growth? Can both ideas be true? Which one do you find hardest to understand? Cope with? Respond to? Share your thoughts with others.

3. Should we deliberately seek sickness and suffering (persecution for our faith) as a way to grow in faith and goodness?

4. What response can you give when people refer to their sickness as the cross they have to bear? Is this the meaning of taking up the cross as a follower of Jesus? See Luke 14:27; Matthew 10:38.

5. What is God's answer to the problem of suffering and pain in the world? How does God's answer help us in dealing with the problem of suffering and pain in our lives?

6. Nowhere do the gospels suggest that Jesus was physically sick. How do you respond to the church's tradition that Jesus was always healthy — physically, emotionally, and spiritually? Is it important for our understanding of healing that we never see Jesus as "sick," or doesn't it matter?

7. In what ways are the followers of Jesus called on to suffer for their faith today? Think of your own social and cultural situation, but also try to find out other situations around the world where Christians are enduring suffering and persecution for their faith.

8. Investigate in more detail the distinction between sickness and suffering in the New Testament writings. Do you think the distinction between sickness and suffering is a valid distinction? Refer to the references, especially J. Glennon, *Your Healing is Within You*, pp. 154-165, 181-185; and F. MacNutt, *Healing*, Chapter 5.

9. "If it be Your will," *or* "According to Your will and purpose" — Do these phrases mean the same thing? Which phrase do you think is more suitable in praying for healing, or are both phrases valid?

References for Further Reading

Blue, K., *Authority to Heal,* IVP, Leicester, England, 1987.

Carson, D., *How Long O Lord?,* Baker, Grand Rapids, 1990.

Collins, G., *Christian Counseling,* Word, Milton Keynes, U.K., 1989.

Glennon, J., *Your Healing is Within You,* Hodder & Stoughton, London, 1978.

Glennon, J., *How Can I Find Healing,* Hodder & Stoughton, London, 1984.

MacNutt, F., *Healing,* Hodder & Stoughton, London, 1988.

Masters, P., *The Healing Epidemic,* The Wakeman Trust, London, 1988.

Storms, C. S., *Healing and Holiness,* Presbyterian & Reformed, New Jersey, 1990.

Yancey, P., *Where Is God When It Hurts?,* Zondervan, Grand Rapids, 1977.

6

BY MANY MEANS: METHODS USED IN THE MINISTRY TO SICK AND TROUBLED PEOPLE

Frank has become involved in the healing ministry because of the healing he experienced in his *own* life as a result of concerned friends praying for him. He now realizes that God gives his healing power in many different ways and he is keen to understand the various methods used by those involved in the healing ministry, especially prayer and the laying on of hands. Some of his friends claim to possess a special gift of healing prayer so that God responds when they lay their hands on people. They urge Frank to be open to God so that he too can use this method effectively. But Frank feels rather confused, for two reasons. One is that he doesn't feel as if he has any special prayer gift. In *fact,* when he prays, he struggles to get words and thoughts in order, and usually doesn't know what to pray for. Also, he doesn't feel any special power in himself, and therefore assumes that he would not be effective if he laid hands on sick people. Secondly, he is aware that many non-Christian groups also use methods like touching, laying on of hands, and meditation, and he wonders whether their approach is the same as Christians who seem to use similar methods. Is there any real difference? Frank comes to talk to you about which methods are correct and which are not correct from a Christian perspective. *Briefly* write down the main points you would make in your response to him.

Along with many individuals and groups involved in the healing ministry, OSL recognizes many different methods as ways through which God may bring healing to people's lives. No one method is regarded as special or essential. In fact, any method which ac-knowledges that healing is from the activity of God, Father, Son and Holy Spirit, and is centered on Jesus Christ as the focal point of healing, is acceptable.

This chapter aims to:

- Study some of the methods used in the healing ministry, and suggest reasons why these methods are used.

- Clarify some of the differences between Christian and other use of some of these methods.

Some Basic Assumptions about Healing

The use of different methods in the healing ministry rests on some basic beliefs about healing. Healing is given by God and ultimately derives from His activity rather than from any human skill or method, such as ritual, prayer, action, prescription. One writer says:

> Healing of any kind is necessarily divine. The physician does not heal, nor medicine, nor a scientific diet, nor an improved environment, nor anything else that may be named. All creation, or re-creation, is from God, and hence in every instance of healing He is the one who heals, whether He acts directly through unknown laws or indirectly through known laws.[1]

This does not lessen the importance of human skill and care, but correctly affirms that the complex healing mechanisms of body and mind which can be triggered by illness, injury, disease or other upset, are a gift from God. So also is sunshine, rain, fresh air, vita-mins, proteins, and the many human skills involved in medical sci-ence, counseling, prayer, faith, love. These can all be described as the ingredients of health and healing, and all are ultimately God's good gifts which he uses to maintain and restore health.

It is God's normal purpose to heal, and each method can be used as a way to allow this to happen. The methods are used to counteract disease, to prepare the way to receive healing, and to remove barriers which could prevent this from happening. Each method can be seen as a channel through which God's healing activity moves into needy lives and situations. Christian healing is focused in Jesus Christ and any method used must be evaluated by the extent to which it acknowledges His authority.

While methods are important, and should be carefully studied and practiced, they need to be activated by the power of love which is given by the Holy Spirit and which provides the essential climate for healing to occur. This necessity of caring love does not excuse sloppy or naive methods, but it is a reminder that God's healing is not confined to the correctness of any particular method. Methods are the means to an end, like the framework or scaffold used in a building, but they are not the end themselves. Healing will occur as a result of people being surrounded by loving care even though the methods used may not have been the best way to follow in that particular situation.

A Variety of Methods in Healing

God is not restricted to any one method, however successful it may appear to be. In his healing ministry, Jesus used many different methods; for example, sometimes healing came by touch; sometimes instantaneously; occasionally in stages; sometimes at a distance; or in response to a plea from the sufferer; at other times through the faith of friends; and at times by using some material thing like saliva or mud. However, it is clear that these various methods were not the cause of the healing, rather they were the means used by Jesus to bring the healing he desired. In one healing incident Jesus seemed to divert the faith of a distressed woman away from a particular method; that is the touching of his clothes, to faith in himself as the source of healing (Mark 5:21-34).

Methods may be either natural, through the normal process of recuperation and restoration without any input from medical science; or medical/scientific, through the use of medication or other treatment; or supernatural, through the use of prayer, faith, and the laying on of hands. However, the use of terms such as natural/super-natural, spiritual/non-spiritual, create problems because they suggest that some methods are from God and therefore truly *spiritual,* while others which are based on human skills are therefore *non-spiritual.* This is a false distinction which is often based on an inadequate theology of God, man, and creation, and which can lead to distortions in any understanding of the total healing ministry. (See Chapter 9 — Healing and Medical Science — Pills or Prayer or Both?)

Similar methods — such as relaxation, visualization, and meditation — may be used in Christian and non-Christian healing, so discernment is needed. Secular, alternative, and New Age healing often uses similar names but the focus and ultimate purpose of the methods are different. Many groups and people use the method of healing touch, but the aim may be to draw on some universal energy or psychic power rather than to symbolize the healing touch of Jesus; or in meditation the aim may be to move into an altered state of consciousness and thus come into contact with the god within, rather than to focus on the word and action of God the Father, Son and Holy Spirit. Because of the possibility of confusion, discernment is needed to understand the differences in the use of similar methods.

But the Christian should not vacate these various methods or therapies because they are used in non-Christian systems. Many of these methods which are now being used by physicians and psychologists as adjunct therapies in treating illness — like relaxation, meditation, and visualization — were actually pioneered by the founders of healing prayer movements long before these new therapies were being recognized and hailed as new discoveries. The writings of leaders like Glenn Clark, Frank Laubach, John G. Banks, and Agnes Sanford (published from the 1920s through the 1940s) promoted these methods within a Christian theological context which is completely lacking in the contemporary humanistic versions recognized today. The Christian healing ministry has the task of reclaiming some of these legitimate and valuable methods while at the same time pointing out the differences in approach which can lead to confusion, and the tendency by some Christians to discard and dismiss all such methods as "New Age," or "Satanic." (See Chapter 11 — Christian Healing and Alternative Healing Movements.)

The methods used may be directed to the individual where the person needing help is the focus of the ministry, or they may be used in the more public way as in a healing service or group. Certain methods may be especially applicable to particular healing needs. Just as there are different types of sickness, so there are different methods which are used. Francis MacNutt suggests that there are at least three different kinds of sickness which require different responses or methods.[2]

- Sickness of the spirit caused by personal sin which requires repentance, confession and prayer.

- Emotional sickness caused by emotional hurts of the past, requiring prayer for inner healing and often accompanied by prayer counseling.

- Physical sickness caused by disease or accident, requiring prayer and medical care.

All three of these may also be caused or aggravated by demonic oppression which may require prayer and exorcism. Prayer, the laying on of hands, anointing, confession, the blessing of the eucharist may be involved in healing all or some of these kinds of sickness. Sometimes one method will be used by itself, but it is more common to combine several methods in any healing ministry.

Such variety in methods of healing ministry means it is not possible to describe each method in detail. The following brief explanations suggest some of the main aspects of the various methods. These include prayer, laying on of hands, anointing with oil, sacraments, confession and absolution, deliverance and exorcism, prayer counseling, and co-operation with medical science. In many of these there is an effective use of spiritual gifts, so this also must be included in any catalogue of healing methods.

This chapter deals specifically with prayer, laying on of hands, and anointing with oil. References to other methods are included in later chapters.

Prayer

It is impossible to adequately explain the significance of prayer in a few sentences. It is one of the most discussed subjects but probably one of the least practiced. As a gift of grace, prayer cannot be presented in any stereotyped package for it is one of the most simple and yet most profound responses to the activity of God, and is experienced by people in all cultures, ages and generations, from the stumbling yet piercingly accurate words of the honest small child to the mature reflections of the elderly. It can be formalized in set ritual and liturgy, and it can be free and extemporaneous in expression. It covers a wide gamut of human needs and responses which are often expressed in the ACTS formula — *adoration, confession, thanksgiving,* and *supplication.*

One description suggests that prayer is a conversation with God in which God and a person or people talk together just as friends share and talk with each other. This correctly emphasizes the sense of fellowship. However, it can cause us to think that talking is the essence of prayer; that is, us talking to God. This is in fact how many people actually pray, by continually talking to God in a one-way monologue in which we bring our shopping list of needs and problems to God (perhaps prefaced by some words of praise and thanksgiving), and then, having placed our order, we wait eagerly for God to supply what we have asked. If God chooses not to answer our requests then we easily lose our desire to pray because it doesn't work! This consumer approach to prayer is often found in relation to the need for healing, because we naturally want to be freed from our problem, and we see God as there to supply our need.

Prayer can also be used as a form of magic in which God is seen as the source of something we desire; for example, power, healing, or wisdom, and prayer is seen as the key to unlock the storehouse and get what we want. To ensure this will happen, the correct words and forms of prayer must be used, so an element of demand is present — because we have done what is required, therefore God is obliged to respond in our favor. We have kept our side of the agreement, now it is up to God to respond in our favor, hopefully on our terms. There are many variations of this attitude which make human needs rather than God the focal point of praying. This self-centered attitude is really the opposite of true prayer, which at its heart is a relationship with God who is Father. In instructing his disciples to pray, Jesus emphasized that the focal point of prayer is "Our Father" (Matthew 6:9).

Prayer is a symbol of a relationship in which the covenant God is present with and active for His people. The covenant God is also the creator who continues to act in His world where His creative sustaining activity is experienced. Prayer is being with this creating and saving God who is revealed to us as Father, Son and Holy Spirit. It is the relationship of a child going for a walk with his or her father, each being in the other's company because of the love they share. That relationship includes our moods, words, pains, hopes, joys, concerns, failure — all that we are, and is expressed in various patterns of prayer: in thanksgiving, praise, confession, intercession, and often in silence. The basis of this relationship is what God has done and continues to do for us rather than what we can offer to him. God is the initiator who invites us to share with Him in this covenant relationship and to become involved in His world. Prayer is the means by which the relationship is deepened and experienced in our lives. Within this love relationship we are encouraged to share our lives with Him — to offer thanks, to seek forgiveness, to ask Him to meet our needs, to intercede for others, to receive strength for service — in fact to bring everything to God in prayer. And we do this not just to gain what we want, but to express our trust and confidence in the goodness and loving purpose of our Father (Matthew 6:9-13; Philippians 4:6-7; Hebrews 4:14-16). This does not mean that this relationship will always be light and sunshine, easy to explain and understand. Sometimes it may be strained, dark, and painful, and prayer will be difficult. Often we will not know how to pray; often we will not want to pray; but the invitation remains for us to come, to seek, to knock, to ask, to bring our requests, to find grace and mercy, and to walk humbly with our covenant God.

On this basis healing prayer will include the following: aligning ourselves with God's purpose to heal; offering to Him people and situations where healing is needed; making ourselves available to be agents of healing; asking for His blessing on all those involved in the healing process; trusting Him in confidence to do as He has promised, to raise up and heal the sick and to put down and defeat the powers of evil. It is not so much a matter of asking God to intervene in a needy situation as if He were absent, but rather it is a means of creating an environment or climate in which God's creative love and power may be released in healing. It is becoming open and attuned to the God who is always there; it is clearing the decks so that the healing which is wholeness may be experienced and God's purpose for each person may be realized.

Prayer for healing then is not only a matter of asking for a cure to a specific problem, although it will include this, but rather a seeking and a desire to be with God and open to His will. One of the leading theologians of the twentieth century, Paul Tillich, writes:

> Generally speaking, one can say that a Spirit determined prayer seeks to bring one's own personal center, including one's concern for the health of someone else, before God, and that it is willing to accept the divine acceptance of the prayer whether its overt content is fulfilled or not. Conversely, a prayer which is only a magical concentration on the desired aim using God for its realization, does not accept an unfulfilled prayer; for the ultimate aim of the magic prayer is not God and reunion with Him, but the object of the prayer, that is, health. A prayer for health in faith is not an attempt at faith healing, but an expression of the state of being grasped by the spiritual presence.[3]

An essential part of healing prayer is faith (Mark 11:22-24; James 1:6, 5:15). And the prayer of faith is basic to any effective healing ministry. However, it is not so much our great faith which will ensure that healing is given, it is rather our trust and confidence in God's great faithfulness and promises. We can believe that we will receive blessing and healing because we have trust and confidence in who God is; so the prayer of faith depends first of all on God's faithfulness, and we are linked to that through our trust in what He has promised to those who believe. The object of our faith is God, not the power of faith. Sometimes when healing is not experienced even though believing prayer has been offered, the reason given is lack of faith. Whilst this may be true in some situations, as in Matthew 13:58, it cannot be applied to all situations; the healings in John 5, John 9, and Mark 5:1-20 do not mention faith at all. If a lack of faith is over-emphasized, then people may become guilty and confused and try to work harder to have greater faith. It then becomes a human performance which is really the opposite of what faith is — a restful but active trust in God's faithful promises so that we can take Him at His word. Confident assurance and a relaxation in the power of God to meet our needs for healing are the basic criteria. Praying in faith has been described as "resting in the conviction (literally being conquered by the conviction) that in God there is a power of love sufficient for all my needs. I put myself in His hands without wishing to force any outcome, or even necessarily believing that I know best what the outcome should be."[4] This aspect of faith is studied in more detail in Chapter 7 — The Prayer of Faith.

In the healing ministry there are many variations in the actual methods of praying for healing. The content of prayer will depend on the situation and the time available. Two examples of ministry are given to illustrate the different patterns of prayer which are offered.

• In a more formal situation, such as a healing service, prayer is offered and laying on of hands is given to those who come forward or indicate in some way their desire for healing. There is usually insufficient time for any in-depth counseling in relation to personal needs. Those offering the prayer usually ask the person concerning their need (or they may be coming on behalf of another person), then these are gathered up into a prayer which may include the following: acknowledging God's power and presence, recognizing our dependence on Him, and our need for wholeness in body, mind and spirit and the blessing offered in the name of the Lord. The prayer may be all encompassing, asking God to touch all levels of a person's life, or it may be more specific in relation to a particular need. It is usually accompanied by the laying on of hands. There may be time for the expression of the gifts of discernment and knowledge, but sometimes there is insufficient time for this to take place as there is often a need to conclude the service. In a more informal setting, sometimes the period given to the ministry of prayer can be extended, thus allowing for a greater flexibility where there are no constraints of time, and there is greater opportunity to listen carefully and to spend a longer time in prayer.

- In a more informal or non-service setting, such as a healing group, or two or three people meeting together, there is often greater time available to allow different methods to be followed.

In this type of situation the first step is one of listening to the person who asks for healing so that they can explain what they feel is the problem, but also listening to God who often gives some special insight concerning the problem. However, there is a prior step which is also involved and that is listening to God to find out whether or not to pray in this particular situation. This suggests that some people may not be ready for healing, or perhaps this may not be the best time to pray, or I may not be the best person to pray in this situation. In other words, we should not assume that we must pray for everyone who asks for prayer, or that we must pray in every situation. Sometimes it may be best to say "no" to requests for prayer to prevent overload stress. Agnes Sanford has these wise words to say:

> It is not the duty of every Christian to pray for everyone. Our prayers will help some and not help others, for reasons beyond our understanding or control. Only the Holy Spirit can safely direct our healing power, and if we will listen to the voice of God within, we will be shown for whom to pray.[5]

What if there is no clear guidance as to whether to pray or not? We can go ahead and pray for those who ask for prayer, assuming that God has moved them to ask for help; also we should pray when our compassion urges us to pray for someone who is sick. Again, Agnes Sanford has some helpful words:

> God directs us most joyfully through our own desires. The impulse of love that leads us to the doorway of a friend is the voice of God within, and we need not be afraid to follow it.[6]

Listening, to know what to pray for. What type of healing is needed?

Physical? Emotional? Is there need for repentance, or forgiveness? It may take time to clarify the situation so that we can decide which way to move forward in prayer.

Presuming that we are confident to move ahead in prayer, what is to be the content of prayer? The prayer for healing usually involves an acknowledgment of and thanks for God's presence and power in the situation, and a request for God's healing in relation to a particular need.[7] As far as possible the prayer should be:

- **Specific** — stating the need clearly if this is known, without a detailed and lengthy explanation.

- **Positive** in looking forward in hope to the healing rather than focusing on the problem.

- **Confident** that God hears and answers prayer.

- **Inclusive** — recognizing the needs of others involved in the healing process; relatives, friends, medical personnel.

- **In the Spirit** — under the control of the Holy Spirit. This may be in a special prayer language (in tongues), or it may be waiting in silence, believing that the Spirit Himself is praying according to God's will and purpose (Romans 8:26-27).

Even though these guidelines may be helpful, there are many times when prayer will be quite unstructured and may often be in silence, with perhaps none or a bare minimum of words. The situation may be such that words are superfluous, and we simply offer the person and the situation to God, trusting in Him to bring about His will and purpose. Thus, simple words like, "Lord, the one whom you love is sick, please help," or other brief sentences are all that is necessary.

There are several therapies which are often used as part of healing prayer; such as relaxation, affirmation, visualization, meditation.

Relaxation is allowing the body and mind to wind down and become calm in the presence of God. It may include measured breathing, physical movement, rest, letting go of tension and of stress, so as to be able to receive healing.

Affirmation is focusing on the positive aspects of faith in relation to God's grace, and promises; for example, by repeating some of the promises of scripture, "I can do all things through Christ, who strengthens me"; or some aspect of faith, such as "I believe in God the Father"; or it may be the constant affirmation of personal significance; for example, "I am loved by God and I can do this as His child"; or "My Lord is with me this day. His presence is around me and within." It is the spoken affirmation of the positives which molds the mind and influences behavior and action.

Visualization is the use of the imagination in seeing the person as healed or in the process of being healed, rather than focusing on the problem of sickness. It is holding something in the mind's eye and using this positive mental imagery to stimulate hope in the struggle against sickness. Two examples are given:

- As we pray with people we are helping them to open their hearts to receive the love of Jesus, and then to pour out their hearts to him in return. We may use the picture of their opening the windows of their hearts to let in the sunshine of his love. We may use the simile of basking in the warm sun on a summer's day. We may indeed tell the person to picture themselves being like a beautiful summer flower in a garden. Drinking in the life-giving light of the Lord is a necessary part of prayer.[8]

- Make a picture in your mind of your body as well. Think especially of the part that most needs to be well. See it well and perfect and shining with God's light, and give thanks that this is being accomplished.[9]

Another writer, Glenn Clark, suggests that the secret of Jesus' healings lay in his ability to look through the facts (the symptoms of the illness) to the reality of that person in the Father's eternal kingdom (whole, happy, loved). Sometimes visualization is used where writing and art is the process by which this mental imagery is allowed to operate.

Meditation is related to affirmation and is focusing attention on the love and the power of God. It is stretching the mind to take in all of God. It is not a denial of the facts of the situation, but rather recognition of the larger realities which give a new perspective by seeing the problem in the context of God's presence and power. It may involve focusing on scripture, or positive affirmation, such as, "Be still and know that I am God." It is not a focusing on ourselves but it is a way of re-educating our minds to be more aware of divine realities and resources by focusing on God.

The use of these therapies in healing prayer is a controversial area for some Christians because these and other techniques are also extensively used in secular and non-Christian healing, in medical science, and more especially in New Age and Spiritualist healing. The use of such therapies therefore requires discernment and careful explanation to those involved in the healing situation. (See Chapter 11 — Christian Healing and Alternative Healing Movements.)

The Laying on of Hands

At almost every healing service there is a time when people ask for prayer and others come and lay hands on them and pray for them. In the church as a whole, especially where there is a renewal and charismatic emphasis, there is now an accepted use of touching and laying hands on others, often not connected with healing, but rather as an expression of every member ministry, or symbolizing the blessing of the Holy Spirit, or a sign of fellowship. In recent years there has been a steady increase in the use of laying on of hands, and it has become an accepted part of the healing ministry.

However, this increase has not always been accompanied by clear thinking as to its meaning and practice, resulting in several areas of confusion:

- That laying on of hands is about the transfer of some invisible psychic or spiritual healing energy, variously named as life force, prana, odic force, orgone energy.

- That each person possesses an invisible energy field which can be tapped for healing.

- That this action is part of the general increase in understanding of the significance of touch for personal growth, awareness and healing, both in its orthodox and alternative expressions, and that the use of the laying on of hands within a Christian setting is only one example of this renewed understanding.

As with all other areas of healing, the Christian understanding of the laying on of hands relates to biblical teaching and practice within the church. The reason why this method is used is because there is clear biblical support; it has been the continuing practice within the church throughout history (although the meaning has not always been the same); and because it has been recognized as offering blessings to those who receive this ministry — blessings which are physical, psychological and spiritual.

Laying on of Hands in Scripture

In the Old Testament, laying on of hands is a symbol of:

- Commissioning to a particular task involving the transfer of authority for that task or office (Numbers 27:22, 23).

- Transfer of strength, power, and life (Deuteronomy 34:9). Joshua was full of the Spirit of wisdom for Moses had laid his hands on him.

- Blessing (Genesis 48:14ff), and where individual blessings were impractical, the whole group is blessed by raised hands (Leviticus 9:22).

- Dedication, as when people laid hands on the Levites to dedicate them to God (Numbers 8:10-12).

- Sacrifice, as when animals were offered (Leviticus 1:4), for the sin offering for the congregation (Leviticus 4:15), and on the scapegoat on the Day of Atonement (Leviticus 16:20-22). This contains the idea of dedication to God, representation of the sacrifice to God, and transference of guilt to the scapegoat. There was also the use of touch to heal, but not in the form of laying on of hands (1 Kings 17:21, 22; 2 Kings 4:32ff). There is no use of the laying on of hands as a specific healing ministry in the Old Testament.

In the New Testament, laying on of hands is a symbol of:

- Blessing, as with Jesus and the children (Matthew 19:13-15), and the blessing of a group (Luke 24:50, 51).

- Commissioning or ordaining to a particular task (Acts 6:6, 13:1-3).

- Initiation and blessings of the Holy Spirit (Acts 8:14-17, 19:2ff; 1 Timothy 4:14).

- Healing, as the laying of hands and touch were important aspects of Jesus' ministry (Mark 6:5; Luke 4:40, 13:13); laying on of hands is also used in the early church (Acts 9:17-19, 28:7-10; James 5:13-15). There are also several instances of touch which are not specifically described as the laying on of hands (Acts 3:7, 14:19, 20, 19:11, 20:10).

In both Old Testament and New Testament the blessing through the laying on of hands was seen as God's provision and activity. It was the hand of the Lord: His power and grace, which accepted, blessed, sent forth and healed, and not some magic power inherent in those who performed the actual action; for example, Peter disclaimed any power to heal (Acts 3:12), and it was clear that it was the hand of the Lord which healed (Acts 4:29-30).

In the history of the church the laying on of hands continued to be used as a means of healing for the first three centuries, and it has continued to be used by individuals in all ages of the church as a means of ministry to the sick. However, from the fourth century onward there was a decline in its official and formal use in healing and it became mainly restricted to ordination and baptism. The use of the laying on of hands and anointing with oil became more a preparation for death than for healing — a practice which was strongly condemned by many of the Reformers. Throughout much of the history of the church, the laying on of hands for healing actually declined in importance and it is only in the last century that it has been officially recognized by the church and used again as an essential part of the healing ministry.

The Significance of the Laying on of Hands

The laying on of hands is a physical act of touching which God uses to bless and heal people at different levels of experience and need. Touch is recognized as an important part of helping people in a wide variety of problem areas: in physical healing, psychotherapy, pain control, and in personal growth awareness. There are three main areas which are affected.

Physical. There is considerable evidence that contact through touch does have some effect on the experience of physical pain, and in fact contributes to pain relief as the result of the stimuli of nerve fibers; hence, the natural comforting act of touching a painful area. The use of what is known as therapeutic touch recognizes this fact and the practice has become an accepted part of modern nursing practice.

Psychological. Laying on of hands can have a significant effect on helping people to reduce anxiety levels, to re-order thinking, to relax, to lessen depression and feelings of rejection. It is an effective way of non-verbal communication in which people can enter into deep experiences of acceptance, forgiveness, and sharing.

Spiritual. This is the most important aspect because the laying on of hands is both a symbol and a means of the power and love of God working within the life of the person receiving this ministry. In the gospels there are two incidents where the idea of a transfer of power in healing occurs; that is, power going out from Jesus to heal (Mark 5:25-34; Luke 6:19). It should be noted that the power to heal resides in Jesus and not in the outward act, hence he directs the woman's faith to himself and not to any cultural superstition about the magic of touching clothes.

These three aspects all relate to the use of the laying on of hands in healing. However, the spiritual aspect whereby the power of God is released for healing is the primary meaning.

Two significant meanings are therefore suggested when the laying on of hands is used. Firstly, there is the idea of *identification* by those who perform this action. This involves identification with God in his desire to bring healing to needy people, and also identification with people in their need. Secondly, there is the idea of *impartation* by which the grace, mercy, and healing of God are imparted to people.

There is an important difference between these two aspects. *Identification* is an act in which we share; it is our responsibility and privilege to identify with God and others; it is something we can do. However, *impartation* is different because we do not and cannot impart any healing to people. God is the source of healing, and those who lay hands on others are the instruments or channels of HIS blessing and healing. They have no innate power in themselves which provides an automatic healing. Any power which is present is of God, and not of human origin (2 Corinthians 4:7).

This is the fundamental difference between the Christian ministry of laying on of hands and other forms of touch therapy which are based on the idea of energy transfer from one person to another. By the power of the Holy Spirit it is Christ's touch which brings the blessing and healing which he alone can give. It is therefore Christ who is ministering, and not the passing on of an anonymous power or force.

The Methods Used

There is no one method which is prescribed for all situations. Sometimes hands are placed on the person's head or shoulders, sometimes on the affected areas of the body, sometimes the hands are held close to the person without actually touching. Whatever method is used, there needs to be discretion so that there is no stress or embarrassment or misunderstanding; especially when ministering to people of the opposite sex, or from a different culture. For those ministering the laying on of hands, there needs to be a recognition that the Lord is present to heal and an openness to his love so that there will be a clear channel through which he can work to achieve his purpose in the needy person's life. Those ministering the laying on of hands may experience some physical sensation, such as warm hands or tingling, but these should not be seen as essentials and they are not the source of healing. For those receiving the ministry, there may be various experiences. Sometimes there will be a sense of peace, or love, or relief, or power flowing into their lives. At other times there will be no such emotional high. As the healer, God deals with each person according to their need and so too much emphasis should not be placed on the outward trimmings which may accompany this ministry. What is important is that it is the Lord working to heal and not any outward sign, however spectacular. Sometimes the laying on of hands is accompanied by the act of anointing with oil and the difference between these two ministries is explained in the next point.

In summary, to avoid possible confusion in relation to this ministry, it is essential to stress in every situation that it is the touch of the Lord, and the stretching forth of his hand, that brings healing. We should recognize that it is possible to bring changes by human psychological and psychic forces, and some people do seem to possess "green fingers" in relation to people just as some possess "green thumbs" in relation to garden plants. Pain may be reduced and some form of spiritualistic healing achieved. The actions appear to be the same but the underlying understanding of the source of healing power is quite different. Christian ministry through the laying on of hands is related to the activity of God the Father, Son and Holy Spirit, and is focused in Jesus Christ who, through the power of the Holy Spirit, is present to bless and heal. He works through his committed people who use the means of laying on of hands to minister to others.

One leader in the Anglican Church, Canon Bryan Green, gives wise words about the value of this ministry.

> I wish that many more Christian people, not just parsons, would realize that to pray with someone who is anxious and lay hands on them, is a real ministry of healing. I do not pretend to understand the way in which prayer and the laying on of hands works. But experience shows that if in simple faith and belief in the healing love of God we pray with a friend, laying our hands on him if this seems right, then very often some kind of healing power works with him. It is so easy to be complicated in our thinking so that we are not simple enough in our actions.[10]

Anointing with Oil

In the healing ministry people are sometimes anointed with oil as well as receiving the laying on of hands. There are three main ideas relating to this. First, anointing is a more advanced or deeper means of healing, and is for those with very serious or more acute illness and it is ministered less frequently than the laying on of hands. Second, anointing with oil is a sign of a person's consecration to Jesus Christ and the imparting of the Holy Spirit to that person's life. Third, it is a sign of our unity with Christ as the person who is anointed is open to receive God's blessing in a special way, or for a particular purpose.

In the Old Testament anointing was given as a sign of consecration to the service of God, so kings, prophets and priests were anointed (Exodus 28:41; 1 Samuel 15:1). It was not only a human act of dedication, but it was primarily an action by which God consecrated or set apart the anointed one for His service or particular task. When this happened to a king or leader, they were described as God's anointed one. Also the people of Israel are referred to as God's anointed, to be consecrated to His service (Habakkuk 3:13). It is interesting to note that the practice of anointing rulers continues today. When Queen Elizabeth II was crowned, she received anointing with oil as a sign of God's blessing and her dedication to her role as Queen.

In the New Testament Jesus is the anointed one, consecrated to God's service and empowered by the Holy Spirit to carry out his ministry (Luke 4:18-21; Acts 10:37, 38). Also, those who believe and follow Jesus Christ are anointed in him (2 Corinthians 1:21, 22), that is, they are set apart for his service. In 180 AD a writer named Theophilus said, "We are called Christians because we are anointed with the oil of God." 1 Peter 2:9 describes the church as a "chosen people, a royal priesthood, a holy nation, a people belonging to God." There is no actual mention of anointing, but the idea of consecration to God's service is clear. The Greek word for anointed is "Christ," hence the title Jesus Christ means Jesus, the anointed one. Sometimes in church history believers were described as "Christed", or simply "Christ's", emphasizing the idea of belonging to him and being consecrated or set apart for his service.

The New Testament also contains the idea of anointing with oil as a means of healing. The disciples used oil (Mark 6:13), and it appears to be a regular practice in the life of the church. James includes it as a normal part of the healing process (James 5:14, 15). Some suggest that the use of oil in healing is best explained by recognizing that oil was used in many different ways; for domestic purposes, lighting, bodily cleanliness, medicinal purposes (Luke 10:34), and for hospitality of honored guests (Luke 7:46). Oil was seen as a symbol of joy and life, as in the oil of gladness (Isaiah 61:3). Because oil was regarded as a healing agent and was accepted as a valuable medical remedy at that time, it has been suggested that the oil mentioned in James 5 should be understood as a reference to the normal medical means of healing of that day. So when the James 5 passage is used today, oil should likewise be taken to refer to the accepted contemporary medical practice. This is an interesting interpretation and there is no doubt about the health-giving properties of oil. However, there is more to the biblical understanding than this.

When oil is used in healing it should include the idea of consecration to God's service. It is an action which symbolizes an inner anointing by the Holy Spirit and a renewal of the person's life affecting body, mind and spirit. It therefore relates both to sickness and to the total healing of the person as the person seeks to be completely consecrated to God's purpose. The prayer that is offered makes this clear:

> As you are outwardly anointed with this visible oil, so may our Heavenly Father grant you the inward anointing of the Holy Spirit . . . may he forgive your sins, release you from suffering, and restore you to wholeness and strength. May he deliver you from all evil, preserve you in all goodness, and bring you to everlasting life.[11]

Other prayers also give this meaning:

> I anoint you with oil in the name of our Lord Jesus Christ. May our Heavenly Father make you whole in body and mind, and

grant you the inward anointing of his Holy Spirit, the Spirit of strength and joy and peace.[12]

A further longer prayer emphasizes the same point:

As with this visible oil your body is outwardly anointed, so may our Heavenly Father grant of His infinite goodness that your soul may be inwardly anointed with the Holy Spirit and filled with strength and comfort. May the Almighty God restore to you bodily health and strength to serve Him. May He send to you freedom from all your pains, troubles, and diseases, whether of body or mind. May He pardon you all your sins and offenses, and grant you strength to serve Him truly; that aided by His Holy Spirit you may have perfect victory and triumph over Satan, sin, disease and death. Through Jesus Christ our Lord, who by his death has destroyed death, and now with the Father and the Holy Spirit evermore lives and reigns, God, world without end. Amen.[13]

In the actual anointing, oil may be applied to different parts of the body — the forehead, the hands, and often the diseased area if this is appropriate. It is a sign of offering these completely to God.

It is important to understand that when a sick person is anointed with oil they do not receive something abnormal and extraordinary because they are ill. The oil is used to restore and renew the sick person's unity with God and to receive His blessing, life and healing through the anointing of His Spirit. It is therefore an action which involves confession, forgiveness, consecration, renewal — all part of a total healing. It therefore should not be given casually and is only appropriate for those who sincerely wish to make this renewed commitment. In the history of the church, particularly within the Catholic Church, anointing with oil came to be associated with death rather than life, and for many centuries it was used as part of the Last Rites (Extreme Unction), preparing people for death. Today, however, there is a renewed understanding of the true meaning of this symbol, and it is now recognized and administered as relating to our present daily life and commitment to God's service.

Whether anointing with oil should be done only once during an illness (because it is a sign of giving the entire situation to God, and the consecration of the person's life), or whether it should be done more frequently is an open question. The present practice in OSL is to limit its use as a special consecrating symbol; whereas the ministries of laying on of hands, prayer, and the Sacrament of Holy Communion are seen as continuing sustaining ministries in the healing process. However, some leaders in the healing ministry suggest a more frequent use of anointing, for example, Morris Maddocks (UK). This is supported by Canon Jim Glennon who invited people in the regular healing service at St. Andrew's Cathedral in Sydney to receive anointing in these words:

> If you have received the laying on of hands . . . and you would like to be anointed with oil as a sign of your consecration to God and the endowment of the Holy Spirit in a special and relevant way . . . one of the clergy or deaconesses will minister to you. Remember these words, "Samuel anointed him and the Spirit of the Lord came mightily upon David from that day forward" (1 Samuel 16:13). I believe that when this ministry of anointing with oil is faithfully carried out there will be that same blessing on those who partake of this aspect of the healing ministry.[14]

Sharing and Discussion

1. (a) This chapter suggests that all methods are a means to healing and none of them are the actual cause of healing. Do you think that is true?

(b) If healing is the goal, then does it really matter what methods are used as long as healing occurs; that is, does the end (healing) justify the use of any means?

2. Share with others your experience of the laying on of hands — when you have laid hands on others, and when you received the laying on of hands for yourself. What significance did this have for you?

3. Should anointing with oil be more regularly practiced with the laying on of hands, or offered less frequently to ensure its real significance?

4. How important is faith in praying for healing?

5. How do you respond to Frank Wright's description of faith:

"Resting in the conviction (literally being conquered by the conviction) that in God there is a power of love sufficient for all my needs. I put myself in His hands without wishing to force any outcome, or even necessarily believing that I know best what the outcome should be."

In what ways is this description helpful or not helpful to you?

6. Reflect on some of the explanations or symbols of prayer given in this chapter — for example, talking/walking with a friend; relating to the Covenant God. Which of these do you find most helpful? Are there other symbols of prayer which you find helpful in praying for healing? Share these with others.

7. Study some of the prayers for healing offered by past and present writers on the healing ministry, including the prayers contained in various orders for healing services used in churches, for example, the prayers used in OSL healing services. What are the main ideas in these prayers, and how helpful are these prayers for your own involvement in praying for others, or being involved in a prayer ministry for the sick? Adapt these prayers for your own use.

References for Further Reading

Gunstone, J., *Prayers for Healing*, Highland Books, Crowborough, East Sussex, 1987.

Headley, C., *The Laying on of Hands in the Parish Ministry*, Grove Worship Series No. 104, Grove Books, Bramcote, Nottingham, 1988.

Maddocks, M., *Twenty Questions About Healing*, SPCK, London, 1988, Chapter 13.

MacNutt, F., *Healing*, Hodder and Stoughton, London, 1988, Chapters, 8, 9, 20.

Richards, J., *The Question of Healing Services*, Daybreak/DLT, London, 1989, Chapters 6 and 7.

Richards, J., *Faith and Healing*, Network No. 6, Floreat Flame Books, Mirrabooka, undated.

7

THE PRAYER OF FAITH

Marcia and Harold are keen members of the church and are moving into a healing ministry. They are learning to pray for healing, but have become aware of different interpretations and styles of ministry. They are confused as to how they should pray because they see many different models or examples of prayer. They notice that different leaders and people in the healing ministry have their own interpretations and practice. Harold is especially attracted to one of the more charismatic-type leaders who prays very loudly (as if the Lord is deaf), and who claims to know with great certainty the outcome of his prayers. The leader describes his way of praying as "the prayer of faith." For Harold, keen to be successful in the healing ministry, there seems to be so much power in this man's praying, which appears to come from his faith. So, when Harold prays, he tries to be forceful (especially in commanding the power of evil to depart and claiming healing from God). He does this to emphasize his faith in God's power to heal, and to give others greater confidence in seeking healing. Sometimes, however, while he is praying or afterward in reflecting about his prayers, Harold feels awkward. He wonders whether he is a phony because, within himself, he isn't very confident despite his strong words. Is Harold pretending to be someone else? Is he giving the appearance of having a sure faith when often he is very unsure about the whole deal? If Harold admitted to these feelings, wouldn't this weaken people's trust in him and curtail the development of his ministry?

Marcia, too, is unhappy with the local healing ministry. Marcia feels uncomfortable with the "claiming" attitude which Harold and others take in prayer. They seem to be so bold in affirming God's promises, and there does not seem to be very much humility or any possible thought that they may be mistaken. Marcia would love to be able to pray with great confidence and assurance that people would be healed. But she cannot honestly do this. Often Marcia has doubts about healing, is not sure what God's will is, and just can't put words together properly — certainly not in the super-confident way that some leaders do, and in the way which Harold is now using in his own prayers.

Both Marcia and Harold are asking questions. Is Marcia a failure in praying? Is it that she just isn't bold enough to claim God's power and to stand on His promises? Is Harold really beginning to pray effectively? Is Harold onto the secret of effective prayer for healing? Has he in fact understood and begun to practice the principles of the prayer of faith? What is this prayer of faith anyway? Marcia and Harold come to talk to you about their different understanding and questions. They ask for your opinion and advice. How would you respond?

This chapter aims to:

- Clarify the meaning of faith and its significance in healing.

- Respond to the question — Is faith essential for healing? — and grapple with questions asked about the prayer of faith.

- Outline some of the interpretations of the prayer of faith.

- Clarify some issues and tensions relating to these interpretations.

- Suggest some responses to be worked out in our lives.

Faith and Its Significance for Healing

Whenever prayer is offered some form of faith is present because prayer is always directed to something or to someone, that is, to some form of reality. The faith which produces the prayer may be more like fear, but it is still prayer toward some person, power, or object which is recognized as a higher reality.

In Christian healing there is often a close link between faith and healing, but this does not apply in every situation. In the ministry of Jesus it was apparent in many situations that faith was an important factor in the healing process. At other times faith does not play an important role (see examples below).

But what is *faith*? The word "faith" incorporates several ideas. Faith can mean a set of beliefs, as in the Apostles Creed — "I believe in God the Father Almighty." Faith can mean *adherence to a tradition*, the faith given to the church (Jude 20; I Cor. 15:1-3). Faith can mean *an attitude of trust* in someone's reliability and judgment, and goodness — I have faith in my doctor's ability to perform this operation, so I am ready to trust myself to his skillful care. Or, I have faith in the advice of my financial adviser, so I am prepared to invest my money in the way he suggests.

In the New Testament the main meaning of faith is *to trust in, rely on, have confidence in, respond to*. It is an attitude which involves the mind, the emotions and the will. So, faith accepts the reality of God (Hebrews 11:6); faith believes that God responds to those who seek Him (Hebrews 11:6); faith accepts the reality of God's resources and promises as real facts, even though they are not seen by human sight (Mark 11:24; Hebrews 11:1); and faith, in relation to healing, trusts in the power of God to heal and then acts on that trust (Mark 5:34).

In relation to healing, Francis MacNutt suggests that faith means a trust or confidence in:

• God's faithfulness in His promises to hear and answer prayer whether we see the desired results or not.

• God's wisdom to do what He knows is best in each situation.

- God's power to do what He wishes to do.

- God's goodness to do what is ultimately the most loving thing.[1]

So, the object of faith is God's faithfulness rather than our human effort to be "trustful" or "full of faith." This *objective* foundation for faith in God's nature and character enables the person praying to trust themselves to Him, producing the *subjective* experience.

Thus faith can be described as abandoning all reliance on our own efforts and giving ourselves in total surrender to God's will, whatever it is; being "willing to accept whatever God wishes to do at whatever timing He wishes to accomplish it."[2]

This raises two important questions: Is faith essential to healing? And if we have faith will God automatically heal us?

Does God Require Faith Before Healing?

The answer to this question may be both "yes" and "no." As already mentioned, some scripture records people being healed in the absence of faith (John 5:2-18). The sick man did not even know who Jesus was (John 5:13). Also, when Jesus raised the son of the widow, no faith is mentioned and certainly the dead person was not able to exercise it (Luke 7:11-15). If it were true that God requires faith before He heals, then this puts Him at the mercy of our faith, and therefore God would be no longer the sovereign Lord. But faith is not our power or ability. Ultimately, faith is God's gift to us.

Also, if God automatically heals according to a certain amount of faith, then faith becomes a magical transaction — if the person seeking healing has sufficient quantity and quality of faith, the answer must come. In that case, God has no choice! But experience shows that those who sincerely trust in God are not always healed in the way expected. Sometimes the failure may involve *lack of faith*, but often healing fails to occur even when there seem to be *great amounts of faith* being offered in prayer. Compare Paul's thorn in the flesh (2 Corinthians 12), as an example of non-healing in the midst of great faith. Failure may seem to fly in the face of another important New Testament practice which is basic to the healing ministry, and that is the prayer of faith.

The Prayer of Faith

Sometimes translated as "the prayer offered in faith" (James 5:15), the prayer of faith is an important aspect in our understanding of God's promises of healing and blessing, and indeed of our relationship to Him. The prayer of faith is based on the words of Jesus in Mark 11:22-24 — that you will receive what is asked for, provided it is asked in faith without any doubt as to the fulfillment of God's promises. The answer may not be apparent, but faith claims the answer *before* it is received. This is a general principle which applies to all areas of prayer, including healing.

In relation to healing, James 5:15 affirms that the prayer of faith *will* make the sick person well, and the Lord *will* raise him up (restore him/her to health). There is definiteness about the answer — not "could" or "may" or "if it be your will," but "*will make*" and "*will raise.*" This confidence and certainty is different from the more general "trust in God's wisdom" approach described above. This confidence and certainty raises two important questions:

• Is the prayer of faith a special way of praying which removes all doubt as to God's response, and is therefore superior to the general prayer which trusts the outcome to God's wisdom?

• Does the prayer of faith apply to all those who pray? Are all those who pray capable of the prayer of faith, or is it a special gift from God, given only to particular people who then exercise this special gift?

In other words, the question becomes: are there two kinds of prayer — a *general* prayer of trust and reliance (available to all who pray), and a *special* prayer of faith which guarantees results (available to those especially gifted by God)? The following material considers different perspectives on the prayer of faith from people involved in the healing ministry, and then seeks to clarify some of the issues which cluster around this idea.

Perspectives on the Prayer of Faith

The perspectives of four significant authors are presented.

Jim Glennon[3]

Glennon's understanding of the prayer of faith is built on the following ideas:[4]

- By the death and resurrection of Jesus, Satan's rule has been broken and a new order has been established — the kingdom of God.

- The kingdom of God is both a present reality and a future hope. It will be revealed in its fullness only at the end of this age when the kingdoms of this world become the kingdoms of our God and of His Christ (Revelation 11:15).

- This kingdom rule and blessing is also a present reality within the lives of those who respond to God's grace in repentance and faith: "The kingdom of God is within you" or "in the midst of you" (Luke 17:21).

- The blessings of this "here and now" kingdom are contained in the divine promises which God has made. These promises reveal God's will for us and are to be appropriated and experienced now as present and available blessings (2 Peter 1:4ff).

- One of the promises of the kingdom is healing. It is part of

God's present provision for us, part of the perfection of the kingdom "within us."

- Therefore the experience of healing is not something to be prayed for as if it were not available and we have to plead with God for it. Rather, we already have the experience of healing as one of the blessings of the kingdom (along with forgiveness, adoption, and so on). Since we already possess it, or it is within us, why ask for what we already have?

Let us have a big picture of what that means for us now, and what it means so far as the reality of divine healing is concerned . . . . Divine healing is part of that greater reality called the kingdom of God, and the kingdom of God is among us. This is the immediacy of healing; this is the sureness we have of healing. This is why you can believe so that you do not doubt, because it has been given . . . . Why ask for what you've got? . . . It doesn't have to be asked for . . . . Why ask for what you've got as far as the reality of the kingdom and the reality of divine healing is concerned? IT IS WITHIN YOU.[5]

- The way to appropriate healing as a present blessing of the kingdom is through the prayer of faith which accepts the promise and then experiences the actual healing being worked out in our lives. We must believe that the prayer of faith is being answered and we accept the answer even though the outward circumstances may not seem to change. So we have what we accept and we do this to the point where we do not doubt in our heart (Mark 11:22-24).

- An analogy to understand this meaning of faith is the experience of conversion. Conversion occurs as we accept Christ as Savior and give thanks to God for His grace given to us. This acceptance of Christ is by faith, and there may be little or no immediate change in our feelings or experience. However, because we have believed, we continue to thank God for His grace and we trust in His faithfulness and not in our feelings. We have been accepted, we are saved by faith.

In the same way we accept the grace of healing even though there may be no immediate experience in our lives. Glennon affirms this principle in these words:

> The person who would become a Christian must accept Jesus and what that means, so that Jesus is now theirs from here on; tomorrow, he is still there. They "wear him," as it were, and when they think of him they are grateful to God. That is exercising what the Bible calls the prayer of faith.

> So it is in appropriating the kingdom of God and that part that we call divine healing. The kingdom of God is available; indeed, it is within you. If it is to be effective in your life for this need or that, you must accept it as a gift so that you are sure that you have it, so that from here on you have it. This is a new kind of reality. You have exchanged the old for the new. If you want one word which explains what I want to say about the prayer of faith, it is the word "accept" — you *have* what you *accept.*[6]

- The problem for most people is that they accept not the healing offered by God which they already have within them, but the problem or the sickness which is readily apparent and may be very painful. By accepting the problem (the sickness), rather than the solution (the healing), they remain unhealed because they are not accepting God's provision which is within them. They are to see themselves as healed rather than as remaining in the state of sickness or pain.

- The actual experience of healing becomes a reality as praise is offered to God for the healing He has already provided as a blessing of the present kingdom. This may take some time, but the affirmation of thanks for healing received must replace any doubt as to whether God has granted or will grant the blessing.

So:

- Your healing is within you as a blessing of the reality of the kingdom of God. There is no need to ask for what has already been given.

- We accept the reality and do not doubt in our heart, and then the blessing will be experienced in reality.

The prayer of faith is believing in the promises of God as a reality, claiming and then experiencing them in our actual living. This is a general principle which applies to all prayer and to any matter about which prayer is offered. This is the standard way in which the Bible presents this type of prayer (Matthew 18:19; John 14:13, 14).

Who is able to pray the prayer of faith? Because the prayer of faith is a general principle of prayer it is not restricted to any particular subject, nor is it a special gift given only to selected people. Rather the prayer of faith is for all those who believe in Jesus Christ. It is one of the foundations of effective prayer and when applied to healing is the *key* to experiencing the blessings which God desires to give as part of the present reality of the kingdom. Healing therefore should be prayed for with assurance that it is going to happen. There is no need for provisos to be added, such as "if it be your will," because God's will *has* been revealed: healing is part of the kingdom's blessings which are now available.

Understanding the prayer of faith is a challenge to radical trust in God's provision of healing. It focuses on the fact that prayer is essentially a response to God's blessing (the foundation of prayer is divine grace), rather than a striving to work up more faith as a human effort. It is also an encouragement for all believers to be involved in this approach to prayer. It is not something for the "super-spirituals" or those with a special gift.

However, this understanding is not without its difficulties, the main one being that sometimes healing does not occur even though all the conditions of the prayer of faith seem to have been fulfilled.

Glennon responds to this difficulty with an honest awareness of human limitations:

> I do not go out on a limb and speak about the promise of healing in an unqualified way. This is not to say that God cannot heal, but the size of the mountain has to be taken into account as do the limits of our faith.[7]

He notes the possible limitations resulting from our human understanding of the situation.[8]

> There is no limit to what God can do, but there is a limit to what His servants can do, so there is a need to recognize our limitations and know when we can pray in faith and when we can only relinquish the matter to God.

- When it is a long-standing problem or when the sickness is very advanced and has a strong hold on the person.

- If the disease or sickness is lethal from a human perspective and this diagnosis is accepted by the sick person.

- Where bodily structure is severely affected, then healing is much more difficult; for example, it is not reasonable to believe an amputee could grow a new limb.

- When there is need to recognize that the time has come for the person to die. Death is to be accepted as God's ultimate healing. However, until this point is reached, healing is available in the same way as medical resources are available, and the prayer of faith should continue to be offered to God.

How can one know when the point of ceasing to offer the prayer of faith is reached? The point of ceasing is reached only by discernment from God, which comes through the ministry of the Holy Spirit as He makes His will clear to those involved in the healing situation.

Francis MacNutt[9]

MacNutt affirms the necessity of faith in prayer and emphasizes the need to trust in God's wisdom and goodness rather than in the quantity or quality of our faith. To concentrate on our faith focuses on our inadequacy and produces a struggle to achieve faith, which may give rise to anxiety, guilt and confusion about our inability to pray effectively. God is responsible for answering our prayer; our part is to pray and leave the result to God. MacNutt encourages the continuation of prayer even though there may be no assurance of healing.

> If I cannot force myself to believe that this particular person will be healed right now, does that mean I do not have faith in God's promises? No, it simply means I am willing to admit I do not know all the factors involved in this situation unless God chooses to reveal them to me . . . My faith is in God, His wisdom, goodness and love . . . To claim more than this, unless it has been specifically revealed that a given person is going to get well, is to make ourselves into a counterfeit trying to play God.[10]

To pray in faith is to turn to God in complete trust that He knows what is best, that He loves us more than anyone else, and that He has the power to accomplish whatever we need. This involves accepting our doubts about our own adequacy and what is going to happen, and to leave the results to God.

Everyone in the healing ministry should be involved in this sort of prayer, which is described as the *virtue* of faith; a confidence in

God's faithfulness, wisdom, power and love. This is one level of prayer which is available to all.

However, there is another level of prayer which involves a special *gift* of faith. "The gift of faith is a ministry gift which God imparts to help us pray with confidence and no hesitation in our hearts for a given intention." This confidence comes from God as He reveals His will, usually through a special word of knowledge.

> Through the word of knowledge God intimates to the person(s) praying that His will is to heal a particular person at a particular time. The gift of faith lies in accepting this inspiration without hesitation and praying with absolute trust, believing that this person will be healed.[11]

This *gift* of faith is only given to certain people whereas the *virtue* of faith is possible to all Christians.

Thus there are two models of prayer for healing. Both are valid, but one is *deeper* than the other. For ordinary Christians in ordinary circumstances the usual prayer for healing is a prayer of petition, asking God to help others in the name of Jesus. If unable to pray with the special gift of faith the ordinary believer can affirm that God loves the sick person and that He has power to heal, but we are unable to know exactly what will happen so the results are left to God.

For the believer with a special gift of healing the prayer for healing is one of special confidence: "God loves you and will heal you NOW." There is no element of doubt because the person praying knows the mind of God and can speak in the name of Jesus. It is as if the person praying is actually standing with God and speaking for Him.

MacNutt illustrates this point with the following diagram and explanation.[12]

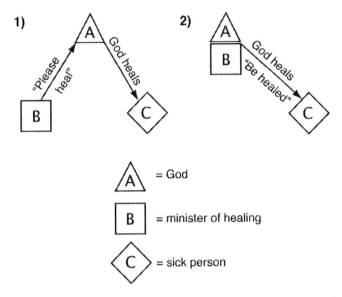

A = God

B = minister of healing

C = sick person

The diagram illustrates the difference between two types of prayer. In 1) the person praying is not sure what God's will is in asking for healing of this sick person at this time. He or she is speaking TO God asking Him to heal the person. In 2) God has revealed His will to heal at this time; therefore the minister of healing is not only praying to God, but is actually speaking FOR God to the sick person.

MacNutt concludes by suggesting that both styles of prayer are valid, that both are based on faith, but are very different. Each person should learn to pray in the style that suits their particular ministry. If there is no exceptional gift of knowledge, we must continue to pray for the sick and desire to grow in our understanding, and be open to this special gift of faith from God. We have to develop an extreme *confidence* in God's power, and literally *go for healing* with keen determination. MacNutt confesses that in his own prayers he often does not have any special sense whether the person prayed for will be healed; he feels that he lacks the special gift of faith, but he continues to be faithful in prayer believing that God will do what is best for each person.[13] Other prominent leaders in the healing ministry also make the same comment about their ministry; for example, Kathryn Kuhlman.[14]

It is not clear whether MacNutt's special gift of faith in prayer is the same as the prayer of faith because he has both a wider general meaning and also a special limited meaning. Yet he seems to put his main emphasis on the wider general meaning rather than the specialized and limited *gift*.

> Faith is not an extraordinary version of what you believe, but is rather the courage to pray for the sick person. Like Abraham setting out for the Promised Land, faith lies in setting out on the journey, not in being sure of exactly where we are going. God is faithful, and faith is obedience and the willingness to risk, not an absolute certainty about what is going to happen on the journey.[15]

C. Samuel Storms

Storms defines the prayer offered in faith as

> Not just any prayer prayed at any time, but a unique and divinely motivated one, literally the prayer of faith. God enables the person (or elders) to pray this prayer only in exceptional circumstances. It is therefore not just an ordinary prayer, however good and sincere it may be, but the prayer prompted by the Spirit-wrought conviction that it is God's will to heal the one being prayed for.[16]

Most of the time we are not able to know whether it is God's will to heal, and we may not always sense whether the special gift of faith is present. Faith is not something we manufacture, but a work of grace, not a product of our own efforts however earnest we may be. Only God can produce this special prayer of faith in our hearts and we can only exercise this kind of faith when God wills that we do so.

Peter Masters

Masters is very critical of those who claim that healing will definitely follow when both the healer and the sick person possess absolute certainty that the illness will be cured.

So confident of this are the more exhibitionist leaders that they have made the prayer of faith the executive instrument of healing, but often their prayer is no more than a command to the illness to depart.[17]

For Masters the prayer of faith does not mean that healing will result as long as the right amount of quality faith is present, rather that healing will certainly occur if it is God's will to heal in a particular situation. In other words, the prayer of faith is not a special sort of prayer, but along with all other types of prayer is subject to God's will. The fact that there are no *qualifying* words about the will of God when the prayer of faith is mentioned, as in James 5:15, does not mean that this prayer is exempt from this general principle. Masters suggests that James takes it for granted that his readers will add this qualifying statement for themselves because it is an over-riding principle of the scriptures that ALL prayer is subject to the sovereign will and wisdom of God (1 John 5:14). Masters notes that the word translated "prayer" in James 5:15 is the humblest Greek word for prayer; from the verb to beg, plead, request, ask, petition. On this basis he describes the prayer of faith as:

Not a demanding, claiming, insisting kind of word, but one which recognizes and is ready to bow to the higher wisdom and authority of God. It is a pleading word, the prayer of one who hopes to prevail upon the Lord but who recognizes that He may have a higher plan. This kind of prayer cannot be offered by someone who has made up his or her mind how God must answer. It is not the prayer of someone determined to get his own way, come what may. It is not a form of will power which attempts to bend circumstances to our own will.[18]

He concludes that

The prayer of faith is not the prayer of people who have convinced themselves that the healing is already accomplished. Such an attitude is mind-power, not prayer. The prayer of faith is a prayer offered by those who recognize that God is supreme and perfect and that He will bring things to pass according to His perfect will and timing. The true prayer of faith NEVER takes God's sovereignty away from Him.[19]

This does not mean that all incentive for prayer is destroyed. Rather, it is the realization that God invites appeals and petitions, and promises to listen and respond and applies His supreme wisdom to each request. With deep conviction and urgency we believe that God hears our appeal and therefore make our requests on the ground that God promises to take the fullest account of them. We pray in confidence that God is ready to be moved and persuaded by our cries unless in a given case He has something better in mind, or some higher purpose to achieve through the illness.

Clarifying Some of the Issues

It is clear that there are different interpretations of the meaning of the prayer of faith. For some the prayer of faith is part of the general ministry of prayer but without the doubt and uncertainty which often accompanies prayer. The prayer of faith is a prayer which accepts the reality of God's promise, and does not doubt. For some, the prayer of faith is a special prayer in which faith is given as a gift from God but is only to be used in exceptional circumstances. This gift brings a certainty that healing will occur. For others, the prayer of faith is the same as other prayers: it must be subject to God's sovereign will and purpose, and God may or may not reveal this in a special way to particular people. The following points may clarify some issues:

- However we define the prayer of faith it is clear that the two most destructive agents of all prayer are doubt and fear — doubt as to the reality of God's promise, power and presence; and fear as to the consequences of either claiming too much or too little. The prayer of faith is a challenge to "go for it" with a much more intentional attitude than is often present in our prayers.

- There could be some danger in suggesting various levels of prayer; namely, that the general faith prayer is all right for ordinary Christians, whereas the special gift is only for particular people. This may easily discourage those who feel they have no special gift of faith. On the other hand, some suggest that this can act as a challenge to deeper faith, to spur on ordinary believers to more definitely "go for it."

- Rather than suggesting different levels of prayer it may be more helpful to think of different types of prayer. Must all prayer have this deep conviction that God is going to do a specific thing so that the result is absolutely certain? There are prayers of rest, of praise, of quiet communion with God, of affirmations, of thanks, and there are also times when we do not know what to ask for and so wisdom is needed (James 1:5) and the help of the Holy Spirit is given (Romans 8:26). An over-emphasis on certainty in prayer can suggest that we only pray effectively when this certainty is present, and this further suggests that any effectiveness in prayer will only be as far as our faith stretches. But Ephesians 3:20 affirms that "God is able to do far more than we ask for or even think of."

- There are differences about the emphasis on God's will. Those who suggest that the prayer of faith is subject to the sovereign will of God are affirming an important principle, that ultimately everything is subject to God's will. However this emphasis can include the idea that we cannot truly know God's will in relation to healing. But other writers affirm that God's will and purpose for healing can be known because this is clearly revealed in the teaching of Jesus and the practice of the church; namely, that it is God's normal will to heal unless it is clear that there is some countervailing reason. This debate will continue and depends on where you start on the prayer-faith-will of God relationship. Several writers see the use of the phrase "if it be Thy will" as a positive rather than a negative in prayer. J. Motyer writes:

The effect of this petition is to take away from our prayers the limitations imposed by our knowledge of what our needs are; by our proposals of what will meet them, and by our sense of what is best. Its effect is to place ourselves and others unreservedly into the hands of that infinite wisdom, love and power, which belongs to our Heavenly Father. To say "thy will be done" does not impose a restriction on what we ask, rather it lifts all earthly restriction. The disposing of the welfare of the child of God cannot be left with greater confidence anywhere else than in the Father's hands, nor can any solution of the plight be more fitting, beneficial and glorious than that which He has in mind.[20]

- There is both a true confidence and a danger of imbalance in the faith formula idea, which suggests that because healing is part of the present kingdom blessing we can therefore "name it and claim it." On the one hand we are encouraged to take God at His word and come boldly to the throne of grace, and claim the blessings He wants to give to us (Hebrews 4:16). On the other hand, we are to come in humility and with the awareness of our human limitations and proneness to misunderstand the purposes of God. Both of these aspects are true and our emphasis will depend on which we see as the most significant, both in our general approach to the healing ministry and in particular circumstances. A helpful comment is offered by J. Motyer:

Such promises are intended to bring us with confidence into the place of prayer. They speak to us of a God who can do all things, who is so generous that He will not withhold from us anything that is good, and whose ears are open to our every word. But the one thing the promises do not encourage or allow is that we should come into the place of prayer in a stubborn insistence that we have got it right and that our will must be done . . . In the prayer of faith our faith is not that the *promises* will be fulfilled just like that; it is the faith which rests trustfully in the will of the sovereign, faithful and loving God. Neither the sick person nor any of the elders is there to insist that his or her will must be done, but to put the sick one within the total eternal security of the unchangeable and unchanging gracious will of God.[21]

- There are obvious limitations to the prayer of faith (as suggested by Glennon), and there needs to be a balance between the limitless power and resources of God and our ability and openness to receive His blessing. Overall we are probably too timid in our response, and we therefore limit God's healing work by our lack of faith.

- There is danger of theological imbalance in either over-emphasizing or under-emphasizing the present reality of the kingdom blessing. Some so emphasize the future blessings as to almost deny the reality of the kingdom here and now; while others so stress the present kingdom reality that they seem to forget that the blessings are only partial and will not be fully experienced in this life. There is an obvious tension between the now and the not-yet of the kingdom. Whilst substantial healing may be experienced now, it is not full or total healing. Because of our limited perspective and a genuine desire to affirm the reality of healing today, it is possible to become unrealistic in claiming absolute healing in our present lives. At best, the healing we experience now is limited by the boundaries of our physical existence and the surety of death. So any promises of healing must take into account the interim nature of the kingdom's blessings, whilst at the same time affirming their reality and power in our lives. There is an inevitable tension in keeping the balance between the now and the not-yet of the kingdom, but living in this tension is an essential aspect of the healing ministry.

- This partial and provisional nature of the kingdom of God, on this side of the coming of Christ, means that we live in the confidence that God does heal today, but we also wait for the full experience of that reality tomorrow in the future. Both today and tomorrow, the present and the future, belong to God, and therefore the prayer of faith must also be the prayer of hope which accepts the reality of God's healing both in the present and the future. Thomas Smail offers this wise counsel:

> When the prayer made in faith is not answered, and the healing for which many have sought does not come, we are not to look for someone to accuse of failure in faith. Rather we are to remember that beside faith there is hope. Hope has to do with God's promises that are still future and hidden, just as faith has to do with God's promises that are here and now. To the person who has believed for today but has not seen the answer come today, there comes the call to hope. Hope says tomorrow also is God's. Enough has happened already to assure you that the rest is on the way:[22]

Some Practical Implications

If there are such different ideas about prayer and faith, how can the ordinary believer come to some conclusions which will be helpful in the actual work of praying for healing? Some suggestions are:

• Respect and try to understand different approaches to this question. Determine to grow in faith so that the prayer of faith becomes an important principle in your prayers. Be open to any particular gift or blessing God may give you and encourage others in growth also. Be challenged by the prayer of faith and "go for it" in your own prayers!

• Realize that there are many different ways to pray, so pray in the style which is suitable for you. Do not try and copy any of the prayer "gurus" in an obsessive way.

• When your faith is limited, ask others to add their faith to yours, so together the total faith is strengthened, and you are enabled to believe and accept God's promises and blessings.

- Be open in seeking to understand each situation from God's point of view. This may involve using the prayer "if it be your will," not in the sense of doubt, but rather of humble submission and acknowledgment that our understanding is limited. Note the following diagram from J. Richards.[23]

Do not try to manipulate God under the guise of having faith in Him.

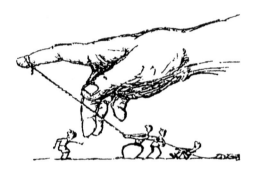

Faith is not getting God to give His attention to what we are focusing on, but giving our attention to what He is focusing on.

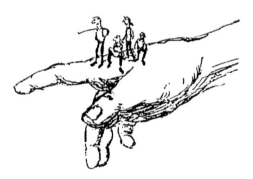

- Remember that in all prayer and ministry, faith is not the greatest thing, but love is. This means that if our prayer ministry is offered in a deep love for God and for those to whom we minister and for whom we pray, this climate of love overcomes many of the shortcomings and limitations of our faith. Read 1 Corinthians 13, especially verse 2.

Sharing and Discussion

1. Discuss the diagram by Richards. In what ways does it help your understanding of faith? Can faith be used as a way to manipulate God?

2. In an earlier chapter we discussed the use of the words "if it be Thy will" in prayer. Note the words by J. Motyer and respond to this positive use of the phrase. What is your thought about "if it be Thy will" now?

3. What are the positive points about the idea of "name it and claim it"? Are there any dangers in this approach?

4. How can we grow in faith so that we feel confident to "go for it" in our prayers?

5. Refer to the story of Marcia and Harold. Now that you have worked through this chapter, share how you would respond to their questions about prayer and faith.

6. Write out a brief statement about faith and prayer which you feel summarizes the different aspects mentioned in this chapter.

7. What can we do when we are faced with a very big "mountain"; that is, a very severe sickness or condition which seems to be beyond our faith and ability to respond?

- Throw up our hands in despair?

- Back off because we don't know what to do?

- Give up praying for healing?

- Hand it over to the "expert" healers, or those with the special gift or knowledge?

- Leave it with the health professionals to solve?

- Call for help?

- Or what?

References for Further Reading

Blue, K., *Authority to Heal*, IVP, Illinois, 1987.

Glennon, J., *Your Healing is Within You*, Hodder and Stoughton, London, 1978.

Glennon, J., *How Can I Find Healing?* Hodder and Stoughton, London, 1984.

Glennon, J., *The Theology of Healing*, OSL, Australia, undated.

MacNutt, F., *Healing*, Hodder and Stoughton, London, 1988.

Masters, P., *The Healing Epidemic*, The Wakeman Trust, London, 1988.

Kraft, C., *Confronting Powerless Christianity*. Baker, 2002, Chapter 5.

Motyer, J., *The Message of James*, The Bible Speaks Today, IVP, Leicester, 1985.

Richards, J., *Faith and Healing*, Network No. 6, Floreat Flame Books, Mirrabooka, undated.

Storms, C. S., *Healing and Holiness*, Presbyterian and Reformed Publishing, New Jersey, 1990.

8

INNER HEALING — HEALING OF THE MEMORIES

It was *Jan's* thirtieth birthday. She has everything she needs materially. Add to this the fact that she has been a Christian for twelve years and we would expect to see a radiantly happy person. But on the evening of her birthday Jan was feeling most depressed.

For a number of years Jan was happily engaged in Christian service, and had been very successful. Then came the "breakdown", as she called it. Although she had partially recovered, she was subject to frequent fits of depression, when she found herself worrying about everything that happened to her or around her. She had withdrawn from her friends, and had given up her Christian work. At the age of thirty she felt that there was nothing worthwhile left in life. She sought help from various people but had found no lasting relief. Was there no answer?

Jan knew all about confessing her sins to her Lord. Jan did this often and accepted God's forgiveness. Quite frequently she suffered pain from various physical illnesses which her doctor was able to relieve, but no sooner had she gotten rid of one pain than another appeared. Surely this was not what her Heavenly Father would will for her! Surely there must be a way to be free! She had confessed her known sins, but was still conscious of a deep need which was almost a constant yearning for relief and for the lifting of the cloud of depression.

Jan's whole outlook was being affected by memories of happenings of the past, some even before she was born. Her early childhood had not been a happy one. Lying deep in her unconscious mind were emotional stresses that had been passed to her from her mother. Jan had caused great disappointment to her mother simply by being born a girl. A son had been wanted, and Jan's mother had convinced herself she would have a son. When a daughter arrived, though no fault could be found with the attention given to her, there was no expression of joy or satisfaction. No bond of love was evident, and, as Jan grew, the little girl was constantly made aware that she was a "scrap of a girl" instead of being a strong healthy boy. This estrangement left a scar on her mind and as an adult she still felt unwanted and inadequate. This was the chief cause of her depression and this had led to her breakdown. Though some of these happenings from her early life were not consciously recollected, they were deeply embedded in her unconscious mind and were now affecting her in a most harmful way.

As so many do when they are bound by depression, defeat and unhappiness, Jan sought help from many places and people, but experienced what many have found when they go from counselor to counselor. Jan became more confused than ever, because each counsellor gave her a different reason for her depression and each one offered different advice. Jan's condition worsened as she continued to search earnestly and almost frantically for the help she felt she must have before it was too late.

At last she found relief. A Christian counselor was able to tell her that the Lord Jesus Christ has the power to heal the whole person. The one whom she had known as her Savior was also the one she could trust to heal her. This counselor had the gift of discernment and realized that her deep depression had a deep-rooted cause. He explained to Jan that the Lord Jesus who healed all kinds of people during his earthly ministry is the same *yesterday, today* and *forever.* Time does not limit Jesus, and because of this, he could go right back into the deepest area of her life and deal with the root cause of all that was hurting her and causing such sorrow.

Jan found that Jesus could uncover those things that had been suppressed for so long and could free her from the pain they caused.

It is God's will that she should be whole and free, and it is God's desire that she would be fully healed. Jan's eyes showed the first glimmer of the hope that was dawning.

It took some time of patient guidance, but Jan came to the place where she was ready to allow the Lord Jesus to take over and share life with her. From the first moment the counselor prayed with her she began to relax. In faith, she prayed that the Savior would go right back into the deep places of her mind and reveal what needed to be known. At this point Jan became aware that something was happening. The prayer continued, asking that Jesus now heal the hurt and remove the scars. Healing commenced right then.

Each day Jan followed the advice of her counselor and, in faith, thanked the Lord Jesus for entering the depths of her unconscious mind to heal the hurts of the past. She did not plead for healing; she just kept telling the Lord that she was trusting his healing power.

If any sign of depression, defeat or unhappiness appeared, she simply asked the Lord to perfect the work of healing he was doing, and she gave thanks.

Three weeks went by, weeks during which Jan says she started to live again. She was being healed! She was experiencing inner healing. She was a new creature in Christ Jesus. The change was obvious to all, as she took up her Christian work again.

Reflect on this story and respond to the following questions: What were the reasons for Jan's depression? Comment on what you think are the key sentences which point to the problem.

- What did Jan do to solve the problem? Can you suggest why her efforts failed?

- What was the secret of release for Jan? How did this release become a reality in her experience?

- If Jan was a Christian for many years, according to 2 Corinthians 5:17 she already was a new creature in Jesus Christ. Why then did she need this inner healing? Was this not part of the blessing she received from Jesus when she first became a Christian?

- Is inner healing an essential part of the blessings of conversion, or is it something which often comes afterwards?

This chapter aims to:

- Clarify the meaning of inner healing and healing of the memories.

- Understand the place of memory in our lives.

- Examine the principles on which this ministry is based.

- Outline the process through which healing is possible.

- Suggest some reasons why and situations where this ministry is needed.

- Evaluate whether this ministry is biblical.

- Understand and evaluate some criticisms of this ministry.

- Suggest some values of this ministry.

Inner Healing and Healing Memories

Inner healing and healing of the memories are often given the same meaning by some writers; others refer to either one or the other; and some speak of inner healing through healing of the memories. Some recent books show the close connection between the two ideas:[1]

Inner Healing Through Healing of Memories

Healing the Wounded Spirit

Healing For Damaged Emotions

One definition gathers together these ideas and describes inner healing as "the healing of the inner person; the mind, the emotions, the painful memories, the dreams."[2]

Another writer describes inner healing as "a process wherein the Holy Spirit restores health to the deepest aspects of life by dealing with the root cause of hurt and pain . . . this involves the breaking of the power of evil in a person's life and the healing of past hurtful memories."[3]

The idea of inner healing began in the 1960's through the work of Agnes and Edgar Sanford who described it as "healing of the memories" or "memory healing". Since that time it has become widely accepted as an important part of the Christian healing ministry. In this chapter "healing of the memories" will be used to describe various aspects of inner healing.

Healing of memories refers to two particular areas of sickness: the sickness of the spirit, brought about by one's own personal sin; and emotional sickness, caused by the hurts and traumas of the past. Through the medium of prayers and counseling and the ministry of the Holy Spirit, past memories can be healed and emptied of their negative power. David Seamands sees healing of the memories as "a form of Christian counseling and prayer which focuses the healing power of the Spirit on certain types of emotional/spiritual problems." Aware of the dangers of abuse he warns:

It is one, and only one of such ministries, and should never be made the one and only form, for such over-emphasis leads to exaggeration and misuse. It is very important that Christian workers possess both sufficient knowledge and Spirit-sensitized discernment to know when it is the right tool of the Spirit for healing.[4]

The Significance of Memory

What is memory and why is it important?

Memory is the power to retain and reproduce thoughts and feelings which we experience, either to keep them in our minds or to recall and remember them. Memories are like pictures on the screens of our minds, arising from our experiences, ideas, attitudes and feelings.

The Bible contains few references to the noun *memory*, but more than two hundred and fifty references to the verb *remember*, or *call to mind*. Many of these refer to God. He is a God who remembers His covenant promises (Genesis 9:15; Exodus 2:24; Psalm 106:45.). In His kindness He remembers human frailty (Psalm 103:14). He also forgets and does not remember our sins and failures (Jeremiah 31:34). People are urged to remember the Grace of God in bringing salvation and the need to be obedient to God (Deuteronomy 5:15; 1 Chronicles 16:12; Ecclesiastes 12:1; 1 Corinthians 11:24, 25).

> In scripture, memory is considered one of the most important aspects of both God's mind and ours. Memory is central to God's nature as well as to forgiveness, salvation and righteous living. God's ability to remember or not remember is part of the divine mind or knowledge which filled the biblical writers with awe. Since we have been created within the Divine image, we too have this ability, though ours is limited. Biblical writers considered this human facility a reason for wonder and praise.[5]

Memories are more than mental pictures. They also involve actions and feelings. When people are commanded to remember the

Sabbath or to remember their creator, it is more than having a mental picture of God, or a mental picture of a place of worship. Rather, it involves thinking, reflecting, and living according to certain spiritual principles of worship and action. Because memories are active and dynamic, they bring both pleasure and pain as we remember and recall happy events, or as we are hurt and wounded by painful memories.

Again, because they are active, memories exert a great influence on our lives, especially painful memories of failure, neglect, abuse, or trauma. Time may heal many wounds of the past, but often painful memories remain and may continue to affect our lives like an untreated wound which infects other areas of the body. While this may especially apply to early childhood and later adolescence, painful experiences at any time in our lives have the power to strongly influence or even control our behavior. People can be crippled emotionally and spiritually by the painful memories of past events which continue to haunt them. Sometimes a painful memory can be repressed and stored away in a part of the brain where it is not consciously recalled; however, it may suddenly break out of this hiding place and reappear to cause deep pain and trauma. Such painful memories may be the result of our own actions and attitudes, but in many cases (especially if they occurred during childhood and adolescence) they are caused by the actions of others toward us. Whatever the cause, the healing of memories is seen as a way to bring healing to these damaged emotions.

Understanding of Personality

Healing of the memories is based on the belief that there are three areas in our minds — the conscious, subconscious and the unconscious.

- The *conscious mind* functions all the time. Thoughts, plans, and ideas are formed as we use our minds to explain our present experience, to reflect, to argue, to communicate; all the things that enable us to be aware of the world, ourselves and others.

- The *subconscious mind* is like a storehouse or memory-bank, where thoughts, reflections and responses to life are stored. These can be recalled by the use of our memory, sometimes easily, and at other times with more difficulty. We are able to recall both good and bad memories. Sometimes, however, we do not wish to recall painful or unpleasant memories, so we try to push them into the deeper inner areas of the mind and suppress them so that they do not reappear to cause pain.

- The *unconscious mind* is the greater storehouse which contains memories of all that has ever happened to us. We may not be aware of these things, but they are there, as if they were recorded on a great tape recorder. If the tape could be played back, it would faithfully reproduce every experience in our lives, even though we may be quite unaware or unconscious of their existence. The memories in the unconscious mind are often beyond our conscious recall, but they can be recalled through various methods of probing and counseling.

This general picture of the personality, or something similar to it, is common to those who seek to help people deal with the hurts and traumas in their lives. Some prefer to speak of only two areas in the mind, that is, the conscious and the subconscious/unconscious. Others prefer the threefold model, but the basic idea is the same. Selwyn Hughes uses the illustration of an iceberg to describe the mind or psyche and explains where painful memories come from and the damage they can cause.

> The psyche is like an iceberg with the part above the water representing the conscious mind and the huge submerged portion representing the subconscious or the unconscious mind. Scientists have discovered that by probing differing areas of the brain, memories long forgotten can be recalled . . . (this is) because all the experiences of life are recorded on memory tapes and stored intact in the deep chambers of the unconscious.

During the developmental years, some people experience great pain; such as sexual abuse, rejection, brutality, deep disappointment . . . and often these painful experiences are too awful for the conscious mind to carry. What do they do? Usually they push them down into the unconscious and clang heavy doors on the vaults, believing that what is out of sight is out of mind.

The unconscious however, is like a tidy housewife who cannot tolerate anything unseemly or disorderly within these chambers, and occasionally throws up to the conscious mind . . . these stored up memories, and shouts: "Here you take care of this for me." But what does the person do when a horrific memory from the past flashes through the conscious mind? Most people resort to the same mechanism as before, and press the pain back down again in the unconscious and lock it behind another closed door (psychologists call this defense mechanism, repression).

But not only is the unconscious mind like a tidy housewife, it is a persistent one also, who finds other ways to get the conscious mind to share some of the burden. She "whispers" to it in the symbolic language of dreams, or introduces it in such an oblique way, that the person concerned is not really aware of it and wonders why he or she is suddenly plunged into depression or caught up in illogical anger or hostility. If these signals are ignored, the unconscious mind can help spread the load by producing physical illness.[6]

Breaking the Control of Past Memories

This control can be broken and memories healed because of three facts:

- Jesus Christ is able to heal both past and present because he is the Lord of time. "He is the same yesterday, today, and forever" (Hebrews 13:8), and is able to move back into the past in people's lives and bring release from any painful situation.

- Jesus Christ is able to empty the memory of the pain and to fill the vacuum left by the pain with love and forgiveness. Forgiveness is given by Jesus from either the guilt of one's own sins or the sins of others, and the person is no longer controlled by this memory.

- Jesus Christ is able to reclaim the person's Christian inheritance so that they can become more integrated in their lives and continue to grow in their Christian life, without being constantly dragged back by emotional and spiritual problems.

So the healing of memories offers release from the binding control of those painful memories which derive from particular situations in our lives. Through this ministry, Jesus brings release to the captives and also binds up and heals the brokenhearted (Isaiah 61:1).

How does this actually work out in a person's life? What is the process by which the healing of memories moves from the realm of theory to the realm of experience, to actually produce inner healing?

The Process of Healing the Memories[7]

There are several steps in the process as described by those involved in this ministry. Whilst there may be variations as to the number of steps, their exact description, and the particular order in which they occur, the following outline would reflect the general approach.[8]

The whole process occurs in an atmosphere of openness to the Holy Spirit in which prayer, counseling, silence and speech are intertwined. There is no set order in the sense that prayer comes first, then counseling, then silence; but rather a waiting on the Holy Spirit to give the appropriate means to keep moving forward into healing.

- The person seeking healing is asked to reaffirm his or her faith in Jesus Christ as Savior and Lord. This is the foundation on which all the following steps are built.

- They are then invited to bring to light the hurts and pains which continue to dominate, and relate them to specific situations in the past. This is done through sharing and counseling with the help of the counselor or prayer partner. Sensitivity is needed to be able to discern the problem area. This may come through the person's own recollection of events, through a word of knowledge, or some special insight given by the Holy Spirit. Sometimes questions can be asked which may help to reveal the basic wound; for example, "When did things start to go wrong?" "Do you have any idea why or what caused the problem?"

This process of recollection enables the person to "uncover" broken relationships, hurtful actions, and traumatic experiences which may be the cause of the pain. If the person cannot respond to these questions or cannot remember anything which seems to point to the cause, then the Holy Spirit is asked to reveal this.

Not all past experiences are negative, so it is not a matter of dredging up everything; rather it is asking the Holy Spirit to bring out the memories or situations that he knows are relevant. It is also important to uncover and bring to light the painful experiences because any incomplete or twisted or undealt-with situations can block growth in the various stages toward emotional development. Rosemary Green, a Christian psychologist, refers to a particular insight gained from counseling: "You cannot move satisfactorily on to the next stage with incomplete agenda from the previous stage."

She then adds:

> Imagine a child building a tower with wooden bricks. If a few bricks are out of line, the tower may grow tall without

mishap, but it will still be less steady than one with bricks wholly in line. It is when the tower of a person's life is seen to be unsteady that we need to ask what experience is contributing to the present instability.[9]

- The Counselor then affirms the unconditional love of Jesus Christ as the source of healing and his ability and willingness to deal with the painful situation. Jesus is confessed and trusted as the Savior who has a complete knowledge of every person and situation, and is therefore able to respond in the exactly appropriate way. He is also recognized as the one who has shared our human lives and identified with our pains and sorrows, so he acts toward us with understanding and sympathy (Hebrews 2:18, 4:14-15). He is also the Lord of time and space and is always the same, so his love can reach back into the past as well as being available in the present (Hebrews 13:8). So we can be confident to come to him and find grace which is effective for both our present and our past lives (Hebrews 4:16).

- The painful experience is revisited or relived but this time with Jesus present. As he walks back with us into our lives, the painful situation is "re-imagined" or "visualized" and Jesus is asked to bring his healing love to that deep hurt: to move back into that experience and heal the person of the wound and pain that has resulted from it. Francis MacNutt describes how Jesus is able to accomplish far more than human counseling:

> Jesus as Lord of time, is able to do what we cannot. He can heal those wounds of the past that still cause us suffering. The most I was ever able to do as a counselor, was to help the person bring to the foreground of consciousness the things that were buried in the past so that he or she could consciously cope with them in the present. Now I am discovering that the Lord can heal these wounds, sometimes immediately, and can bring the counseling process to its completion in a deep healing.[10]

Another leader in this ministry, David Seamands, describes this time of healing prayer as one of the distinctive features about the healing of memories:

> So that the Holy Spirit may actually touch the barriers to health, a full use is made of conversational prayer with emphasis on visualization, imagination, the pinpointing in time of the specific situation(s) which produced the painful memory, and a deeply empathetic faith on the part of the praying partner.
>
> In this special prayer, we allow the Spirit to take us back in time to the actual experience(s) and to walk through those painful memories with us. It is then, through the use of our sanctified imagination, that we pray as if we were actually there at the time it took place, allowing God to minister to us in the manner we needed at that time.
>
> This prayer time is the very heart of the healing of memories. It is in prayer that the healing miracle begins. Without it the whole process may simply be a form of auto suggestion, catharsis, or feeling therapy. This special time of prayer cannot be bypassed, if there are to be lasting results.[11]

- As the painful wound is healed, the person is encouraged to repent of and renounce any sinful attitudes which may be present in relation to the past events; for example, resentment, anger, revenge, and unforgiveness. Then Jesus is asked to fill any void in the person's life with his love, so that the person is able to experience the fullness of the Holy Spirit in daily life and to know the love of Christ which is beyond human understanding (Ephesians 3:16-19).

Because one of the basic needs of life is for love, full healing cannot occur until the person is given the love that was denied to him or her in the painful situation. For some people, this part of the inner healing may be more difficult than the healing of past wounds. Francis MacNutt suggests how to proceed with the person who is so accustomed to being without love that he or she does not know how to receive it.

> If the person says he does not feel the love of God, Jesus is asked to speak to the person at the depth of his soul and to call him by name. Since the nature of the wounds is known to the healer, he or she prays that God will provide the specific kind of love the person did not have.[12]

• The final step in the process is to maintain this healing because it is possible for any release from the past to fade, and the person fall back into captivity again. So there needs to be an integration of the whole person toward new attitudes and actions which will encourage the person to continue to grow in the grace and knowledge of Jesus Christ (2 Peter 3:18). This includes regular prayer, Bible reading, praise, fellowship, commitment to Jesus Christ as Lord, and a constant readiness to forgive others.

It is important to recognize the central place of repentance and forgiveness both for the beginning and for the continuation of true healing. D. A. Seamands states:

> Forgiveness is the very crux of the healing of memories, forgiveness in the sense of forgiving and being forgiven. It is impossible to exaggerate its importance in the healing process. It is at this point where the greatest struggles of prayer will take place . . . this is usually where the battle is won or lost . . .

> Forgiveness (and being forgiven) is the key relational issue in the Bible. This is true for all our relationships with God, others and ourselves. God has built this supreme principle into the very structure of all interpersonal relationships. It is based on the nature and character of God Himself, and since

we are made in His image, it has been built into us. So we are talking about a basic biblical and psychological principle. Every experience of memory healing confirms this. If we want forgiveness without forgiving, we are asking God to violate His own moral nature. This He cannot and will not do.[13]

The reason for this basic principle is that the first step to forgiveness is to acknowledge feelings of resentment and hate which are usually part of the painful situation.

When people experience severe hurt they usually end up hating the person who caused this hurt. If they then bury the hurt, they also bury the hate. But God has so structured our personalities that we cannot do this and get by with it forever. We cannot long ingest and integrate hidden resentments any more than our stomach can incorporate bits of broken glass. In both, we are going to feel a lot of inner unrest and pain! Both require serious operations. The healing of memories is therefore a form of spiritual surgery and therapy.[14]

David Augsburger sums it up in a beautiful way:

Forgiveness is acceptance with no exceptions. It accepts not only the hurt you have received; it accepts the one who did the hurting; and the loss caused by the hurtful actions or words . . . Forgiving is self-giving with no self-seeking. It gives love where the enemy (the one causing the pain) expects hatred. It gives freedom where the enemy deserves punishment. It gives understanding where the enemy anticipates anger and revenge. Forgiveness refuses to seek its own advantage . . . it brings new life to our withered hearts, new energy to our paralyzed emotions, and new understanding to our frozen feelings.[15]

When is Healing of Memories Needed?

We have seen that healing of memories makes sense because it focuses on a deep human need. We are deeply affected by what we do, and also by what happens to us through the actions of others, and the evil in the world. But the gospel is the good news that we can be freed from the evil that burdens and controls us, and that this freedom relates to our past, present and future experiences. Not only is this an important aspect of the gospel, but it also clarifies some insights of psychology which are of value in pointing to the possible causes of emotional problems. However, while these insights clarify, they are often not able to give the answer required to meet the deep needs.

When is healing of the memories needed? Is it something which should be applied in every situation? To some extent we all carry hurts from the past which have the potential to make us emotional and spiritual cripples. D. A. Seamands warns against a *blanket* application of this ministry to every person, and using it as a sort of gimmick or easy answer to emotional and spiritual problems.

Memory healing is one and only one form of spiritual therapy. Let me say it with unbecoming intensity: the healing of memories is not a cure-all for every emotional and spiritual hang-up. In fact, under no circumstances should it be used with certain types of problems and personality types. (Extremely emotional and hysteric types of people who surround themselves with all kinds of fantasy emotions relating to hundreds of minor incidents, rather than deep-seated repressed emotions and memories. These people need help to control their *unruly* emotions rather than their *unexpressed* emotions).

. . It is most useful and successful with people who have severely repressed the memories of their most painful experiences and have then tended to become closed and unable to express their true feelings about God, others and themselves. As a result they have become withdrawn and unable to form close and intimate interpersonal relationships. With such persons, sometimes known as "God's frozen chosen," it can bring release from buried resentments, forgiveness, and the freedom to move on to genuine emotional and spiritual maturity.[16]

What are the indicators that such healing is needed? Francis Mac-Nutt offers a general guideline when he suggests:

Inner healing is indicated whenever we become aware that we are held down in any way by the hurts of the past. We all suffer from this kind of bondage to one degree or another, some severely, some minimally.

Any unreasonable fear, anxiety or compulsion caused by patterns built up in the past can be broken by prayer, provided we are also doing our best to discipline our life in a Christian way . . .

MacNutt refers to Christians whose lives are weakened by a sense of worthlessness, erratic fits of anger and depression, compulsive sexual drives, and anxiety and unreasoning fears; and who are unable to cope with these through repentance and a decision to change. He concludes that healing is required when:

. . We find that the powerful memories of the past rise to fill us with fear and anxiety whether we wish these fears or not — and we cannot wish them away by an act of the will.[17]

Other practitioners suggest that healing of memories may be needed by any Christian especially if there are recurring mental pictures and dreams of a disturbing and disruptive nature relating to:

• Hurts which lead to a strong sense of rejection and a weakening and lowering of our ego or self image.

- Humiliations which lead to a sense of shame.

- Fears and horrors of many different kinds.

- Hates and resentments directed toward others and toward God.

Another area which suggests the need for such healing is when a Christian has a distorted picture of God which gives rise to the following:

- Inability to feel forgiven.

- Inability to trust in the goodness of God and being able to surrender to Him.

- Very strong doubts about some aspects of faith and inability to come to any positive response to these.

- Problems with neurotic perfectionism.

Many of these attitudes are related to concepts of God as a stern judge, a demanding perfectionist father figure, or to ideas of faith as strict dogma shackling any independent thought, or to experiences of domination and control in the church.[18]

The fact that healing of the memories is widely accepted and practiced in the church could suggest that there are no concerns about this ministry, and that it receives widespread support by all Christians. However, this is not so, and in reality, this ministry is strongly criticized by many people. What are these criticisms, and are they valid?

There are several criticisms, but two main ones. One is that this ministry is non-biblical in its approach and that it is imposed on the scriptures (by use of selected texts and doubtful interpretations), rather than emerging from scripture. The other is that it is over-dependent on doubtful psychological models and makes use of techniques which are prominent in New Age and occult teaching and philosophy. These two criticisms need to be examined.

Is the Healing of Memories Scriptural?

After careful consideration of the issues, Selwyn Hughes concludes that whilst such things as prayer, love, support, and forgiveness are true to scripture and commanded by scripture, many of the techniques used are not.

> In my judgment the ministry of inner healing as it is generally practiced in today's church, is a ministry that is imposed on the Bible rather than exposed from it. Certain elements of the ministry . . . such as prayer, love, empathetic support, encouragement, forgiveness, confession and so on most certainly have the commendation, even the command of scripture . . . (but) some of the techniques do not.[19]

Another writer, Don Matzat, strongly opposes this ministry.

> The inner healing teaching is not based upon or drawn from the content of scripture. The New Testament does not teach that the traumas of childhood, often inflicted by others and buried within the subconscious or unconscious mind, hinder the sanctification, spiritual growth and maturity of believers in Jesus Christ. The Bible offers no promises and gives no examples of Jesus being available to heal the hurts of the past by "playing a little game in the imagination." Neither the understanding of inner healing, nor the methodology of inner healing is drawn from, based upon, or even remotely suggested in the Bible.[20]

Matzat's position is that the scripture teaches that "all things relating to life and godliness" are provided for us through Jesus Christ

(2 Peter 1:3), and that there are no New Testament promises or precedents which offer any experience such as that offered in the healing of memories.[21]

These criticisms suggest that this ministry relies for its rationale on extra-biblical sources, especially theories from psychology and other social sciences rather than the scriptures, which do not contain or endorse any of the techniques used.

> The Bible fairly bulges with accounts of people who were traumatized, slandered, rejected, beaten, abused, even tortured. Hebrews 11 contains a long list of such people. But not once do you ever read that someone came alongside them and said, "Look, what you need is the healing of memories."

Nowhere in the Word of God is there any record of anyone, not even Christ Himself, adopting this approach to human problems. If it were integral to Christian growth and development, the Holy Spirit would have laid down both the concept and the process clearly in the scriptures.[22]

The issue is whether or not it is essential to be able to establish actual scripture references to validate a ministry, that is, explicit statements which provide specific scriptural authority for this ministry; or whether it is sufficient for any ministry to be in line with biblical principles without having to validate it by specific references.

Those who support the healing of memories as valid, respond to this "non-biblical" argument by noting that there are many areas of knowledge and experience which are not mentioned in scripture, but which are accepted and used as part of our daily lives. For example, there are no verses referring to modern surgery, air-conditioning, cars, airplanes, computers, TV and many other modern facilities and practices; but this does not mean that we should not use them. What is important is not being able to locate specific references, but to ask whether any particular ministry or practice is consistent with general biblical principles of thought and conduct.

Rosemary Green states:

> We do not specify chapter and verse for every counseling tool. We need to submit to biblical attitudes and to submit to God, as authority in every way; we need to discover as much as we can of His purposes for mankind and His ways of fulfilling those purposes; we must avoid opening ourselves to any spiritual power that is not the power of the Holy Spirit. We fly in un-biblical airplanes, we keep our food fresh in un-biblical freezers, we are glad of un-biblical anesthetics when we undergo un-biblical surgery . . . we ought to be soaked in scripture and in God Himself. When we are, we have no need to copy the Pharisees in nit-picking while remaining on guard for Biblical truth.[23]

This response, which represents the general approach of those involved in healing of memories, is based on the axiom that "all truth is God's truth, wherever it is found." It accepts the Bible as the revelation of God's purposes and His great design of salvation in Jesus Christ, and recognizes it as a sufficient revelation of all that we need to know for issues of faith and conduct. As the record of God's special and unique revelation of His will and purpose for the world and His salvation in Jesus Christ, it is the ultimate criteria by which all knowledge is to be evaluated. But the scriptures are not seen as an exhaustive revelation of everything that can be known, and the scriptures themselves do not claim to cover all areas of knowledge.

There is also a more *general* revelation in nature, reason and conscience, through which God makes known to us the mysteries of the universe, and from which we are able to formulate an understanding of science, art, medicine and all the various areas of knowledge open to us. An adequate philosophy of knowledge acknowledges many sources of truth which have been given different names in different thought systems, but all remain as God's truth.

> Christians have been grateful for every new truth . . .
> Calvinists have believed in common grace, Wesleyans in prevenient grace, Roman Catholics have the concept of natural theology or general revelation. All truth is God's truth wherever you find it.[24]

To say that all truth is God's truth means that all truth has its ultimate source in God and is therefore to be gratefully accepted as one of His natural gifts. It does not mean that every idea or aspect of knowledge which claims to be true is actually true from a Christian perspective. Much knowledge is neutral in relation to Christian perspectives, whereas some knowledge clearly supports and supplements a specifically Christian world-view. Other areas of knowledge contain a mixture of truth and error in their understanding of God and people, and therefore need to be evaluated by the standard as given in scripture. The task of responsible thinking Christians is to separate truth from error, and incorporate truth into our overall understanding of God's purposes. Truth is therefore not divided into *secular* and *Christian* — all real truth is from God but needs to be carefully evaluated.

As one of the foremost leaders in healing of memories, D. Seamands insists on the need to "keep our balance by continually running all truths through the sieve of God's Word," especially knowledge which derives from psychology and other social sciences. Where any system or method actually contradicts a Christian perspective on people and the world, it must be rejected. Therefore in rejecting the claim that this ministry is not based on scripture, Seamands reiterates the approach that "all truth is God's truth" and also outlines what he sees as a valid biblical foundation for this ministry.

It is of utmost importance to understand that the healing of memories has a solid foundation in the scriptures which is our final authority in all matters of faith and practice. Some people have totally rejected all forms of inner healing because precise definitions do not appear in the Bible. If we applied that reasoning to everything . . . we would actually be denying that all truth comes from God and that we have a spiritual obligation to use every new insight and discovery in any area of life for God's glory and human good. The real question is not whether a practice appears in the Bible in the specific form or language we use today; rather the question is whether it is contradictory to, or consistent with, principles stated in scripture. In accordance with this basic tenet, Christians are grateful for all new truth, insight and discoveries . . . As we look at the biblical teachings, we find the principles upon which we base the healing of memories.[25]

These principles are:

- Putting away "childish" things (1 Corinthians 13:11). This refers to any childish behavior which can be disruptive and destructive. People may be grown up chronologically, but be children psychologically and emotionally — lacking spiritual and emotional maturity because of inner hang-ups which keep them in a bind. These "hang-ups" need to be put away (the word used in 1 Corinthians means "made powerless," "released from," "rendered inoperative," "inactive") through their healing.

- Accepting Jesus Christ as a present helper (Hebrews 13:5, 8; Matthew 28:20). As the eternal contemporary, Jesus transcends all time and space and is made real to us through the power of the Holy Spirit. It is not self-hypnosis or mental gymnastics to imagine that he is present, for the Holy Spirit assures that he is truly alongside us. The form by which we visualize his presence is from our imagination, but the fact of his presence is not from our imagination, but from the promises of scripture.

- Honestly facing our sins, failures and needs through specific prayer, rather than covering them before God, others and ourselves. It is the work of the Holy Spirit of truth who brings conviction of the truth and enables us to confess our need and be open to receive grace (John 14:15-17; 16:7-14; 1 John 1:5-10).

- Ministry to others as members of one Body of Christ, the church, through confession and prayer, bringing about restoration and healing (James 5:15, 16). The significance of confession, forgiveness and restoration is clearly recognized in scripture (Psalm 32: 1-7), and is now being confirmed by the latest findings in medicine and psychology as an important aspect in protecting against damaging internal and physical stresses.

Is Healing of Memories Dependent on Non-scriptural Psychological Understanding?

Selwyn Hughes practiced the healing of memories for many years, but now believes that this ministry is inadequate in its use of techniques derived from psychology. He views psychology with great respect, but asserts that it cannot provide the ultimate answers concerning human need because it is not consistent with biblical principles. He contends that much counseling in the contemporary church is scripture plus psychology, and that it is accepted because "it works, rather than because it is right." He opposes the ministry of the healing of memories because:

- It separates emotional need/sickness from spiritual need/ sickness. For Hughes, all non-organic personal problems have ultimate spiritual roots. They may be reflected in the emotions but the real issues underlying all human behavior are invariably spiritual.

- It does not adequately deal with the deep-seated and sinful determination of every person to depend on themselves, rather than on the grace and strength which God offers in Jesus Christ.

It does not take realistic notice of human self-centeredness which always tries to preserve its own soul and shift the blame on to others. It treats people as victims (which is often true) but frequently fails to tackle the sinful responses which people make to past experiences; responses which in themselves bring further problems and must be regarded as sinful.

• It too easily seeks to release people from the pain of the past, rather than encouraging them to accept the discipline of the experience, and through this very experience come to a deeper knowledge of God. He cites Jeremiah as an example of one who remembered his affliction, bitterness and depression, yet in the midst of these he was able to remember God's compassion and mercy, and find strength in His faithfulness (Lamentations 3:19-25). He suggests that by releasing the person too quickly from these painful experiences, the person is thereby robbed of an opportunity to understand the grace of God more deeply.[26]

We need to recognize that we are dealing with a deep issue which divides Christians and for which there may be no clear answer. Different attitudes to the scriptures and the use of psychological insights and techniques produce different responses to human problems. Those who practice the healing of memories would not accept Hughes' criticisms, believing that they do not err in the way he suggests, and that their understanding is equally biblical. They insist that they do not subject the Bible to psychological theory, but always attempt to ensure that any insights or methods from psychology are subject to the scriptural principles.

Another area of concern relates to the use of imagination or visualization as a healing method.[27]

Those who criticize healing of the memories claim that it is an occult practice which attempts to create or manipulate reality through mental processes, that is, if your imagination is strong enough, it will create reality. So a person is asked to imagine or visualize Jesus being present in the past, whereas in actual fact Jesus was not literally there. He did not literally walk with the person. Critics further contend that the use of visualization is not found in scripture, but is derived from the work of the psychologist Carl Jung (1875-1961); and can lead to involvement with spirit guides, which is a road into the occult. Those who walk down this road risk being controlled by powerful unseen forces which may be unleashed. Jesus becomes another spirit guide like Moses, Buddha, and a host of others. The real Jesus is not encountered through our imagination and visual images, but rather through the preaching of the Word. It is through the declared Word that faith is born, not through any game in the imagination (Romans 10:9-17).

In responding to this critique, it is pointed out that the use of the imagination or visualization is a normal part of Christian activity; such as in singing hymns, or visualizing scenes from the Bible stories, or in such fictional poetry as "Footprints," where a person who has just died imagines talking to Jesus and learns how Jesus had been with him all through his lifetime. Much of the music and teaching in the church evokes images which help us to reflect on and understand God's love for us. The scripture itself is not given only in the form of word propositions, but in flesh and blood stories which project pictures in our minds. So imagination is an important way of understanding the meaning of the gospel. It is true that it can be misused and become a means of occult involvement, but the method itself is neutral and can be used to point us either to God or to evil. Its use in New Age and occult systems does not invalidate the method itself — it simply shows the essential difference between a Christian and a non-Christian use of this facility. To turn away from something good in itself because it can be corrupted is a denial of the original giver of all good things. Our imagination is one of God's good gifts which separates us from the rest of creation.

Those who defend the use of imagination or visualization as a legitimate way to experience the reality of Jesus' healing point out that when a person is asked to visualize Jesus being present in a past experience, this is not something that never took place. Jesus *was* there, but the person did not realize his presence. Picturing Jesus as present helps to understand and apply what the scriptures have declared. This is not creating the reality of his presence, it is *realizing* the reality that was already true. So, to see Jesus standing with us at the time of any tragedy, or feel him comforting us or laying our pain and resentment at his feet for him to take away, or sensing him smiling at us or walking with us, all of these are valid ways of entering into the reality of his love. All of these imaginative dimensions are regularly used in Christian education when stories are told to children. Why is it right when we are young, but wrong when we are older?

However, because this is a potentially dangerous area, there is need to understand and deal with the essential difference between Christian imagining and the kind of visualization found in New Age and secular self-help programs. There are four warning guidelines to help clarify this difference.[28]

- Proper Christian imagining is always based on specific biblical truths, never on the invention of truth or the idea that we can bring reality into being by simply imagining it.

- Let God be sovereign in the process; that is, recognize that the Holy Spirit is the leader in the process and trust in His guidance to lead us to Jesus. Robert Wise emphasizes this important point:

  In the inner world, it is not always clear what is good,
  demonic or redemptive. The only sure guide into our past
  is the Holy Spirit. Jesus Christ is Lord of the present and
  the past and is the perfect one to help us. In contrast to
  the use of inner guides, prayer involving reconstruction of
  experiences is not talking to oneself. Jesus Christ is objective
  reality who comes in from the outside . . . and leads us to

specific content of actual past experiences . . . When we pray in the name of Jesus, we are asking for God to be with us and to make us whole. No one who reaches out to the Spirit of God and seeks contact with His Holy person will ever be misled . . . As we ask Him by the power of the Holy Spirit to speak healing words to us we can be assured that the voice of Jesus has integrity.[29]

• Make sure it is the Jesus of scripture that we seek. Healing does not come simply through the exercise of imagining, but through the Jesus who is revealed in scripture, who is the only one who can truly bring holiness. To imagine or seek help from other spiritual entities could provide an opening for evil and demonic forces to enter our lives.

• Check the truth of any vision, word or experience against the scripture. Thoughts from our sub-conscious minds, ideas from others, and evil impressions may come to us as well as genuine communications from God. Therefore do not accept anything without making sure it squares with what God has given in the scriptures.

So while there are risks in the use of this method, it can be effective provided that it is used carefully and prayerfully, always being subject to what has been given in the scriptures, and always focusing on the *Jesus* who is revealed there. This avoids the danger of being seduced by New Age and occult counterfeits, but does not throw out a method which has been used extensively in the history of the church. M. Pearson offers this helpful summary:

A close familiarity with the history of Christian spirituality will teach us the difference between the proper, legitimate, time-tested, Christian mystical experiences, and the New Age, magical occultic variety. We must be careful we do not fall off either end of the table — rejecting all imagining, or accepting any imagining without careful discrimination.[30]

Some Positive Values of this Ministry

After noting some criticisms, H. N. Maloney concludes that:

> All in all, inner healing should be looked on as a unique and powerful form of therapy, currently held in wide respect by a large part of the Christian world. Christian psychotherapists should study it deeply and attempt to learn from its bold use of Christian resources in the helping process.[31]

The following emphases arising from this ministry show its powerful contribution to the overall healing work of the church.

- A re-affirmation of the healing power of Jesus Christ in human lives bringing release to many held in captivity by past experiences, and to many broken-hearted as a result of past traumas.

- An emphasis on the possibility, necessity, and releasing power of forgiveness.

- The recognition of the value of counseling and prayer as one means by which healing is made possible.

- The recognition of the value of some psychological principles in understanding human behavior, and the use of some methods as they are applied according to the principles of scripture and the ministry of the Holy Spirit.

- The recognition that help is available to the "captives" beyond what is possible through the insights of psychology. While psychology is to be respected because it helps to give understanding of the situation, it must remain subservient to the gospel of healing love, through which alone the deepest human needs and hurts can be met.

- The recognition of healing gifts in the church, and the important role of the church as an accepting fellowship where healing love can be experienced, and those who are released from the tyranny of the past can be helped to grow in faith and love. Christians have the privilege and gifts to minister to each other, so that the church can play a leading role in bringing healing to the human personality.

Yet having noted these positives, it is perhaps wise to conclude this chapter on a note of caution. The fact that this ministry is strongly criticized by many Christians who are skilled in the area of helping, who are concerned for true biblical interpretation, and who desire that the healing power of Christ be experienced more deeply in people's lives, should alert us to the possible dangers in this ministry. As with the ministry of meditation and other healing aspects which use insights from the Bible and the social sciences, there is often a fine line between these two resources. Also, because this ministry often deals with emotionally frail people, there is always a danger of causing deep emotional and spiritual harm if some of the methods are used unwisely. Having noted the cautions of one of the leading practitioners in this ministry, it is wise to heed the warning that the healing of memories is not a cure-all for every emotional and spiritual hang-up, and it should not be used as a "quickie" emotional cure-all. It is not for novices or mavericks and should only be undertaken after training from those experienced in the ministry. There remain several unknowns to some issues, so it is wise to proceed cautiously. David Seamands offers sound advice, as we continue to think about the healing of memories:

> There are some things we know about healing of memories; there are some things we do not know. Certainly there have been enough positive and miraculous results in people's lives to encourage us in seeking further truth about it. There are also enough negatives to make us issue cautions. No one will ever fully fathom the mystery of memory, any more than we will ever fully understand the mystery of God in whose image

we have been created. So let us walk humbly before the Lord asking His Holy Spirit to keep guiding us into the truth which sets us free. In the meantime, let us use the wisdom He has given us in the spirit of Moses who said: "The secret things belong to the Lord our God but the things revealed belong to us and to our sons forever, that we may observe all the words of this law"(Deuteronomy 29:29).[32]

Sharing and Discussion

1. Read Isaiah 61:1 and Luke 4:18-19 and respond to the following:

(a) Who are the captives that Jesus releases:

• In the gospel stories?

• Today?

(b) What are some of the hang-ups and traumas which bind people today and from which they seek release?

(c) "To bind up the broken-hearted"

• Describe some of the things which break people's hearts today.

• How can the material in this chapter help people who are "broken-hearted?"

2. Read the outline of the process of healing of the memories. Discuss with others any points needing further clarification.

3. Study the reasons why some people criticize, or are very cautious about the healing of memories. Do you think these are valid?

4. Because there are areas of mystery about this ministry, is it wise

to suggest the healing of memories to hurting people? Should we not wait until all the questions about this ministry have been satisfactorily answered?

5. Is inner healing or healing of the memories a significant part of the preaching and experience of the gospel in your congregation? Should it be? How could you begin to encourage this understanding in your church?

6. Have you experienced healing of the memories?

(a) Can you share this experience; how it happened; what is happening now in relation to your past?

(b) Have you helped others to experience the healing of the memories? What did you learn from that experience?

7. "He breaks the power of cancelled sin; he sets the prisoner free; his blood can make the foulest clean; his blood availed for me." — *Charles Wesley.*

(a) What does Wesley mean? (b) Is this an aspect of inner healing?

8. A person struggling with painful memories and seeking healing is bothered by your comment that they need to forgive others and repent of their wrong attitude before healing is possible. They ask, "Why should I have to forgive and repent, when it was their fault — they were the ones who caused the pain, so why should I be asked to forgive them? Surely the problem is with them not me? I feel angry and hurt and I just cannot forgive them." How would you respond?

9. Someone asks you to give some guidelines as to how to evaluate whether the healing of memories is okay from a biblical perspective. How would you respond?

References for Further Reading

Amano, J. Y. and Geisler, N. L., *The Infiltration of the New Age,* Tyndale, Illinois, 1987, Chapter 6.

Augsburger, D., *The Freedom of Forgiveness,* Moody, Los Angeles, 1970.

Cosslett, N., *His Healing Hands,* Hodder & Stoughton, London, 1985, Chapter 9.

Glennon, J., *Your Healing is Within You,* Hodder & Stoughton, London, 1978, Chapter 4.

Green, R., *God's Catalyst,* Hodder & Stoughton, London, 1991, Chapters 11 and 12.

Hughes, S., "The Healing of Memories — is it a valid Biblical Ministry?" *The Christian Counselor,* C.W.R., Farnham, Surrey, Volume 1, Numbers 1-4, 1991.

MacNutt, E., *Healing,* Hodder & Stoughton, London, 1988, Chapter 13.

Maloney, H. N., "Inner Healing" in D. Benner (Ed), *Baker Encyclopedia of Psychology,* Baker, Grand Rapids, 1985.

Matzat, D., *Inner Healing — Deliverance or Deception,* Harvest House, Oregon, 1987.

Pearson, M. A., *Christian Healing,* Chosen Books, F. H. Revell, New Jersey, 1990, Chapter 6.

Seamands, D. A., *Healing of Memories,* Victor, Scripture Press, Illinois, 1985.

9

HEALING AND MEDICAL SCIENCE — PILLS OR PRAYER OR BOTH?

Liz is a physician in her early 30's. She was raised in a Christian home, she received an excellent education, and she went to a top-notch medical school. Liz has devoted herself to family practice, and she finished medical residencies in both pediatrics and psychiatry. Liz believes that the first line of defense against illness is a medical doctor. She does not pray regularly, she does not attend church, and while she believes that prayer can be useful practice for some people, she believes that prayer is a "placebo".

Liz's father *Bob* is a pastor in his mid-50s. Bob was raised in a Christian home, he received an excellent education, and has been happily married for many years. Bob has consulted doctors whenever he has been sick, but he has fortunately never been injured or in a terrible accident of any kind needing hospitalization. Bob went through a bout of depression fifteen years ago when he was urged by his wife to see the family doctor who referred him to a psychiatrist. The psychiatrist put Bob on a series of pills, and at one point Bob was taking three different kinds of medicine. His moods got better, but Bob did not like the way he was feeling. He told the psychiatrist he was going to quit all the medicines, and rely on daily exercise and prayer. The psychiatrist reluctantly let Bob go. Bob now resists taking any medicine, and believes that many doctors tend to push medicines rather than listening to patients, and also do not give sufficient attention to other healing resources like faith and prayer.

Liz's mother *Lucy* is a hospice nurse in her mid-50s. Lucy was raised in a Roman Catholic home, she attended parochial school with compulsory daily mass, and she saw her mother praying the Rosary nearly every day. Throughout her career Lucy has been with many people when they are dying. Her main job is to look after patient's comfort, which includes their physical and emotional care. She is an excellent nurse who as the case manager works closely with a health care team, including a physician, a social worker, and a chaplain. When Lucy visits a patient, she talks to them primarily about their illness, and the management of that illness wherever the patient lives, often either in their own home or a nursing facility. Lucy is interested in the patient's whole life context, primarily their health care, but also their moods, their family support system, and the other resources which sustain and support life. Lucy does not bring up discussions of God, but patients often do so. She is not often asked to pray with a patient, because the chaplain comes to do so when requested. But Lucy finds that it helps her as a nurse to pray actively for her patients when she is coming to see them, and after she leaves. She does not know if her prayers are effective, but she trusts that God will hear her prayers and answer them.

Consider the cases of Liz, Bob, and Lucy. How would you describe their attitudes to the use of medical care and other resources like prayer and faith in healing? Which attitude do you think is the most helpful?

When anyone becomes sick where do they look for help? Do most people you know tend to try pills or prayer or both? When your family, friends and acquaintances become ill or injured, do they first call go to the doctor or the emergency room of the hospital, or do they go see the minister/pastor/priest/church as in James 5: 13-15? Should our family, friends, and acquaintances be encouraged to seek help from various sources, not as a form of insurance policy in case one does not work, but rather because all are channels through which God's healing can be experienced? Do all of these channels have a role to play in helping people to become whole or is this the work (jealously guarded) of one group only? Who is responsible for healing? Whose task is it to heal? Write down your response.

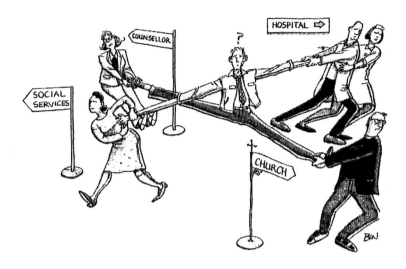

This chapter focuses on the relationship between the healing ministry offered by the church and the healing offered through medical/health services, and aims to:

- Clarify the different attitudes which people have about the relationship between healing and medical science, and understand how these attitudes developed.

- Note the criticisms which are made from the different perspectives, and clarify the need for co-operation among the various approaches.

Co-operation, Ambivalence or Opposition?

Co-operation

The Order of St. Luke sees no conflict between medical science and the healing ministry of the church. Medical science and healing ministry are seen as complementary, with each perspective having something to offer. One objective of OSL is "to encourage complete co-operation between the spiritual ministry of the church and the healing professions."

A similar approach is taken by the Lambeth Conference of the Anglican Church which affirms that the work of the medical and caring professions are integral to the healing ministry. The latest Lambeth statement encourages the church "to work in partnership with doctors, nurses, and all involved in the care of the sick and to encourage medical research and the study of related ethical issues." The Lambeth statement urges "support [of] the church's medical mission work throughout the world as a vital arm of its ministry and outreach." In OSL and many churches involved in the healing ministry there is strong support for the work of chaplains in hospitals and other health agencies. There are many organizations and ministries which offer both the insights and methods of spiritual healing and the treatments for sickness and disease which medical science offers: for example, in the UK such groups as the Churches' Council for Health and Healing; the Institute for Religion and Medicine; many Healing Guilds and homes. In Australia there are groups like the College of Chaplains; the Australian Institute for Religion and Medicine (Western Australia); and other groups of chaplains and health workers; for example, Monash Medical Centre, which offers professional training in chaplaincy and pastoral care services. All these groups recognize the immense contribution of medical science to the healing of sickness and seek to work in co-operation with professional health services.

Ambivalence and/or Opposition

For some Christians, co-operation between medical science and healing ministry is unacceptable, and they have a very negative attitude to medical science in relation to healing. They regard healing as the prerogative of the church, available through prayer, laying on of hands, and especially faith in the promises of God. They see the work of the medical profession as based on purely secular and human skills which generally ignore spiritual factors, and therefore fall short of the healing offered in the gospel. At best, they believe medical science offers a second-best option in healing and is ideal only for those who lack sufficient faith to believe in the availability of God's healing power. In answer to the question, "Should the believer in divine healing take medicine, or should he trust entirely to the power of the healing Christ?" one writer responds,

> The answer to this question depends entirely on the stage
> of spiritual development we have attained. If our personal
> experience of the abiding presence of our Lord is as real to
> us as his visible presence was real to those who beheld him in
> Galilee, then I cannot see that medicine should be any more
> necessary to us than it was to those who were healed by his
> touch or by his spoken word alone . . . The use of medicinal
> aids depends upon the stage we have reached in spiritual
> development.[1]

This may suggest that it is a sign of a weak faith or no faith in the promises of God if we seek to be healed through medical means. To the question, "pills or prayer?" the answer of this writer would seem to be "prayer, but if your faith in the power of God to heal is weak then pills are okay."

The same writer also recognizes medical science as one of God's gifts to suffering humanity. He also sees the medical and nursing professions as fellow workers with God in fighting against evil, and he urges co-operation between doctors and clergy. He recognizes that vaccines and serums have been powerful allies in the fight against disease. However, alongside this positive attitude another question is posed:

> Is it not a strange thing that we should have to fight disease
> by inoculating diseases when the healing Christ is willing to
> cast it out by the power of his love? Which would you rather
> have — the divine life of the Son of God filling spirit, soul
> and body, or goodness knows how many millions bacilli forced
> into your blood? Which think you is God's way? Will the
> Father be offended if you turn from the bacilli to accept the

divine life of his Son? Is healing through Christ less his gift than the drugs?[2]

This type of argument is carried much further by some healing groups who affirm that the healing power of Christ is available by faith alone, and therefore forbid any use of medicinal aids. In this line of thinking, medical science is viewed as a human response to sickness which does not address the real spiritual issues involved, and in no way can medical science substitute for the healing power of Christ. If death comes as a refusal to use medical help then this may be explained as a lack of faith in the promises of God.

These two approaches (co-operation and opposition) illustrate the difference in attitudes to conventional medical means of healing — everything from very close co-operation to lukewarm acceptance to complete opposition.

In Actual Practice

In theory most Christians in the Western world probably support the co-operative approach, but in practice often recognize and use spiritual or religious methods of healing only as an accompaniment or even as a last resort. One writer suggests:

> The vast majority of contemporary Christians respond
> to illness and healing in ways which are probably
> indistinguishable from those of their non-Christian neighbors.
> That is to say that most Christians see illness and healing
> primarily in organic terms and seek cure from medical
> methods. Perhaps they will see a theological significance in
> their disease. Possibly they may give thanks to God for the
> gift of modern medicine. Resorting to sacraments, prayer, or
> any other distinctively religious healing method will however
> usually be very much an accompaniment, a second thought,
> or indeed a last hope. Modern Western Christians, like their
> forebears and non-believing contemporaries, are pragmatic

in their responses to illness and healing. Where there are well-developed and scientifically-based and effective organic healing methods, there is no need to give the supernatural or faith element in healing a prominent place.[3]

So the question remains, "What is the relationship between healing and medical science?" We will pursue the question by examining in more detail the practical issues involved, and then suggest some ways forward in thinking about this issue.

Faith and Medicine in History

Biblical perspectives

No organized medical profession existed in biblical times, but the work of the physician was recognized. Whilst there were some negative attitudes there was general respect given to physicians. The emphasis on the skill of the doctor, the use of medicines, and the need for prayer and repentance are recognized as important in Ecclesiasticus 38:1-14, written toward the end of the Old Testament period. The book of Ecclesiasticus is included in the Apocrypha, and is usually found in Roman Catholic versions of the Bible. Today many Protestant versions also include these books.

Honor the doctor with the honor that is his due in return for his services, for he too has been created by the Lord.

Healing itself comes from the Most High like a gift from a king. The doctor's learning keeps his head high, he is regarded with awe by potentates.

The Lord has brought medicines into existence from the earth, and the sensible man will not despise them.

Did not a piece of wood once sweeten the water, thus giving proof of its virtue.

He has also given men learning so that they may glory in his mighty works.

He uses them (the medicines) to heal and to relieve pain. The chemist makes up a mixture from them.

Thus there is no end to his activities and through him health extends across the world.

My son when you are ill, do not be depressed, but pray to the Lord and he will heal you.

Renounce your faults, keep your hands unsoiled, and cleanse your heart from sin.

Offer incense and a memorial of fine flour, and make as rich an offering as you can afford.

Then let the doctor take over — the Lord created him too — and do not let him leave you for you need him.

Sometimes success is in their hands, since they in turn will beseech the Lord, to grant them the grace to relieve and to heal that life may be saved.
(from *The Jerusalem Bible*)

In contrast to this positive attitude there are references where physicians are seen in a negative light; for example, in 2 Chronicles 16:12, King Asa is condemned for seeking help from the physicians rather than the Lord. However, his sin was not so much in turning to the physicians but in failing to seek God first (2 Chronicles 15 and 16). In the New Testament physicians are unable to help in a particular illness (Mark 5:26). Again, this statement is not so much anti-medical but rather indicates the severity of the illness. In both Old Testament and New Testament there were those who were not healed by either medical or spiritual means, but overall there is no consistent teaching which suggests that medical means should be despised; rather they are to be used as God's good gifts. Jesus himself used the title of *physician* to describe his *own* ministry, thus suggesting his general respect for their work (Luke 4:23; 5:31); whilst also recognizing that he offered a much deeper healing than those who could only work through accepted medical means. One of the leaders of the early church was "Luke the beloved physician," described as "our dear doctor."

There is also an acceptance of natural remedies which are accepted as good gifts of God's creation and used as aids to health and healing. These include food and eating (Psalm 103:2-5), wine and drinking (Psalm 104:15), water and washing (2 Kings 5:10), salt for sterilizing (2 Kings 2:19-22), soap for washing (Jeremiah 2:22), oil for cleansing (Psalm 23:5), balm probably used as a sedative (Jeremiah 8:22,46:11,51:8), figs for poultice (Isaiah 38:21), leaves for healing (Ezekiel 47:12), and bandages (Isaiah 1:6). In the New Testament we note Jesus' use of natural remedies (Luke 10:29-34); Paul also advises Timothy to use a natural remedy for his "Mediterranean belly" (I Timothy 5:23), and the disciples used oil as a medicinal means (Mark 6:13; James 5:13-15).

In Church History

As the church developed in the first four centuries healing was accepted as a normal part of ministry. However, in the Western church a decline in this ministry occurred as the understanding of sickness and suffering changed. This also involved a change in attitude toward medical science.

In the early centuries there was interest and support for medical means of healing; for example, St. Basil AD 330-379, and Gregory of Nazianzus AD 329-389. Basil founded and maintained a large hospital, probably the first public institution devoted to free care of the sick. At the same time, both of these leaders were equally committed to the reality of healing through Christ. Other leaders also supported the use of medicine in the church's care for the sick. The Benedictine Order, established by Benedict (AD 480-550), gave special attention to the sick as did other religious orders, like The Order of St. John of God. The facilities provided by these monastic orders could not be described as hospitals in the modern sense. They were mainly centers of accommodation, usually attached to a cathedral, church or monastery, and they provided refuge in the form of shelter, food and some amenities. However, some did offer medical care and some centers actually had a staff of trained physicians (especially in the sixth and seventh centuries). These centers were originally called "Xenodochia," meaning a building or a house for strangers. This title was gradually replaced by "hospitia" or "hospitalia" (literally a house for strangers, the sick and those hurt in some way).

Up to the 12th century the use of medical means was supported along with specific spiritual healing. However a change began around the 12th century when the church restricted both medical and spiritual healing. Controls were placed on the healing work of monasteries, including the use of medicine. A church Council in AD 1139 condemned monks who made themselves physicians of human bodies on the ground that this was causing neglect of the care of souls. Surgery was also prohibited due to the shedding of blood, and the use of animals in the study of anatomy was forbidden. In AD 1215 it was decreed that the first duty of the physician was to call the priest, because sickness was associated with sin which must be confessed, only then could medicines be applied. If any doctor did not obey this rule, he was cut off from the church. From AD 1566 onward, Roman Catholic doctors were prevented from seeing patients who had not confessed their sins. Commenting on this development Kelsey notes:

> For continuing to care for patients who had not confessed their sins, the 18th century Catholic physician was permanently removed from the practice of medicine, ejected from medical societies, and bore forever the stigma of infirmary.[4]

As a result of these attitudes, medical science began to move away from the church and develop a non-spiritual view of the human condition which was seen as strictly material. This was supported by the new philosophies which saw the human person in mechanistic terms (as a physical machine functioning according to certain scientific laws), and neglected both the psychological and spiritual aspects. Thus a sick person was like a machine which had malfunctioned for some reason, and the task of medicine was to understand the malfunction and then to use the developing skills of diagnosis and treatment to restore proper functioning again. This began a tragic polarization between medicine and the church which has lasted for many centuries and continues in some measure today, although there are many encouraging signs of better understanding and co-operation.

One interesting aspect is that whilst this polarization continued, the church was foremost in establishing healing centers, and medical missions were an accepted part of the church's missionary outreach. This suggests that the church recognized and used both medicinal and spiritual means in healing, and expressed this in its own institutions. Overall, however, the tension between medicine and the church remained, and this limited co-operation and produced ambivalence in the relationship between church and medicine. This ambivalence is evident in contemporary attitudes toward medical science as a means of healing. Whilst there is a grateful acceptance of the tremendous advances in medical science and the benefits that this has brought to people's health, there remains concern about some of the attitudes and practices of medicine.

Critical Response to Modern Medicine[5]

Over-emphasis on Technology & Neglect of the Person

Today there is an enormous range of medical services available, at least to those who live in Western developed countries, and the overwhelming majority of people look to medicine as the way to healing. The doctor, nurse, hospital, and other health agencies are the symbols of healing in the popular mind. Any influence which the church may give through its ministries of prayer and counseling seems rather puny compared to the vast technology of modern medical science. It should be noted that this does not apply in many countries where people are less dependent on Western technology, for in these situations the church's ministry of healing is accepted much more widely than in Western developed countries. It has been suggested that the Western world-view has become so mentally and emotionally dependent on scientific and technological solutions that it is no longer able to seek and use spiritual and communal resources for healing.

Over-dependence on technology can create a danger for the medical profession, hospital administrations, and staff. A tyrannical rather than a humane use of the new technologies can reduce the patient to something like a broken-down car — a malfunctioning machine whose parts only need to be replaced and repaired. One hospital chaplain suggested that many hospitals and medical professionals function on the following unspoken assumptions, which actually determine what happens in the treatment of sick people, especially in a hospital setting.[6]

• The cure of the patient is more important than the care of the patient.

• The staff assume power over the patient.

• Individuals are separate from each other.

• The provision of health is a task for the experts.

• Every problem has a solution.

• Death is the worst thing that can happen to a person.

Where these assumptions exist they may be reinforced by support structures and services within their own hierarchies, internal competition, and systems of communication. The whole medical system often seems the domain of the expert — far removed from the understanding of the average person. The patient becomes the tool of the system rather than the one for whom the system exists.

Dr. Lewis Thomas, Chancellor of the Memorial Sloan Kettering Cancer Center in New York, writes that if he were a medical student today he would be:

> Apprehensive that my real job, caring for sick people, might soon be taken away leaving me with the quite different occupation of looking after machines. This has resulted from the availability of a vast range of technology which can remove the health worker from the patient and make medicine no longer the laying on of hands, but more like the reading of signals from machines?[7]

So, while the great gain from the new technological advances is recognized and supported, the aspect of dehumanization is seen as a real danger.

Over-emphasis on Cure rather than Total Healing

Over-emphasis on cure rather than total healing is seen in several ways, for example, in the disproportionate allocation of resources to spectacular organ transplants rather than basic health care and disease prevention programs; the over-concern with short-term palliatives; the acceptance of a purely secular and materialistic approach to people, and a corresponding neglect of the spiritual dimensions of life. Then there are the unrealistic expectations placed on medical personnel who are given (and sometimes take and enjoy) a God-like status in relation to patients; the lack of effective communication between doctors and patients; and the overwhelming sense of mystery which effectively prevents the lay person from understanding or even attempting to question the apparent omni-competence (all-powerfulness) of the medical world. One doctor comments that many in the medical professions

"Have seen in society a developing secularism with its emphasis on materialism; the pressures of time demanding cures rather than true healing; the trivia of minor complaints; the apparently disproportionate use of resources; and the real danger of a loss of respect for the dignity of human personality in the pursuit of scientific advance.[8]

Another doctor writes:

We are increasingly conscious of growing factual evidence that our patients go away from our consultations feeling dissatisfied with what we offer them, if all we offer them are pills and potions. People have a gut reaction that health is more than a physical problem, and that their reaction to their illness, and their relationship to their other problems, is an important factor in their recovery and adjustment to life.[9]

Whether these criticisms are valid is a matter for discussion, but it is clear that there is a high level of dissatisfaction and disillusionment with current medical systems. Many people who are concerned for a wholistic understanding of healing have heard these criticisms, and look for ways to bring change. They believe that the true malaise of modern medicine is the failure to understand modern medicine's relationship to total healing. This failure to understand the true nature of healing as an experience of the total person, and the general neglect of spiritual realities, has led some Christians involved in the healing ministry to ignore medical means of healing and to put their trust completely in spiritual healing. This has often further broadened the gulf and resulted in deeper suspicion from both sides — from those within the healing ministry, to the medical scene, and vice-versa.

Medical Critique of Healing Ministry

Some expressions of the healing ministry are seen by many within the medical profession as either naive or dangerous to good health. These criticisms arise from a background of intensive and prolonged training in modern medical skills which focus heavily on physical aspects of healing, and are often accompanied by an explicit or implicit prejudice against non-physical methods of healing. When the medical professional does not profess or practice religious faith, there can be misunderstanding of spiritual issues and also feelings of anxiety and inadequacy which lead to rejection as the safest way to respond. This may be expressed by the medical professional in a confrontational stance (either verbal or non-verbal), which communicates the attitude that spiritual issues are irrelevant; or a patronizing attitude which implies that "although prayer won't do any good, it won't do any harm either, so go ahead if you feel it's important." On the other hand, there can be a genuine desire to co-operate, even when insights of faith and religious understanding are not shared. Sometimes the non-Christian medical worker genuinely wants to understand more about spiritual healing but is put off by the approach of Christians who do not offer to explain the purpose of what they are doing, or the implications of their approach.

The following are examples of criticisms healing ministry from medical workers:

• The healing ministry lacks scientific credibility. Medicine is an exact science building up its knowledge by careful methods of observation, testing, and diagnosis, which leads to varied forms of treatment. Where diseases are not conquered, or new diseases are not identified, a determined effort is made to identify and conquer them. The exacting nature of medical research and medical practice gives hope and confidence to those who are sick, and the best available science is constantly being used to promote good health.

In contrast to this, the common idea of spiritual healing is that it often seems to be unreliable, unpredictable and the province of those who have had no medical training, who do not accept the discipline of scientific method, and who often make claims which cannot be verified by independent scientific processes.

- There is skepticism about claims for healing. Medical assessment is based on careful diagnosis and evaluation, whereas many claims to healing appear to lack this rigorous procedure of controlled experimentation.[10]

- There is often a lack of understanding of established medical procedure and systems and a careless attitude about the norms of medical practice. This is an affront to the professional status of the medical worker, and reflects a failure to appreciate the complexities of modern medical practice.

- There is often a very simplistic and dogmatic faith in religious and spiritual power which ignores the fact that God can and does use the insights of modern medicine to achieve His healing purposes. There is no understanding that modern medicine is one of God's good gifts.

- There is sometimes a smug arrogance in the healing ministry, because there is always a fallback explanation if healing does not come; for example, it is due to a lack of faith. The medical worker does not have this cop-out and has to struggle with the problem of non-healing.

- There is sometimes a refusal to accept the realities of the situation, in the case of incurable and terminal disease, for example. And sometimes there is a desire to give only hope to patients and families, even if it is false and unrealistic hope. This escape into fantasy brings turmoil and frustration in patients and their families, and can prevent those involved from accepting the reality of suffering and death.

- There is little understanding of the redemptive value of suffering and sickness as the way through which new insights can be experienced by the sick person. In the same way that some medical workers see death as an indication of failure, so do some in the healing ministry see non-healing as a failure for which a reason must be found.

Whilst some of these criticisms may be seen as caricatures of a true healing ministry, there is sufficient truth in them for taking them very seriously.

Having looked at the negative response to healing ministry from the perspective of medical science, we must quickly add that there is also a very positive response which leads to a positive relationship of mutual respect and cooperation, as discussed below.

Signs of Co-operation and Support

The majority of groups and individuals involved in the healing ministry gratefully accept the insights and contributions of medical science and do not see any opposition between spiritual healing and medicine. The majority of those involved in healing ministry recognize that there are areas of tension which arise from different perspectives on sickness and health, but they urge co-operation, mutual understanding and acceptance of the distinctive contributions from each perspective. To the question, "pills or prayer?" the answer would often be "pills **and** prayer"; that is, a *combined* effort to overcome the problem until such time as a change of approach is needed. Both represent legitimate ways of healing as expressed in the words of a practicing psychiatrist Dr. Ruth Fowke:

> We need to work for a truly functioning partnership of all that modern practice has to offer, utilizing sound psychological principles, and working with the rich, though often neglected, resources of the church. Healing is not the exclusive domain of either medicine or the church; rather it is a joint task in which

both disciplines complement each other.[11]

There are three reasons to support this partnership, one arising from the concept of wholeness, and two others from a Christian understanding of God and creation.

Co-operation is important because true healing is wholeness which gives significance to all aspects of life, not just physical wellness. This has often been expressed by both the medical profession and the church. For example, in 1983 the British Holistic Medical Association was formed to place emphasis on whole-person medicine and to incorporate other insights into their understanding of healing. The following principles form the basis of this approach:

- The human organism is a multi-dimensional being possessing body, mind and spirit; all inextricably connected, each part affecting the whole, and the whole being greater than the sum of the parts. There is an inter-connection between human beings and their environment which includes other human beings, and this inter-connection influences each person.

- Disease or ill health is a result of imbalance, either from within the human being, or because of some external force in the environment, family, work, or community.

- We each possess an innate and powerful capacity for healing ourselves, in our attitudes, responsibilities, and actions.

- One of the primary tasks of the healer, doctor, nurse, or priest is to encourage this self-healing of the individual.

- This primary task can often be achieved through helping each person to understand the meaning of health and sickness, and their own part in this, rather than through exclusive reliance on drugs, surgery, or other procedures.

• Each healer needs to be aware of his or her own life, and be working toward achieving a state of balance and harmony within themselves (compare the biblical idea, "Physician, heal thyself," Luke 4:23).[12]

Along with the re-emergence within science of a more wholistic view of the universe, there has also been a renewal of the idea of wholeness among Christians, and this has encouraged the coming together of medical and spiritual factors in healing. Christians see spiritual therapy as a necessary component in giving a sense of meaning and purpose in relationship with God, the source of all wholeness. This relationship takes bodily form in Jesus Christ, who is the norm for what it means to be whole. So while there may be differences between medical science and spiritual healing as to the meaning of wholeness, there is sufficient common ground to enable recognition and cooperation to become a reality.

The Christian understanding of wholeness and the role of medicine also come from a theological understanding of healing in relation to God and the creation. A basic premise this theological understanding is that God is the healer, and the source of all true healing. The experience of healing of whatever sort is part of His purpose, and He heals through whatever resource is appropriate to a particular illness or disease.

Natural healing. As creator of the universe God formed us with means of healing within our bodies, by making living forms with the capacity to renew damaged tissues and combat invading organisms and toxic substances. The ability to recover from injuries and sickness is part of the in-built healing system. As well as putting healing systems within our bodies, God has placed healing properties within "nature," or creation. The animal, vegetable, and mineral resources of the earth, together with human skill in research, experiment, manufacture, and application, provide the basis for much medical and other natural healing. Human beings are unique in their creation, made in the image of God. Many humans do not recognize God as the source of these resources, knowledge and skills but that does not alter the fact that He is. Perhaps the use of the words *nature* and *natural* has helped to distance these things from God in the thinking of many people. Nature is something general or abstract, and the Christian does not think of nature but rather of "creation" which presupposes a creator responsible for this. The important point is that God is at work in His creation — sustaining, providing, renewing, as part of His continuous ongoing creative activity.

God within the normal or natural. Some Christians tend to locate God and the power of God only in the extraordinary or miraculous, as if He could only operate in a spiritual compartment without reference to the rest of creation. John Richards asks the pertinent question:

> Where do we locate God? In the normal processes of creation or distant from it? When we say that God is involved in healing through normal or natural means, we mean that he is *within* that process. He acts in the normal because He is normally in the normal. He is not to be located only in the abnormal or supernatural from where he has to be summoned to intervene in our normal lives. The message of Christmas and the cross is that God is involved with us in the normal.[13]

Richards suggests that one of the dangers of an over-emphasis on signs and wonders is that we tend mentally to locate God only in the extraordinary, the super-natural, and the abnormal; that is, it is a mental, not a geographical positioning. He warns that:

> When we do this, the ordinary, the natural, and the normal seem to be spiritually desolate, and void of God. This is bad news, not good news. This denies the creation and the incarnation and undermines any conviction that God might use bread, wine, water, oil, touch and word (all normal means) to communicate with us. This is the danger inherent in signs

and wonders and why we are discouraged from seeking them. It is right that signs should follow the leaders, but when the leaders identify God exclusively with them, then it is that the leaders start following the signs.[14]

This does not dismiss signs and wonders as one way in which God works. What they mean is that God has chosen to step into his creation in a particular way, and to work within it, but it does not mean that He only works in this way. Richards also notes how different reactions to healing and non-healing arise from these different perspectives as to where God is *located*. An example is the different reactions which surrounded the death of David Watson, a leader in the healing ministry who died of cancer despite prayers for healing all round the world. Many who tend to locate God only in the *extraordinary* and in *signs and wonders* believe that the absence of any healing miracle in David's life suggested that his death was a tragedy in which God was somehow absent or had been defeated in some way. This then produced various theories as to the reasons for this; disobedience, lack of faith, Satan triumphing, and so on. But for those who did not locate God only in the extraordinary but also in the normal and ordinary, it was also a tragic loss of such a valued leader, but it was a tragedy in which God was trusted to be present and not absent! The pain and paradox of the situation was not contrary to the gospel but close to its very center in the cross.

However, to locate God and see Him working in the ordinary and normal spheres of life does not mean that He is confined only to this sphere and unable to act in supernatural or abnormal ways. God is always able to act in extraordinary or miraculous ways which overflow the normal. He is not bound by what *we* see as normal. So signs and wonders are legitimate and valid, and those who see God at work in the normal also rejoice when they see Him acting in the abnormal, because both of these spheres are reality and belong to Him. The problem comes when God is seen in only *one* of these spheres. If He is only seen in the extraordinary or ab-normal, then this produces distortion and imbalance and a refusal to accept the reality of His work in the ordinary or natural spheres. He is confined to extra-spiritual areas and concerns. On the other hand, if God is only seen in the normal, we are not open to the possibility of His acting in any way beyond this, and this also is a distortion. We limit *His* extraordinary and miraculous acts, *His* signs and wonders, because we cannot cope with this in our limited understanding. In both cases, our conception of God is too small for the reality of who He is and what He can do.

This forms the background for thinking about the role of medical science in healing. If God is only located in the abnormal or extraordinary, then His healing will not be accepted or expected in the ordinary human sphere, so all human skill including medical science will be suspect. It will either be rejected outright as being anti-spiritual or anti-God, or it will be only grudgingly accepted as second best. If however God is seen to be at work, located in the natural and normal, then He will be seen as working through medical science, and it will be affirmed and valued.

Another difficulty for some Christians is how to think about the contribution of those who are not Christian or may even be followers of another faith. Granted that God may use medical science as one way to heal — but is this invalidated if those through whom He works are either non-believers, or antagonistic to Him? In other words, can those who do not recognize Jesus as Savior and Lord in any way be His instruments in healing, and be linked with Christian ministry?

The answer is that the Holy Spirit is not bound by a Christian confession of faith, as if this was the only avenue through which he can work. The scriptures show how God used those who did not know or acknowledge Him; for example, in Isaiah 45 where God chose Cyrus, a pagan king, to carry out the divine purposes "although you do not know me" (v. 5). As the Lord of creation and history, God works out His purposes through those who do not know Him, and this applies to those in the medical and health field.

If a person is motivated by desire to relieve suffering and to bring health, that is good, and God's common grace is present behind all expression of goodness and concern. It may seem that modern health care is completely secular. But the Christian sees God's creative and healing purposes being carried forward both by those who acknowledge him and those who do not. This understanding also gives support and encouragement to Christians who work in the medical and health fields, confirming that they are part of God's continuing healing work. It also helps Christians who receive medical treatment, to see this as one of God's good gifts, and to pray for those who administer the treatment.

John Gunstone has a helpful comment:

> The highly scientific and busy atmosphere of a modern hospital often seems light years away from the Christian community in which faith is nurtured, and Christian doctors and nurses often have a difficult task not to keep their professional work and their personal faith in separate compartments of their lives.

> Yet if the Lord is our healer, he is also in the wards, in the operating theatre, in the laboratories and other departments of a medical center as well as in the chapel. The Christian in such establishments should not need crucifixes and religious pictures about the place to remind him of this (although they can be helpful in hospitals and nursing homes with Christian foundations). The Lord is present in all that is done through a genuine concern to cure disease.[15]

The Christian also understands the role of medical science in the light of the belief that God is revealed as Trinity — Father, Son and Holy Spirit. This Trinitarian foundation helps us to understand the complementary contributions within healing. John Richards suggests a Christian "map of healing" which, while it does not express everything, does point to important realities.[16] Under a general heading of *God's healing works* he suggests that Christians believe in *God the Father* who made the world, *God the Son* who redeemed mankind, *God the Holy Spirit* who sanctifies the people of God (makes holy).

This short creed shows three related, but different activities of God: making and sustaining the world = creation; rescuing and saving mankind = redemption; making Christ's followers Christ-like = sanctification.

The healing ministry of medicine is closely related to the area of creation, while the healing ministry of the church is closely linked to the areas of redemption and sanctification. Medicine is a human discipline based on scientific understanding of God's healing laws in nature — "the laws of nature." It is not necessary, although it may be desirable, for a doctor to acknowledge the divine source of these laws. The primary task is to know the rules so that he is able to apply them to maximum advantage.

Medicine primarily applies to lessons revealed in creation, while the church primarily applies the lessons revealed in redemption and sanctification.

Building on this foundation we can see God's total healing work as related to each aspect. To undervalue any of these aspects is to weaken our understanding of Christian healing. Much of the problem surrounding healing is that God's work is only partially affirmed by different groups. Those who see God's work most clearly in the world, in creation, give insufficient attention to the need for salvation and holiness; whilst those who emphasize salvation and holiness need to affirm God's work in the natural created world, thus affirming medicine as an important contribution to the healing ministry of the kingdom.

The following statement from the British Medical Association sums up this perspective:

As the person is body, mind and spirit, and health depends on the harmonious functioning of the whole person, so the task of medicine and the church are inseparable: co-operation thus comes into line with Christ's charge to his disciples to heal and preach.[17]

Wholeness is seen as "the blossoming of our creation, our redemption and our sanctification and heaven is the goal of all."[18]

A Mid-way Approach

The negative response to the relationship between healing and medical science can be summarized as *either/or* — either medicine or spiritual healing with medicine clearly a second best. The more positive approach can be summarized as *both/and* — a clear acceptance of, and co-operation between, medicine and spiritual healing. A midway approach can be summarized as *both/but* — an acceptance of medical science as one of God's gifts, but a gift which by itself is not able to bring total healing which is only possible through spiritual healing.

Those who emphasize this mid-way approach recognize and accept the role of medical science in helping to provide diagnosis, leading to a possible cure of the problem. However, by itself medical science cannot offer more than a cure. Medical science cannot go beyond providing a cure to the greater gift of healing and wholeness, because this involves spiritual realities in a relationship with God and others, and it is not the task of medical science to provide this. This is not a criticism of medical science, but an acknowledgment that its sphere is limited to the aspect of cure, be it physical or mental. To be whole, the gifts of creation need to be redeemed and brought into a deep relationship with God.

This approach can be summed up in a statement such as, "Doctors treat, but Jesus heals." Diagnosing and removing the cause of the problem — for example, some malfunction, a diseased organ, or an anxiety state — is not the same as healing the whole person which only the power of God can achieve. So true healing equals medicine plus God, or psychotherapy plus God. For example, in healing of the mind and emotions, a psychiatrist may bring a degree of healing by probing into the past and bringing out an understanding of weak and vulnerable places as well as angry and fearful reactions, but only the Holy Spirit can move into these areas, remove the scars, and bring total healing.

This brings us back to the understanding of people and their basic needs. Only a relationship with God can meet this basic need, and therefore the contribution of spiritual healing is essential. This understanding is summed up by one writer:

> In modern medicine it is recognized that man as the object of medical treatment cannot be understood merely from a material or scientific viewpoint. The scientific work of the doctor is limited to a certain sphere. The Christian doctor's ultimate responsibility to God requires that he may and must use all God-given means in accordance with the gifts he has received. Further, we know how dependent man is on his surroundings and on his fellow men. His illness is part of his historic existence, but the final dimension of man's self-understanding lies in his relation to God, in the dimension of faith.

We are concerned here with healing in relation to salvation which embraces this world but extends beyond it. We can be healed in the fullest sense only through Christ. The Christian doctor may point beyond the restricted spheres of science, sociology and psychology to the healing and salvation which encompass this world and the other. The physical being of man is not thus devalued, but placed in the fuller context. Man in his passing bodily existence, with which the medical profession is concerned, is neither devalued nor over-rated, but taken quite seriously and with Christian realism as the object of God's healing. Furthermore the gospel comes as Good News in a very special sense to the person who is faced by crisis or threatened by death.[19]

Conclusions About Healing & Medicine

- God, Father, Son and Holy Spirit is the source of both healing ministry and medical science. God is present and active in all spheres — the natural and the supernatural, the normal and the abnormal, the ordinary and the extraordinary.

- God uses whichever resources are appropriate to each situation. He is the Lord whose purposes are not bounded or controlled by human understanding, and therefore He does not have to agree with what we want or see or demand as His will.

- Both medical and spiritual means are legitimate; pills and prayer, and the appropriate use of each, should be discussed in each situation.

- God is not bound by either the medical or the spiritual system. There is danger in both of these avenues of seeking power and control — in the medical, through misuse of knowledge and status and neglect of the patient; or in the spiritual, through a super-spirituality which indiscriminately promises signs, wonders and miracles as the only valid way of healing.

- Co-operation is needed and is to be encouraged between all involved in the healing process. The hospital chaplain, the pastoral counselor, and the Christian visitor — both clergy and lay — can be bridges in this co-operation.

- Total healing must relate to God and therefore involves questions of spiritual realities relating to salvation. True healing cannot be limited to physical or mental conditions only.

- Whatever the input of both medical science and spiritual therapy, total healing in this present life is not possible. There may be substantial healing but this will ultimately end in death, and this should bring a sense of humility to all involved.

The following could be used in praying for the joint ministry of church and medicine:

Heavenly Father, we know that all healing comes from you, and therefore we ask your blessing on all who are engaged in the ministry of healing. We pray for . . . doctors, surgeons, psychiatrists, health visitors, district nurses, chaplains, intercessors, hospital staff, parish workers . . . for the local parish priest . . . and the local doctor . . . and for those who nurse the sick at home. Give to them, O Lord, all needful wisdom, skill and patience; and may they know that in ministering to the sick they are fellow workers with you and are furthering your purposes of love, through Jesus Christ our Lord. Amen. [20]

Building on the comment by Dr. B. Lambourne that "both medicine and church are being called to leave their ivory towers, and to adapt a more outgoing, missionary, community concept of care." Morris Maddocks offers the following prayer:

Lord, teach us not to cling to our vested interests, hiding behind the curtain of dogma and tradition; rather make us adventurous, willing to leave our tightly held corners. Give us a wholeness and largeness of view as you demonstrated in your ministry, totally outgoing, for it is the world you came to save, and we are now your hands.

Totally missionary, for it is you who sends us about your business, and we are now your feet.

Totally united in community, for both church and medicine are the instruments of your healing.

Teach us to care as you cared, and send us to preach and to heal so that your people may turn to you and know you to be their health and salvation, even Jesus Christ our Lord, Amen. [21]

Sharing and Discussion

1. Through your experience of the work of medical science as it has affected your life, or life within your family, how do you respond to the idea that we should see it as one of the ways in which God brings healing to people today?

2. Read Ecclesiasticus 38:1-14. Do you think this can be applied to doctors and physicians today? Are there any extra comments you would like to add, either positive or negative?

3. Read again the criticisms of the medical services. Are they valid or not? Are there others you would like to add?

4. Note the criticisms of the healing ministry by those in the medical profession. Do you think these are valid? What needs to be done by those in the healing ministry to respond to these criticisms?

5. Where do you mostly locate God? In the ordinary and normal, or in the extraordinary and abnormal? Does it make any real difference to our lives where we locate Him?

6. What do you think of the Trinity "map of healing" — God as Father, Son and Holy Spirit, with medicine and the church each emphasizing different aspects of His work? Is this helpful? Do you see any problems with the map?

7. If possible, talk to a doctor (perhaps your own local doctor) about his or her understanding of healing and the relationship between medicine and the church, and ask for reasons why they think as they do?

8. Discuss ways in which you can assist doctors and others in the health professions in their work — By praying for them? By sharing your concern about healing? By asking them to explain their work and how the church may be able to help? — and so on.

References for Further Reading

A Time to Heal. House of Bishops, Church House Publishing, London, 2000, Chapters 4-6.

Gunstone, J., *The Lord Is Our Healer,* Hodder and Stoughton, London, 1986, Chapter 8.

Health, Faith and Healing, International Review of Mission, WCC Geneva, Vol. 90, Nos. 356-357, Jan-April 2001.

Maddocks, M., *A Healing House of Prayer,* Hodder and Stoughton, London, 1987.

Maddocks, M., *Journey to Wholeness,* SPCK/Triangle, London, 1986.

Maddocks, M., *The Christian Healing Ministry,* SPCK, London, 1990, Chapter 10.

Pattison, S., *Alive and Kicking,* SCM-Canterbury Press, London, 1989, Chapter 3.

Richards, J., *The Question of Healing Services,* Darton, Longman, and Todd, London, 1989, Chapter 5.

Richards, J., "Gospel and Medicine" and "Healing Gifts and Healing," in *Faith and Healing,* Network No. 6, Floreat Flame Books, Mirrabooka, undated.

What Is Wrong With Christian Healing? Churches Council for Health and Healing, London, 1993.

Wright, F., *The Pastoral Nature of Healing,* SCM-Canterbury Press, London, 1985. *Healing and Wholeness,* The Broadway, Crowborough, East Sussex.

10
HEALING AND LIFESTYLE

Phillip describes himself as being on the fringe of the church, but lately he has become more interested, especially since his wife received help through a healing seminar sponsored by the church healing fellowship. He is curious about the healing ministry not only because of the change in his wife's condition, but also because he often feels below par himself. Phillip is aware of your involvement in the church's healing group. He comes to see you to discuss his own situation and condition. During the discussion you discover that he works very hard at his business, and has little or no time for relaxation. His exercise seems to be limited to walking to and from the car each morning and evening. He is too busy for any planned relaxation with friends and family. He enjoys his cigarettes (at least two to three packs per week), and a regular social drink before he comes home from work. He admits the garden is rather like a jungle, but bemoans the fact that he simply hasn't got the time or energy to do anything about it. When you raise some of these issues with him he acknowledges their reality, but says he just cannot get motivated to do anything about it. In fact, he feels quite depressed, because he is not able to measure up to the demands of his family and business, and what he thinks he should be doing in order to be successful.

What are your thoughts as you consider Phillip's need for healing? Can you suggest any aspects which may need attention?

This chapter aims to:

- Discuss the issue of lifestyle in relation to healing, and clarify what it means to be fit and healthy in body, mind and spirit.

- Apply this to our personal lives and to the life of the church and community.

From a Christian perspective healing can be described as wholeness in all dimensions of life. Healing relates to a sense of harmony: of physical, mental, spiritual, emotional, political and social well-being. It is to be in harmony with each other, the natural environment, and with God. In this harmony all aspects of our being are involved. The resulting patterns of relationships, thoughts and actions can be described as our lifestyle — how we function as individual people and in our social relationships with others.

It is important to understand the various aspects which constitute a person. The biblical understanding is that we are created in the image of God (Genesis 1:26-27), and we express this in various ways — through our body, mind, spirit, emotions, and relationships. We can refer to these different aspects of our beings, but we cannot really separate them in actual day to day living because we function as a unity. Although the various descriptions of the person given in scripture are not written in modern psychological terms, they do give a true understanding of what we are. Some references suggest that there are three aspects to our being, spirit, soul and body (I Thessalonians 5:23; Hebrews 4:12). This is called the tripartite or trinity view. Other references suggest that there are two aspects of our being — body and spirit/or soul — the bipartite view (Genesis 2:7; I Corinthians 6:19-20). Jesus called people to love God with all their heart, soul, mind and strength (Mark 12:30; Luke 10:27). Other references refer to such aspects as the conscience, the flesh, the bowels, the inner being. There is little point in arguing over the exact nature of our being because the Bible does not give a detailed scientific view of human nature. What it does, however, is to emphasize that we are wholistic individuals who can be described in a variety of ways. There is an impressive diversity in a unity of the whole person, so no aspect of the person can be emphasized as being independent of other aspects.

In the tripartite model we are *Body,* by which we relate to the natural environment; we are *Soul,* which describes our inner being and includes the emotions, mind, will, conscience, and personality; we are *Spirit,* which can be described as the God-conscious part of our being. Each of these aspects influences the others in a unity/ diversity which makes us one person. Because of the difficulties in defining "Soul" many writers use the word "Mind" to describe this aspect of our being, and thus many of the definitions of the healing ministry operate on the three-fold model of *Body, Mind* and *Spirit.* This three-fold definition will be used in this chapter. The scriptures make it quite clear that each of these aspects of our being has been affected by our disobedience and pride (and all the other aspects of sin), and so we need to be healed in all the dimensions of our lives. To be truly healed suggests wholeness or health or being fit in each of these areas. This is a responsibility which we must accept, so that we have a strong and healthy body; strong and healthy emotions; strong and healthy thinking (reasoning); a strong and healthy imagination; a strong and healthy will; and a strong and healthy spirit. Christians are sometimes tempted to divide a person and to elevate spiritual concerns, but healthy living involves the whole of life.

The Order of St. Luke thus urges all of its members to adopt and work toward a healthy lifestyle in all areas of life. One of the rules of the Order to which members subscribe is, "I will seek such health of mind and body as will make me capable of a maximum vocation." So, if Jesus asked today, "Do you want to be whole, or well, or healthy?" (John 5:6), the OSL answer would be, "Yes, I want to be truly healthy and fit in all aspects of life. I want my healing to be clearly seen in my total lifestyle. This involves being healthy in body, mind and spirit, in our relationships to others, to God, to ourselves, and to the environment in which we live."

Healthy in Body

Christian understanding recognizes and accepts the physical body as one of God's good gifts, one aspect of creation which is very good (Genesis 1:31). The amazing intricacy of the human body is one of the great wonders of life. Psalm 139:13, 14 declares that we are "fearfully and wonderfully made" (KJV). Three other translations of these verses are worth noting:

Knox Bible: Author of my inmost being, didst thou not form me in my mother's womb? I praise thee for my wondrous fashioning, for all the wonders of thy creation.

Jerusalem Bible: It was you who created my inmost self and put me together in my mother's womb. For all these mysteries I thank you. For the wonder of myself, and for the wonder of your works.

Living Bible: You made all the delicate inner parts of my body and knit them together in my mother's womb. Thank you for making me so wonderfully complex. It is amazing to think about. Your workmanship is marvelous, and how well I know it.

This attitude of wonder is reflected by St. Augustine (5th Century AD) in his words "Men go abroad to wonder at the height of mountains, at the huge waves of the sea, at the long courses of the rivers, at the vast compass of the oceans, at the circular motions of the stars, yet they pass by themselves without wondering."[1]

Throughout the scriptures the physical body is respected and accepted as a good gift from God. It is true that it is often used to express disobedience and evil, but in itself it is to be nourished and cared for. The whole human situation including the human body is acceptable to God, as in Jesus Christ God becomes flesh, takes upon Himself human bodily form and dwells among us (John 1:14; Hebrews 2:14-18). Paul reminds the Christians that the body is the temple of the Holy Spirit, to be kept pure and holy and separate from any sexual immorality (I Corinthians 6:19-20). Jesus clearly showed his concern and love for the body when he healed people who were physically distressed and afflicted, and the church has continued this concern through the work of medical, caring and healing ministries.

However, as the church developed over the centuries this positive appreciation of the physical body was often replaced by an attitude of rejection and guilt where the body was seen as the vehicle of sin (especially in sexual relationships), and therefore to be brought under submission and discipline. To do this, many ascetic rituals and actions were developed to overcome the temptations of the flesh. This rigorous anti-body stance has appeared many times in church history. It correctly emphasizes how evil can control and be expressed through the body, but also tends to forget its goodness and wonder, and to suggest that the spiritual aspects of life are therefore more important than the physical in our thinking and living.

In contemporary Western society there has been a renewed emphasis on the goodness of the human body, and this has been strengthened by new discoveries in science and medicine. There has been a reversal of previous negative attitudes, so much so that for many people today physical health has become an idol and there is little or no attention given to mind or spirit. This unbalanced emphasis which almost worships the physical body has become an obsession, with millions of dollars being spent on drugs and preparations to keep the physical body attractive, fit and functioning effectively. The Christian accepts the wonder and value of the body, and therefore supports the need for health and fitness, but refuses to make it an idol which consumes all time, attention and a large amount of money.

Paul suggests that we are not to hate or despise our physical body, but to nourish and cherish it; to feed and care for it (Ephesians 5:29). This can be done as we aim to be healthy in body, and includes the following:

- Good nutrition and a balanced diet where we seek to consume health-giving foods and drinks which encourage rather than detract from good health.

- Sufficient exercise and rest.

- Avoiding harmful substances involved in smoking, drinking and using other drugs.

- Cleanliness and grooming, without spending excessive time and money on beauty aids, and so on.

- Self-discipline in relation to our food intake, our leisure activities, our sexuality, and so forth.

To be truly healthy we are to glorify God in our bodies, and we must accept this as a personal responsibility (I Corinthians 6:20, and 9:27). We listen to the wise words of St. Francis of Assisi. St. Francis once found a young brother monk who had practiced such asceticism that he was literally dying of hunger. Francis called all the monks together and spread before them all the food they possessed, and then he said:

> Dearest, we must look after Brother Body or he will turn melancholy and become a drag on us. After all, if we want him to serve us in work and in prayer, we must give him no reasonable cause to murmur.[2]

Healthy in Mind[3]

The word *mind* can have a variety of meanings, and can be described in many ways. We talk of brilliant, troubled, mature, academic, creative, dirty, aggressive, and many other minds; of programs which are mind-boggling; and of people who are mindless or mindful. But what is the mind? A general definition is that mind refers to the total of all our mental activities including thinking, learning, problem-solving, willing, perceiving, concentrating, remembering, attending, and experiencing emotions. The mind, however, does not exist in any tangible form but it refers to human thinking, knowing and feeling. It is not something we can see with our eyes, few of us understand it, but all of us know about it and use it.[4]

The question of a relationship between the mind and the brain has been debated for centuries and still remains a mystery. Recent research suggests that the mind and brain are intimately related, but are not the same. The mind refers to a unique set of feelings, ideas, plans, beliefs, and thoughts — an accumulation of ideas about ourselves, others, and our experiences through which we develop an awareness of self; that is, who I am. It seems to have a chemical basis in the brain, but also appears to have an independent existence, so for example, it is possible for brain-damaged people who are unable to talk or walk, to be alert, to be aware of others, and to be able to think clearly. At other times such damage also seems to affect these abilities. A tentative conclusion is that the mind is something based in the brain but is able to rise beyond the actual chemical and physiological structure of the nervous system. Some suggest that the mind is to the brain as digestion is to the stomach; the brain (like the stomach) is what exists, and the mind (like digestion) is what the brain does. Others suggest that the brain is like a computer and the mind is like the computer programmer or operator.[5] However we may describe it, the human mind is amazing and plays a vital role in our daily lives. It interprets our experiences of people and the world; it makes decisions in line with these interpretations, and influences and often controls the way we behave. It is an essential factor in health and healing.

The Bible contains many references to the mind or to the activities and attitudes of the mind.[6] Sometimes these are also referred to as heart, or soul, or attitude; for example, determination (Nehemiah 4:6); memory (Isaiah 46:8; 9; Lamentations 3:21-23); emotional stability (Mark 5:15; Luke 8:35); instability (James 1:8); intellectual alertness (Acts 17:11); commitment (Matthew 22:37). There can be a mind which is lowly and humble (Philippians 2:3-5; Colossians 3:12); sound (2 Timothy 1:7); wholesome (2 Peter 3:1); renewed (Romans 12:2). There can also be negative aspects of the mind, where the mind is described as evil (Acts 14:2); blinded (2 Corinthians 3:14); deceived (2 Corinthians 11:3); corrupt (1 Timothy 6:5); of evil intent (Proverbs 21:27); reprobate and depraved (Romans 1:28); and futile (Ephesians 4:17). There are promises of peace when the mind is focused on God (Isaiah 26:3,4); there is a need to be convinced in our minds regarding our belief (Romans 14:5); there is a call to be united in mind (I Corinthians 1:10; Philippians 2:2); and an encouragement that Christians actually share in the mind of Christ (1 Corinthians 2:16). The mind is also able to affect behavior; for instance, we can make up our minds not to worry (Luke 21:14); anxious minds lead to loss of peace (2 Corinthians 2:13); foolish minds say stupid things and lead to evil (Isaiah 32:6); sinful minds are hostile to God (Romans 8:7); and corrupt minds lead to conflict (1 Timothy 6:5).

The Importance of "Strong and Healthy" Thinking

The above passages refer to thinking, attitudes and mental abilities, and underscore the fact that our minds shape our behavior and our personalities. In other words, the way we think influences the way we behave and determines what we are like. This is summed up in Proverbs 23:7, "As a man thinketh in his heart, so is he" (KJV), or "As he thinks within himself, so he is" (NASB). Modern psychology confirms this biblical understanding; namely, that we can change our lives by changing our thinking, and that the quality of our life is closely related to the quality of our thinking. In other words, how we think and operate in our minds does affect our lifestyle.

The positive application of this is seen in such ideas and movements as Positive Thinking (Norman Vincent Peale), and Possibility Thinking (Robert Schuller). It is the foundation for the positive mental approach to success in business, sport, management of stress and anxiety, and is the basis of a counseling method known as Rational Emotive Therapy (RET).

In this therapy, the basic idea is that our behavior is a direct result of how we think; that what goes on in the mind is the cause of what we do and say. We, as it were, talk to ourselves, or play a tape in our minds, and this affects our behavior. This can be both positive and negative; for example, if we keep telling ourselves such things as "I'm no good;" "nobody likes me;" "God doesn't care about me;" "I'm too old and stupid to learn;" "life is meaningless if I'm not married;" or "money is the secret of happy living," then our lifestyle will reflect this. However, if we keep telling ourselves, "I am able to do this;" "I don't have to be married to be fulfilled;" and "God does care about me;" then these positive affirmations are also reflected in our daily life, so that the self-image we develop, that is, our perception of ourselves, is closely related to our thinking.

It is an accepted fact that the mind has a strong influence in relation to our behavior and it is possible to change our thinking thus leading to a change in behavior. In relation to healing and sickness the belief system and attitude of a person becomes a potent factor in healing or non-healing. Norman Cousins, the editor of a leading newspaper, was diagnosed in 1964 as having a terminal disease with little prospect of recovery. Cousins knew that negative emotions and tensions like stress, frustration, and anger, had definite harmful effects on the body. Could this be overcome and the body's chemistry be equally affected by positive thoughts and attitudes of love, hope, confidence, encouragement, laughter, and joy? He began an experiment where he concentrated on positive attitudes, especially laughter, and over a period of time he recovered completely from his sickness. He then began to lecture and write on how attitudes and emotions can both bring on disease, but also improve prospects for recovery. Cousins' conclusions are as follows:

The belief system represents the unique element in human beings that makes it possible for the human mind to affect the workings of the body. How one responds intellectually, emotionally or spiritually to one's problems has a great deal to do with the way the human body functions. One's confidence, or lack of it, in the prospects of recovery from serious illness affects the chemistry of the body. We must learn never to underestimate the capacity of the human mind and body to regenerate, even when the prospects seem most wretched . . . what the patient expects to happen can be as potent in touching off biochemical processes as any medication? 7

Today there is growing support for an approach to sickness which is described as wellness; namely, an inner sense of well-being, confidence, optimism, security, interest in others, and vitality. One physician describes it in these terms:

High-level wellness means taking good care of your physical self, using your mind constructively, expressing your emotions effectively, being creatively involved with those around you, and being concerned about your physical and psychological environment.[8]

This approach works on the assumption that lifestyle is an important factor in sickness and health and that overall health can be improved by positive thinking. In other words, one good way to change your health is to change your thinking.

From a Christian perspective, it is important that those involved in the healing ministry develop healthy ways of thinking which enhance rather than prevent healing. Some biblical emphases provide a set of guidelines by which we can develop and strengthen a healthy mind.

I Peter 1:13 encourages all Christians to develop minds which are prepared for action. This includes being mentally alert and ready for thinking things through clearly; examining issues of faith and life and being able to respond effectively to those who inquire about faith issues. It also suggests being mentally self-controlled and not being swept away by the latest fad about healing or any other issue. It also implies that we be hopeful and base our understanding of the future on the promises of God as given in the scriptures. Such an attitude allows us to live in quiet expectation that God's purposes are being worked out in many varied ways.

Romans 12:2 urges a transformation or a renewing of the mind in relation to how we think about God, others and ourselves. Renewal comes as we allow our thinking to be corrected by God's truth so that His will and purpose become clear to us.

Colossians 3:2 urges Christians to "set your mind on things above, not on earthly things." This does not mean to ignore issues of daily life and thus become irrelevant and super-spiritual, rather it means to think Christianly about the world and to put on or clothe ourselves, with positive attitudes of love and concern, and discard and put away negative attitudes (Colossians 3:3-14).

Philippians 4:8 sums up what is involved in healthy thinking. It is to think on things which are pure, true, noble, right, lovely, admirable, excellent, and praiseworthy.

The Importance of "Strong and Healthy" Emotions

It has already been suggested that a constructive use of the mind is a vital component in the formation of healthy emotions. What we think and how we feel are often closely related. Our perception of people and situations is an important fact in our emotional responses, and this in turn has a powerful effect on our physical condition. It is also true that a physical condition, such as a debilitating or prolonged sickness, can have a powerful effect on how we think and feel.

Emotional health is a significant aspect of true wholeness, so it is important to briefly consider the place of the emotions as one aspect of a healthy "mind."

Emotions refer to the *feeling* aspect of the mind. The word is derived from "emotio" meaning "to stir up," "to be moved," as in the sentence: "I felt deeply moved and all stirred up inside." Although there may be some technical differences, we usually use "emotions" and "feelings" interchangeably.

We are not only rational and thinking beings, but we are also created as emotional beings, and the scriptures offer many examples of strong emotions being expressed. For example:

Jesus freely expressed many emotions as he ministered and related to people. He is moved with compassion (Mark 1:41, 6:34, 8:2). He expresses feelings of anger (Mark 3:5), amazement (Mark 6:6), indignation (Mark 10:14), gentleness (Mark 10:16), love and disappointment (Mark 10:21), passionate zeal for justice (Mark 11:15-17, John 2:14-17), distress and sorrow (Mark 14:32-36), rejection and desolation (Mark 15:33-34). As the Man of Sorrows, he bears and feels our grief and sorrows (d. Isaiah 53:4-6). As the great High Priest, he sympathizes, enters into, feels with, our human weakness, because he himself experienced the emotional pressure of temptation (Hebrews 4:15).

The Psalms are full of strong emotions, ranging from intense sorrow and depression, to almost unspeakable joy and exultation. (Read the Psalms from this perspective and note the many expressions of deeply-felt emotions.)

Many of the great leaders of faith experienced emotional highs and lows, as they worked through particular situations. One example is how often these faithful leaders of God's people were subject to depression and "inward fears."

When *David* is forced to leave Jerusalem after Absalom's treason, he speaks of tears, disquiet, being cast down, overwhelmed, forgotten, in mourning, experiencing inward physical pain and discomfort (Psalm 42).

Elijah, burdened for his nation, courageously opposes the evil policies of King Ahab, and experiences great joy as God's enemies are defeated. But then he succumbs to fear, depression, and suicidal thoughts as Queen Jezebel threatens his life (1 Kings 18-19). James offers a helpful insight when he reminds his readers that Elijah was an ordinary man "just like us", and therefore subject to the same deep emotions as we all are — an encouragement for those who are easily confused, afraid, and depressed at the pressure of circumstances (James 5:17).

Peter expresses both highs and lows. On a spiritual and emotional high, he boasts of his loyalty, and is then utterly broken by his subsequent denial; his tears of bitterness an indication of his emotional turmoil (Mark 14:27-31, 66-72).

Paul, the great apostle, who seemed able to overcome most difficulties, speaks of being burdened beyond measure, despairing of life, troubled on every side, grappling with inner fears, and experiencing both emotional and physical weakness (2 Corinthians 1:8, 7:5, 11:23-29, 12:9-10).

These examples remind us that God has given to each person a wide spectrum of emotions, with the ability to experience and express such feelings as love, wonder, joy, peace, anger, fear, grief, guilt, depression, and many others. The fact that a person may be a Christian in his or her beliefs, and may have experienced the reality of a new relationship with God, does not mean that they thereby cease to experience deep emotional feelings. They are a "natural" and essential part of our being, and need to be recognized and accepted as one of God's gifts.

Every day we experience situations which set off different emotional reactions. Each person is different in the way he or she reacts, and these different responses have been established as we experience life's changing scenes. Reactions to particular situations are effected by such things as:

- Cultural background and environment, including the authority structure of the society and family in which we live.

- Basic belief patterns and attitudes about the world — what is true and false, what is valuable; that is, our particular frame of reference.

- Influences from childhood and family, especially early training in either freely expressing emotions, or denying them.

- Constitutional makeup and personality "type."

- Physical factors such as fatigue, illness, drug-induced states, and so on.

The way emotions are expressed is also important. Often we are not able to control particular events which trigger off certain emotional responses, but it is possible to control HOW we will express these. For example, if something or someone causes me to feel a deep anger and resentment, I can choose to respond with corresponding anger and violence, or I can express my deep feelings in a more constructive way. An important principle relating to emotional expression is that it is not the actual event which causes the particular emotional response — rather it is our *interpretation* of the event, and our *reaction* to it. Our response may be either positive or negative, resulting in either constructive or destructive behavior. A particular event may determine whether we feel pleasant or unpleasant emotions, but we determine whether our feelings (and our subsequent thoughts and actions), will be positive or negative, constructive or destructive. In other words it is not so much what happens to us which is the crucial factor, but rather how we *respond* to what happens to us.

Often we ascribe our feelings to what has happened to us, and we blame the event, and/or those involved in it. But the event itself, whether good or bad, is really only the "trigger" which sets off possible emotional responses. It is our reaction to the event (what some psychologists call our "interpretation") which determines how we feel, how we respond, and whether we retain good or ill effects.

If wholeness includes "strong and healthy emotions," how can we move toward being emotionally healthy?

The following suggestions provide a basis for our understanding and action:

• Recognize that we are "feeling" as well as "thinking" people, and that these feelings can be either positive or negative.

• Accept the reality of our feelings and do not deny them. Because of our sinful condition, our emotional life becomes distorted, but this fact should be recognized and not ignored. We need to "keep in touch" with all aspects of our lives.

• Recognize the reality of damaged emotions resulting from life's experiences, but do not escape into blaming others for our responses.

• Recognize that emotional harmony and balance does not automatically come as a result of an experience of Christian conversion. If we have been emotionally damaged at some stage of our life, we do not necessarily become emotionally mature or healed through our response of faith and repentance. Growth in emotional maturity is part of the process of growth in the Christian life. Spiritual maturity therefore should not be measured in terms of emotional evenness. (If this were so, then David, Elijah, Paul and many others, would be spiritually immature, because of their experience of emotional highs and lows).

What conversion means is that the Christian has the potential for emotional balance, and is able to draw on the resources of the Holy Spirit so that this becomes a reality in life.

- Keep working on the constructive expression of emotions, relating to feelings of anger, grief, fear, depression, and many others. The expression of emotions in constructive rather than destructive ways is a learned process, and should be governed, not only by what makes us feel good, but by what is going to build up loving relationship with others, so that we are reflecting God's love to ourselves and others. Many will need help to develop positive emotional responses, and this is an important part of the healing process.

- Aim for the emotional development as expressed in the "fruit of the Spirit" (Galatians 5:22-23). When these attitudes are becoming a normal part of our daily lives, then we are well on the way to becoming emotionally healthy.[9]

Healthy in Spirit

There are many components in keeping fit spiritually. Five basic aspects are suggested, all of which are areas for in-depth study so no attempt is made to treat them in detail. Each aspect is briefly commented upon and it is up to each reader to make the necessary application to their own lives. Each of these five aspects involves both personal and corporate action. We do all these things personally and individually. We also become involved with others as we share in these gifts of grace. It is through these gifts of grace that we keep spiritually fit.

Through a sustained and disciplined practice of prayer. Prayer is an important measure of our spiritual health because it indicates our relationship with God which affects all other relationships. There are many different ways of praying and hundreds of books have been written on the subject. Various patterns of prayer have become part of the life of the church and different church traditions follow different patterns. Whatever pattern of prayer we may choose to adopt, we need to recognize the wideness of prayer which reaches to everything that concerns our lives — our bodies, minds, and spirits. It includes all our physical needs of food, clothes, business, family — everything that is a part of life. It encompasses the smallest details of life as well as the political and social aspects of life. So we are called to pray for all areas of life, and for the life of God's kingdom to be expressed in our world.

Any prayer for healing, both for ourselves and others, is based on the relationship which we have with God, and the quality of this relationship is strongly influenced by the significance and importance we give to prayer in our daily lives. Whatever the particular pattern of prayer we follow, it is essential that we see this as the development of a relationship with God rather than as a sort of "money in the slot" transaction. Prayer should not be seen as a conversation with God in which we do all the talking, then sit back and wait for God's answer. In this way of thinking, prayer becomes a performance in which we supply the shopping list and God delivers the goods. Rather, prayer should be seen as our response to God's initiative in coming to us and being present in our lives and in the world. It is responding to His word to us in scripture, in the life of the church, and in the needs of others in the world. It is responding to the work of the Holy Spirit moving in our hearts and minds, by which we are able to come to God and know Him as Father (Romans 8: 14-17). So prayer is an open relationship of trust rather than a one-way requesting conversation. It is often also an experience of vulnerability and weakness because we do not know what to say, or how to say it. This experience of weakness is important because it reminds us that the essential aspect of prayer is the work of the Holy Spirit in us, rather than the correct form of words that we may be able to offer (Romans 8:26,27).

Through regular participation in worship both privately and in fellowship with others. Worship is "the missing jewel" for many people because it is often crowded out in a busy lifestyle, or compressed into one hour per week. Worship does include and may be focused in this regular meeting with others, that is, in the church worship service; but it is far more than just this one event. Worship involves the commitment of our lives to the service of God, described by Romans 12:1 as our act of *worship*. In this total commitment every aspect of our life is influenced; our conscience to evaluate right and wrong is altered and quickened by God's holiness, our minds are fed with His truth, our imaginations are purged by His beauty, our hearts are opened to His love, and our wills are challenged in their devotion to His purposes.[10]

Worship is our total response to the overtures of love from the Father, and is kindled within us when the Holy Spirit touches our spirits; so that we are set free to receive his grace and respond accordingly. It is more than singing, praising, praying, and various forms of liturgy — it is our spirit touching and being ignited by the divine fire of the Holy Spirit. This may be expressed in many different ways and forms of liturgy. These forms are not the worship, but they help to lead and guide into the true worship of God in spirit and in truth. Ultimately, our worship must be reflected in our daily lives as we reflect in our lifestyle our commitment to God and others (Romans 12:1-2).

Through regular reading and study of the scriptures. Throughout the centuries Christians have regarded the scriptures as the most important book to read and study in order to grow in grace and in the knowledge of Jesus Christ (2 Peter 3: 18). The Psalmist asks the question, "How can young people keep their way pure?" He answers his own question, "By guarding it according to your

Word," and then also adds, "I have laid up your Word in my heart that I might not sin against you" (Psalm 119:9-11). Psalm 119 continually speaks of the Word as being the means by which our relationship with God is deepened and this same emphasis is found in many other references (Joshua 1:8; Psalm 1:1-3; Matthew 4:4). The "Word" referred to in these references would be the Old Testament scripture. Christians have rightly interpreted this as referring to the total scripture (both Old and New Testaments). Paul writes of the purpose of scripture as being inspired by God and profitable for teaching, reproof, correction, and training in righteousness; so that everyone who belongs to God may be effectively equipped for every good work (2 Timothy 3:16-17). We come to the scriptures not only to gain information about the purposes of God, but to be transformed into the likeness of Jesus Christ.

As with prayer and worship, there are many different ways of studying the scripture. It can be read at various levels of intensity, from in-depth detailed study to a more general and devotional reading. Whatever the method used, the basic purpose of all scripture study is to hear God speaking to our contemporary situation through the medium of the written word. As far as the healing ministry is concerned, the scriptures provide the foundation for our understanding. Knowledge of scripture is essential for effective involvement in healing ministry. There is also need to understand some of the different interpretations of the scriptures because these greatly influence our actual practice. So, effective involvement requires a commitment to the reading and study of scripture, and this is an essential component in being spiritually healthy.

Through the regular participation in the sacrament of holy communion or the eucharist. Bishop Owen Dowling recognizes the relationship between the eucharist, healing, and living in communion, in the following words:[11]

A eucharist means thanksgiving. In the eucharist we give thanks most especially for Jesus' death and rising again. He died that

we might live. He died that we might know forgiveness. He died
that we might all be reconciled to one another.

He rose again and is with us always. We experience by faith
his death and rising again, as together we eat the bread and
share the cup which brings us healing in body, mind and spirit
— healing in the broadest sense of being made whole.

We can see from Paul's first letter to the Corinthians (1 Cor
11:17-34) that the apostle was concerned that the members of
the church were treating the eucharist too lightly. They were
not discerning its true meaning. Their lives and relationships
were contradicting what the eucharist meant. In not discerning
the body and blood of the Lord, as they ate the bread and
drank the cup, they were not accepting the full strength
of what he had done for them, in dying for them. In fact,
they were setting it at naught by allowing serious divisions,
jealousies and attitudes of superiority and inferiority to come
into their fellowship. Not discerning the Lord's body has a
double meaning. We might not recognize the body of the
Lord in the sacrament, and we might also not recognize the
corporate Body of Christ to which we belong. This means
recognizing our need for communion and unity with one
another. If we refuse to do this and yet continue to receive the
sacrament then Paul tells us that we are eating and drinking
damnation to ourselves, and acting out a kind of blasphemy.
He is so bold as to say that if we eat and drink the eucharist
without discerning the Lord's Body, nor doing something
about our relationships within the Body of Christ, then
sickness may result, and even death (1 Corinthians 11:30).

How can this be? Our relationships are part of our health. If
we have severe divisions and hatred between us; if we allow
hurts to fester and jealousies to be magnified, then there can
be an inner sickness of the soul which can also come out in
bodily sickness, for our outward body is a sounding board for

our inner being. We can know the peace of God which passes understanding if we are reconciled to God and to one another. We can be "forgiven, loved and free," as the hymn writer says; or as one of the older hymns says, we can be "ransomed, healed, restored, forgiven." On the other hand, to be in an unreconciled, resentful, and bitterly hateful state is to be sick — sick enough to die and sick enough to cause another to die.

God is therefore saying something to us about being joyful and living in communion. The two go hand in hand. The art of living in health is to be joyful and live in communion with God and with one another. This could be called preventative medicine — why wait to be sick to discover it? To participate in the eucharist wholeheartedly and with preparation, attending to our relationships and our responsibilities to one another, and expressing our deep communion with one another, is undoubtedly a means of healing.

Bishop Dowling concludes with these three points:

- Going to Communion should help us to live in communion.

- The cross has a vertical arm and a horizontal arm, so the eucharist expresses communion with God and with others. One without the other, and there is no cross.

- In ancient times Holy Communion was called the "medicine of immortality."

This is summed up in a verse from a hymn:

> As you have given, so we would give
> Ourselves for others' healing;
> As you have lived, so we would live
> The Father's love revealing.
> — C. E. Pilcher[12]

***Through the outworking of God's grace in our lives into all our
relationships.*** Healthy relationships are an essential component of
spiritual health and are a test by which we may evaluate the genu-
ineness of our relationship with God. There are many references
in scripture which make an essential connection between the vertical relationship to God and the horizontal relationship to others.
It is in the horizontal relationship that the quality and depth of our
obedience is expressed, rather than in our ability to say and teach
the correct words or doctrine (Matthew 7:24-27; John 13:35; Romans 13:8-10; 1 John 3:11-18, 4:7-11).

This relationship of love will be expressed toward others in attitudes of concern, sensitivity, compassion, listening, praying, and
serving through practical care; and toward the society and environment in attitudes of social concern for justice and freedom
from all forms of oppression and exploitation. The implications
for our lifestyle are very extensive, and require a lot of effort and
thought; so that we are actually living the truth as well as speaking it. The emphasis on the healing of society is often neglected in
the healing ministry, which usually focuses on individual needs.
But individual sickness has social implications and the healing of
society is an essential part of total wholeness. The healing works
of Jesus should be read in this light and the social implications
of disease and healing need to be understood and applied more
strongly. For example, note the healing incidents in Mark 5:1-20
and 21-34, John 5:1-16, and Acts 3:1-10, and think of the social
implications which are involved in these healings. This is a fruitful field of study because it emphasizes the fact that a lot of sickness and disease has its source in social attitudes and conditions
and these must be addressed if true healing is to be experienced.
Perhaps the most poignant contemporary example of the social
dimensions of sickness is in the AIDS epidemic. But the same applies to many sicknesses and illnesses which people experience.
(For further discussion on the wider social dimensions of healing,
in Chapter 14.)

Conclusion

A Christian doctor suggests that "healthy living is really good housekeeping; keeping this dwelling place of God clean and welcoming." This is 1 Thessalonians 5:23 in modern terms. A truly healthy lifestyle is summed up by Jesus in the words, "You shall love the Lord your God with all your heart, and soul, and mind and strength, and you shall love your neighbor as yourself." A commitment to live according to this pattern is a solid foundation on which to build any involvement in the healing ministry, and gives guidelines in observing the rule of OSL that "I will seek such health of mind and body as will make me capable of a maximum vocation."

Sharing and Discussion

1. Reflect on the third rule of the Order as it relates to your own lifestyle: "I will seek such health of mind and body as will make me capable of a maximum vocation." Are there areas of your life where changes need to be made for you to be truly healthy, and capable of a maximum vocation?

2. What is your response to the current emphasis in Western society on physical health and fitness? Is it something to be encouraged, or not?

3. What would it mean to practice Jesus' demand to love the Lord with all your heart, mind, soul, and strength, and to love your neighbor as yourself?

• For your local church congregation?

• For your family relationships?

• For your personal growth and development?

4. Discuss together the strengths and weaknesses of the "positive thinking" approach to life and health.

(a) Does this emphasis on the power of the mind neglect other equally important aspects of our personalities, and therefore give an unbalanced understanding?

(b) Can the idea of positive thinking lead into a world of make-believe and unreality, by affirming something which distorts the actual situation? For example, by claiming healing when the person is still very sick?

(c) Many people are encouraged to affirm their faith in the power of God to heal. For example: "I affirm (I believe) in the power of God to heal my (your) sickness, and I put away any doubts from my mind. I am completely convinced that God will heal." Is this just the same as human "positive thinking" except that it is called faith? Is faith really "religious/spiritual positive thinking," or is faith different from "positive thinking"?

5. Discuss with others your understanding of how the mind affects physical and spiritual health. Share your own experience, or others that you know about through reading and observation.

6. Three related issues to be discussed together: Why is emotional health an important aspect of "wholeness"? Should Christians be concerned for *strong and healthy emotions*, or is it more important to be "spiritually healthy"? Does *spiritual* health inevitably produce *emotional* health?

7. One person wrote a book called "Our Unruly Emotions." How can people with negative and "unruly" emotions be helped toward greater wholeness?

8. How effective is the life of your congregation in encouraging spiritual health? What can be done to improve this?

9. Why is worship so important in the practice of the healing ministry?

10. Reflect on Bishop Dowling's words about healing and the eucharist . . . "to participate in the eucharist . . . wholeheartedly . . . is undoubtedly a means of healing." Is this how the eucharist or holy communion is understood and practiced in your church? Can this way of understanding be strengthened?

References for Further Reading

Bennett, D. & K., *Trinity of Man,* Logos International, New Jersey, 1979.

Brand, P. and Yancey E., *Fearfully and Wonderfully Made,* Zondervan, Grand Rapids, 1980.

Brand, P. and Yancey P., *In His Image,* Hodder and Stoughton, London, 1982.

Crabb, L., *Understanding People,* S. J. Bacon, Melbourne, 1987.

Collins, G., *Your Magnificent Mind,* Baker, Grand Rapids, 1988.

Foster, K., *The Celebration of Discipline,* Hodder and Stoughton, London, 1989.

McMillan, S., *None of These Diseases.* Lakeland. London, 1966.

Pearce, A., *For His Love's Sake,* OSL Australia, undated, Chapter 6.

Pearson, M., *Christian Healing.* Chosen Books, Revell, 1990, Chapter 9.

Seamands, D., *Healing for Damaged Emotions,* Victor/Scripture Press, Illinois, 1981

Minirth, F., Meier, P., and Arterburn, S., *The Complete Life Encyclopedia*. Nelson, Nashville, 1995.

Watson, J., *The Prayer Adventure,* Highland Books, Crowborough, East Sussex, 1989.

Wellock, P., *In Search of Wholeness,* OSL, Australia, 2005. Section 1.

11

CHRISTIAN HEALING AND ALTERNATIVE HEALING MOVEMENTS

Sandra and Colin are members of your church who are interested in the healing ministry. They have also become interested in the New Age Movement, although they don't know much about it, except that some of their Christian friends are against it. To understand more about healing Sandra and Colin have been investigating alternative lifestyle, especially the annual Body, Mind, and Spirit Festival. At a recent BMS festival they were confused and attracted by the variety of groups involved. As they walked around the exhibits they saw everything from awareness techniques to zenergetics; the whole A to Z for personal development, spiritual enlightenment, and healthy lifestyles. There was acupuncture, acupressure, autogenetic training, aura photography, ayurvedic medicine, creative dynamics, crystal powers, dianetics information, natural therapies, kinergy, goddess rising, mother earth massage, reiki, tarot, homeopathy, kirlian photography, meditation, polarity therapy, wholistic pulsing, the center of light, metaphysical development programs, past lives therapy . . . and many more. Books and magazines offered everything you need to be tuned in to contemporary spirituality and to participate in the "New Age" of human freedom and consciousness, which is rapidly replacing the traditional dogmas of outworn, irrelevant and authoritarian religions, including Christianity. A look at some of the titles suggested the possibilities awaiting them in this "New Age" journey:

From Sex to Super Consciousness: Transforming Your Sexual Energies
The Seven Centers of Your Health
Inner Peace — The Beautiful Inner Self

Eckankar — The Key to Secret Worlds
Esoteric Astrology
Your Freedom is a Breath Away
Numerology and Spiritual Growth
Meditation — The Key to Self and God Realization
Video Hypnosis and Subliminal Programming
The Occult Bible
Channelling — The Road to Knowledge
Mind Power
Crystals — The Way to Health and Meaning
The Tarot — A Guide to Your Future
Developing Your Christ Consciousness

As Sandra and Colin sampled this smorgasbord of spiritual delicacies, they began to ask where their Christian understanding of healing fitted in. Was it just another way of tapping into the spiritual energies of the universe, through a "Christian technique"? Was Jesus just one of the many masters who knew the secret? Was the church relevant to this sincere search for meaning and reality? Should Christians be participating in such "New Age" festivals and offering a Christian understanding of the world, and especially the role of Christian healing?

Sandra and Colin talked to their Christian friends about their experience. Some believed that everything about the New Age and alternative healing was evil and warned of the danger of being deceived and deluded by Satan, and said there was no place for any Christian input in such Satanic festivals — very black and white! Others really didn't know much about the New Age, or the festivals, but they had heard it was both good and bad — a shade of grey, so best to ignore it, as "just a passing fad"! Others were attracted to the sense of excitement and discovery and were eager to be involved in the search for meaning and reality, because they wanted to experience a deeper spirituality than was being offered to them in the church.

Sandra and Colin come to discuss the issue with you. How should they think about all these alternatives? Were the "blessings of the New Age" to be experienced in these ways rather than through the healing love and forgiveness of Jesus? Should Christians be involved in meeting and helping those searching for meaning in the New Age? Or is it safer to keep well away? Does the church have any programs to help people understand this new type of spirituality? And would you come with them to the next BMS festival, so you could experience the varieties offered and advise them what to do? How would you respond to Sandra and Colin?

This chapter aims to:

• Recognize and understand the exploding /spirituality/wholistic health/alternative healing/New Age Movements.

• Suggest some reasons why this new emphasis has developed.

• Outline the basic ideas in New Age beliefs.

• Evaluate the New Age from a Christian perspective.

• Clarify the meaning of "health" terms used.

• Offer some guidelines for evaluation of alternative health therapies.

• Suggest some responses to New Age/alternative therapies, and note some recent Christian initiatives.

The "New Age" and "New Spirituality"

New movements focusing on spirituality and wholistic health have been developing at a spectacular rate since the 1960's. In the health/healing area, there has been a huge growth in medical knowledge and health care costs; accompanied by a strong emphasis on alternative medicine, where the "orthodox" medical model of health is often questioned and sometimes rejected and replaced by an openness to many alternative treatments. There is also a deep search for a new spirituality which focuses on issues of personal consciousness and freedom, and a new awareness of the spiritual and mystical realities of the planet. Popular magazines and books offer new "spiritual" insights and experiences. For example, the Golden Age, The Planet, The Whole Person, Conscious Living, Living Now, Nova, Spirit Guides, Witchcraft, and so forth are all designed to help people explore personal development and soul growth. Health and human potential seminars are readily available and offer every possible path to fulfillment and enlightenment. Regular "Body, Mind and Spirit" and "Rainbow" festivals offer a smorgasbord of possibilities to encourage people to embark on this journey. Courses on meditation, yoga, Eastern religions, soul awareness, dream travel, metaphysical realities, karma, reincarnation, and many other theories, open the way for new understandings of the individual and the universe.

These various strands are often gathered together under the umbrella term "New Age." This term has been used over the past 30-40 years to describe this spiritual smorgasbord of spirituality/health possibilities. However, many sincere spiritual seekers and devotees no longer use "New Age," because it has become so diverse and diluted, and has lost much of its original meaning referring to the dawning of a new age, of transformed people and a transformed planet. In much popular usage, "New Age" covers almost any idea or theory which offers some spiritual insight which is different from the traditional religions and spiritualities. For many it is associated with pop psychology, esoteric mumbo-jumbo, horoscope charts, fortune telling, charlatanism, and so forth, and any do-it-yourself idea and practice which offers some sort of "real living."

In the last few years, New Age has been replaced by other descriptions for example, new spirituality, self spirituality, DIY spirituality, to express the search for spiritual meaning and purpose, either in conjunction with or separate from specific religious beliefs and practices. "Spirituality" and "religion" are seen as different. Religion describes a more formal structure of beliefs and practices, as seen in church creeds and organizations, whereas spirituality refers to the individual consciousness of spiritual power and vitality which may be expressed in either religious or non religious ways. But it is essentially a personal and individual search which is free to pick and choose from many sources those insights, experiences, therapies, and so forth, which make sense, and give meaning and purpose to the seeker — that is, "they work for me!"

But the term "spirituality" has also become a problem because of the wide divergences of meaning. It has become a veritable grab-bag, describing a multitude of different spiritual activities and expectations. Amid the confusion, one writer offers this broad description to encompass the many diverse elements in this spiritual search:

> Spirituality in its broad contemporary usage expresses the longing of the human spirit for an experience of ultimate reality, through connecting to the spiritual realm, with a view to achieving inner contentment and a discovery of ones place in the wider cosmos.[1]

"New Age" can be seen as one expression of this new spiritual search. Some observers see it as one example of a new religious movement, along with many other such renewal and revival movements around the world, with "New Age" being seen as a (mainly) western expression of such movements. Other observers make a distinction between New Age and such movements, but all agree that however it is defined and classified, "New Age" or "new spirituality" is part of a global movement which is profoundly affecting human life.[2]

Even though many no longer use the term "New Age Movement"

to describe this spiritual search, this chapter continues to use the term, because it is still widely used and is probably the best known description of the alternative spiritual and healing scene, especially in much Christian understanding.

The New Age Movement (NAM) has permeated many western societies, and is now widely accepted as the true spirituality, offering meaning, purpose, and fulfillment in a fragmented world. It influences millions of people through various ways — for example:

Health and lifestyles festivals, which explore and offer many therapies and techniques to promote health and wholeness in body, mind, and spirit.

Media programs on various subjects offer insight into the new therapies and new spiritualities, with advertisements for crystals, magazines, and many other alternative styles.

Business seminars on marketing, management, mind power, human potential, are often undergirded by NAM ideas.

New Age music offers the way to enlightenment, freedom and self-awareness.

Education courses at Universities and Schools offer Meditation, Physics & the New Age, Value clarification, Tarot reading, and many others.

In medicine, wholistic health programs vie with and often replace traditional medical approaches.

Counseling proclaims that the key to solving human problems is to be found in a new consciousness of spiritual realities and a discarding of older traditional understandings.

Global movements advocate various ways to attain universal peace, environmental protection, and human well-being.

Because of its varied nature the NAM is hard to define. Many people have a vague idea what it means, for others it remains one of the latest fads; others are not aware of its existence (at all!) but it touches our lives in a variety of ways. Many Christians dismiss it as "cheap pop psychology/horoscopes" stuff, or as a dangerous form of occult and satanic deception. However it is described, it is one of the great challenges to Christian faith at this particular time, and must be taken seriously and responded to with discernment, clarity and love. This chapter is mainly concerned with the effects of this movement on the healing ministry of the church, but it is important to understand that healing and health is only one aspect of this philosophy and world-view being offered to people today.[2] But why has the NAM developed at this particular time?

Reasons for the growth of NAM

The NAM flows from several strands which have merged together since the 1960's.

- The search for meaning in people's lives.

- The influence of Eastern religions in Western countries.

- The desire for world peace and global harmony.

- Conservation movements to protect the environment and promote traditional earth mysticism.

- The new understanding of the physical universe (the new physics).

- The drug counterculture of the 1960's.

- Growing interest in the paranormal.

- The desire for meaningful community in a fractured world.

- The belief in the dawning of a new age.

- Rejections of old authorities and belief systems including the various religions, especially Judaism and Christianity.

- Dissatisfaction with orthodox medicine and a renewed concern for wholistic healing, and emphasis on alternative and traditional healing therapies.

Basic Ideas Underlying NAM Beliefs

It is difficult to define New Age beliefs, because there is no formal "New Age" creed or confession of faith, nor is there any registered "New Age" headquarters or company structure. It is like trying to define a mist because there **are** bits and pieces from many different sources. NAM has been described as:

- An umbrella which provides shelter for many diverse views.

- An octopus with many arms and legs — tentacles which reach in all directions.

- A vacuum cleaner which sucks up many different ideas.

- A river with many tributaries flowing into it.

- A smorgasbord offering a variety of spiritual/psychic dishes.

Two definitions of the NAM suggest some of the main emphases:

The New Age is a smorgasbord of spiritual substitutes for Christianity, all heralding our unlimited potential to transform ourselves and the planet earth so that a new age of peace, light and love will break forth.[3]

The New Age is an extremely large, loosely structured network of organizations and individuals together by common values, a common vision, and a new age of peace and mass enlightenment — the age of Aquarius.[4]

From these two definitions, NAM can be described as a very diverse movement which aims to transform individuals and society through a process of mystical enlightenment and bring about a utopian era, a new age of harmony and progress.

Although there is no formal "New Age" statement of faith, there are several basic principles which provide the cement which bonds together these various emphases. These can be summarized as:

- All is one. There is only one essence in the universe and everything is part of it. This essence, or "reality," has several names; energy, force, prana, consciousness, ki, god. Everything in the universe shares in this "essence" or energy — people, plants, animals, god, the divine (variously defined as he, she, it) and all flow together into one, like drops of water into the ocean. So everything is one — god, people, creation. This belief is also called monism (oneness).

- All human beings share in this essence, this oneness with the divine, therefore ultimately we are god. There is no distinction between the divine and the human, for we all share the same essence. We are both human and divine.

- Because we share in the very essence of the divine, we have unlimited potential to develop our understanding and consciousness of this essence. We are able to create our own destinies and to achieve whatever we put before ourselves.

- Human problems stem from the fact that we do not realize who we are (part of the "essence" or god) and therefore we do not reach our full potential. The human problem therefore is ignorance of our true being; not sin and wrongdoing (as in Christianity). Our greatest need is to be "enlightened" so that we understand who we really are.

- This change to enlightenment and self-understanding is possible through various techniques; such as meditation, visualization, self-consciousness, which bring us into relationship with the one, the divine, the essence, and so forth.

- This change can be a long process and may not be completed in one brief lifespan, so we may go through a cycle of a number of lives, until we arrive at our final destination, and are absorbed into God, the One. This process cycle is called reincarnation.

- This personal transformation will eventually lead to global transformation and the establishment of the new age of harmony and peace.[5]

But as we journey through life, we find that we are subject to sickness and disease. What is the cause of this? It is because there is an imbalance in the flow of the universal essence or energy, or ki, prana, force, and so forth, into our lives. This imbalance can be caused by our wrong thinking, and by our wrong choices and lifestyles. Wholeness of body, mind and spirit depends on the free flow of this essential energy. Restoring this energy balance is possible through the use of different techniques and therapies (sometimes referred to as "energetic" medicine or healing).

A simple way to clarify New Age beliefs, is to ask five basic questions which affect our lives and reflect our understanding of the world. These questions are: Who are we? Where are we — what is our place in the world and whose world is it? What's gone wrong with the world? What's the answer to the problem? How will it all end?

The answers to these questions reveal the essential difference between New Age and Christian world-views.

	New Age	Christian
Who are we?	Part of the Universal Essence Evolving into God The same as the created order Unlimited potential	Made in the image of God Related to Creation but distinct from it
Where are we?	In the evolving universe of energy Part of the spirit force, developing ourselves and the world to reach oneness	In God's world we serve as stewards of Creation, but not to exploit Creation
What's wrong?	Ignorance of who we are Wrong use of knowledge A slow evolving to perfection	Disobedience to God's purpose Self-centered and twisted toward evil and not functioning as God intended
What's the answer?	To understand fully our potential To be transformed through this knowledge by using various techniques	Reconciliation and forgiveness in Jesus Christ Repentance and faith in the mercy of God
How will it all end?	In the New Age of Aquarius, the Golden Age, which is evolving toward a utopia of harmony	In a new heaven and a new earth through the judgment and power of God

Evaluating the New Age Movement[6]

There are a variety of Christian responses to NAM. (Evaluation of alternative healing therapies will be discussed later in this chapter). At the risk of over-simplification, it is suggested that four main responses are regularly encountered at the "popular" level, that is, from Christian people who may have limited understanding of many of the issues involved, but who are influenced by the New Age in many aspects of their lives, and who are bombarded by New Age propaganda in the media, and in festivals, and so forth. These responses may be expressed differently from the more scholarly responses given in many books:

"Ignore" This response puts the New Age into the "too hard" or "nonsense" or "latest fad" basket. The New Age is seen as far-fetched or not worthy of serious thought. This response is common among many older Christians for whom the developments since the 1960s are often confusing and intimidating. So, best to ignore it — it too will pass, like every other new sensational idea!

"Embrace" Many see the New Age as an exciting way forward, releasing a genuine spirituality from the often oppressive control of old traditions and institutions (including the church), and promoting a new understanding of the universe and the possibilities of personal and cosmic growth and transformation.

"Reject," that is, focus on the negatives, and categorize New Age as a satanic lie, to deceive people and to draw them away from the truth as revealed in the scriptures. This ranges from a careful evaluation of the differences between New Age and Christian perspectives, to a more "alarmist" position, where every aspect of New Age is part of the "occult web of deceit," even though there may appear to be some positive and helpful aspects.

The above responses constitute the majority of Christian responses (at least as experienced in many years involved in ministry to the "New Age" in the Australian scene). Whilst some of the above reactions are based on careful thought and evaluation, often they stem from an uncritical acceptance of particular viewpoints and theological and biblical interpretations, often resulting in "more heat than light."

The minority Christian response can be described as **"Examine-Explore-Dialogue,"** where there is careful evaluation of the foundations and claims of the NAM, in the light of biblical and church teaching. This evaluation is open to the possibilities of dialogue with other Christians with differing interpretations, and also with those involved in the diverse expressions of this spiritual search. Of course, many churches and individuals refuse to be categorized in any particular group, and would claim that any such grouping is too general, and fails to understand the wide and complex variety of the Christian community.

Given the wide variety of response, it is not surprising that there are considerable differences among Christians as to how to respond to the New Age. It can be a very divisive subject (for example, speaking in tongues, and so forth), and for some churches it is best ignored, in order to "keep the peace."

Positives and Negatives in the NAM

People are attracted to the New Age Movement because it encourages them to see themselves as significant, able to manage their lives, to bring about change, to develop their human potential, and to experience deep transformation and soul growth. Whilst there are many significant differences between New Age and Christian perspectives, it is important to note both the positives and negatives offered in the New Age.

Some positive areas of agreement with NAM

The NAM can make a significant contribution to our understanding by focusing on important issues which Christians have sometimes ignored or undervalued, for example:

- Emphasis on harmony and cooperation in the global village.
- Concern for the environment.
- Promoting the cause of peace in the world.
- Emphasis on spiritual values in a secular world.
- Concern for the whole person.
- Encouraging human potential and a positive self-image.
- Recognition and use of natural therapies.
- Challenging the established ideas and structures where these have been used to restrict freedom and creativity.
- Recognition of the role of the individual.

But whilst there are some areas in which Christians and New Age people can agree and perhaps cooperate and work together, *there is also profound disagreement* which goes to the heart of two radically different philosophies and world-views.

Areas of disagreement

Christians believe that the New Age Movement:

- Ignores the biblical revelation of God and builds on human wisdom.
- Reduces God to man and makes man into God.
- Ignores the fundamental problem of human sin and disobedience.
- Replaces sin with ignorance and salvation with enlightenment.
- Makes Jesus one of the master teachers of the divine light, but not the Lord and Savior.
- Places its hope in human achievement and not in the coming of God's kingdom.
- Erodes distinctive Christian teaching about life, death and judgment.

- Replaces the power of the Holy Spirit with the universal force or energy.
- Gives an emphasis to self-realization and awareness, which leads to an intense "me-ism" and preoccupation with self-fulfillment.
- Accepts all practices and beliefs as legitimate, including the occult, and thus opens the way to confusion and possible deception.

Christians also feel deep concern about the pervasive influence of the NAM in important areas of social and community life. This has grown steadily since the 1960s, and today there are few if any areas of society unaffected. In some areas the New Age has become the dominant philosophy, affecting public policy and the daily lives of people. In surveying this influence, writers trace New Age influence in such areas as ecology, environmentalism, business, entertainment, science, art, history, politics and globalism.

In the particular area of health care, the extent of New Age influence has increased dramatically. There are several examples where New Age concepts and practices are now accepted as part pf orthodox medical/nursing training and practice, for example, the use of therapeutic touch, energy fields, and so forth. Other alternative treatments have also become an accepted part of health treatments, and are recognized by governmental and medical bodies, including the health insurance industry. In summing up this influence, one writer describes the "enthusiastic embrace of alternative medicine" both by the ordinary citizen, and more significantly by many governmental, medical, educational and financial institutions. New Age has become one of the great realities of contemporary western society.[7]

New Age and Alternative Therapies

There are three terms which are often used to describe various healing principles and practice. Sometimes they may refer to specific

"New Age" therapies, but they are also used to describe therapies which do not share New Age perspectives.

Complementary medicine/health refers to therapies and practices which are accepted as valid by the "orthodox" or established medical system in any given situation. They are often included in recognized training courses, and are used *alongside* and therefore *complement* accepted medical practice.

Alternative refers to ideas and therapies which are not recognized by the established medical system, usually because they have not been scientifically validated and there is insufficient evidence to show they have positive health results. They are often treated with suspicion by the many within the medical establishment, who warn against their indiscriminate use which may cause more harm than good.[8]

Wholistic health/medicine or "wholism"

These words are used to refer to health practices which aim to treat the whole person, often described as body, mind, and spirit. It is related to "holism"(introduced early 1900s in South Africa by Jan Smuts), which sees people as more than the sum of their various parts, for example, to be isolated and fixed through focus on each separate part. People can only be understood in the context of their total lives which includes the material and the immaterial aspects of life. Today the term refers to the need to describe people in all their relationships, mind, body, spirit — their emotional, social, physical and spiritual relationships.

Wholistic health principles re used in both orthodox and alternative health systems. They may be used to describe therapies under the New Age umbrella; for example, New Age therapists use the term "wholistic health" extensively to broaden the appeal of their product! Others use the terms in a more limited way and would exclude any therapies deemed to be "New Age."

Many engaged in the healing professions, including many Christians, endorse many wholistic health principles, but do not accept the New Age perspectives. So whilst "alternative" and "wholistic health" are related (and often used interchangeably), and may often travel together they are not the same, and should not be confused.

Why have alternative therapies and wholistic health principles become significant in western societies?

As well as the general causes which underlay the growth of the NAM and new spirituality (as already noted), one of the main reasons for the growth of the NAM is a deep dissatisfaction with orthodox established medical systems.[9] Orthodox medicine and the healing it offers has been strongly criticized in recent years because of:

- an over emphasis on technology, machines, statistics, and the subsequent neglect of the person.
- control by the medical authorities, often producing a feeling of helplessness in the patient.
- emphasis on cure rather than healing.
- neglect of the spiritual aspects of health.
- expensive and sometimes unnecessary surgery, and other procedures.
- pills instead of counseling and advice.
- a fear of hospitals because of the system they control and represent. Hospitals have been described as "a building without a soul, a nightmare of concrete, glass, tubes, fluorescent lights, beeping computers, cardiac monitors, white coated professionals...a frightening scenario." Dr. Samuel Pfeifer, consultant, psychiatrist and physician from Switzerland, comments that:

Medicine, in spite of its claim of helping and healing, is increasingly finding itself caught in the crossfire. Moliere, the French comedian, had an observation which seems more and more accurate in many situations: "Most people die from their medicines and not from their diseases." Modern-day medical critic, Dr. R. Mendelsohn, puts this warning on his book *Confessions of a Medical Heretic*, "Caution: medicine as practiced today may be dangerous to your health.[10]

A similar comment is offered by Ivan Illich who warns... "the medical establishment has become a major threat to health."[11]

It is always easy to show the inadequacies of any system without offering any other positive aspects, and there is a tendency to emphasize the negatives in an unbalanced way. But the very fact that such comments are made and often enthusiastically endorsed by many people, both by professionals and patients in the system, is a cause for concern, and points to some significant problems.

Given this type of response to the established systems, the emphasis on wholistic health introduces new approaches to healing by emphasizing such principles as:

- discussing and offering alternative explanations as to the causes of illness, where this may be applicable.
- the use of natural treatments as opposed to "unnatural" medications.
- time and a listening ear.
- touch, compassion, and understanding, rather than a rush to prescribe some medication.
- an acceptance of the realities of the patients symptoms and feelings.
- an interest in spiritual and relationship issues.
- helping people to feel in control of their treatments, that is, to understand and approve the treatment after adequate discussion, especially as to their possible feelings of fear and apprehension.

Many of these wholistic principles are included in New Age health perspectives. But there are also some dimensions, which relate specifically to the New Age world-view. One writer sees the following characteristics as being integral to New Age/alternative healing:

- health is a positive natural state, for the whole being of the person, and not only rectifying a particular isolated symptom.
- the frame of reference is much broader than the purely physical and encompasses the mental and emotional aspects of health, spiritual values, the search for personal meaning, and the interactive nature of religious beliefs.
- the focus is more on prevention than cure.

People are encouraged to take responsibility for their health:

- the emphasis is on positive promotion of health and prevention of disease.
- illness provides an opportunity for personal growth and self discovery.
- respect is given to ancient and traditional systems of health care, especially in non- Western cultures.
- emphasis is on the capacity of the human organism to rectify imbalances and engage in a self-healing process.
- healing should not be intrusive and should not involve potentially toxic drugs or other unnatural agents.[12]

Many of there characteristics of both wholistic and New Age health share in the "wider world-view" and the basic beliefs of the universe and our role within it (as outlined under New Age beliefs). By locating many of the alternative health therapies within this larger framework, helps to understand respond to them.

Evaluating NAM Healing Therapies

As with the NAM in general, there are different Christian responses to and evaluation of alternative healing therapies. There is no *standard* Christian evaluation, but a wide divergence, ranging from a complete dismissal of all such therapies as spiritually and even physically dangerous, to an acceptance and use of some therapies.

The reasons for negative responses include the beliefs system of the practitioner; the pagan and non-Christian origin of many therapies; the use of "invisible energy fields"; the lack of scientific evidence to support claims relating to some therapies; and the "falseness" of the world-view and beliefs when compared with orthodox biblical Christian beliefs, as given in the scriptures, and traditionally interpreted in the church.

Other Christians are much more pragmatic and their first question about any therapy often is "does it work?" that is, is it effective in bringing the desired health result? If it is effective, then surely this is the most important fact, even though we may be unsure of *how* it actually works, and what is the actual origin of the therapy. It should be accepted "as a good gift from above," from God, who is the giver of every good and perfect gift (as in James 1:17), rather than checking out spiritual issues such as world-view and origins, and so forth. This attitude is reinforced if the practitioner shows knowledge of the problem, offers care and a listening ear, is interested in the patient's total welfare, and comes across as really sincere in their desire to help.

Other Christians offer a more positive response on the basis of their biblical and scientific understanding of God and creation: they accept what is seen to be of value in the therapies, but reject some of the negative aspects.

So we are presented with choices — to dismiss the wholistic alternative scene as satanic and dangerous; or willingly (and often uncritically) embrace everything which seems to be giving benefit; or respond cautiously and adopt a middle way which attempts to evaluate each therapy, so that good practices are not needlessly rejected or neglected, and dangerous therapies are accepted without any careful examination.

Some Christians in their counseling/health ministries use certain therapies to promote whole-person healing, for example, meditation, visualization, guided imagery, acupuncture, and so forth. Other Christians regard the use of such therapies with great suspicion, as opening the way for occult and satanic deception and bondage and possible rejection of the Christian faith. They point out that because many therapies have their origin in non-Christian and pagan world-views, that they are spiritually dangerous, because this pagan background continues to permeate and influence their use and the people who become involved, that is, the two aspects cannot be separated.

Those Christians who do use them affirm that it is possible to separate these two aspects, and that you can make use of the natural health-giving potential of certain therapies without accepting the belief systems on which they are, or were, originally, based. They work of the assumption that the health-giving properties of any therapy are part of God's good creation, and can be used to bring healing. The philosophies which may surround these therapies are the human and cultural explanations which have been given. Some of these may be wrong from a Christian biblical perspective and can be discarded, but they do not affect the validity of the therapy itself. The philosophy is like a shell which surrounds the inner nut or kernel. The shell can be discarded, but the kernel or nut remains. The philosophy surrounding many therapies may be impregnated with pagan or occult ideas, but these can be discarded without affecting the quality and value of the method itself.

Acupuncture is a good example. Some Christian practitioners use this to relieve pain and restore health without accepting the basic Taoist philosophy which underlies it. Meditation, visualization, touch, massage, and other therapies are used in the same way.

This basic issue of separation or non-separation of a therapy from its philosophical origins is an important issue in how Christians respond to and evaluate alternative therapies. It has also led to some

Christian ministries being accused of being "New Age." Two examples are Richard Foster for his use of meditation, and David Seamands for his emphasis on visualization and inner healing. Similar differences apply to the use of other therapies, for example, reiki, reflexology, acupressure, aromatherapy, and so forth.[13]

The debate will continue as Christians clarify their use of, or rejection of, many health alternatives and try to evaluate them in the light of their understanding of scripture and their Christian experience.[14]

How should we think of this issue? Is it legitimate or possible to *separate* a particular therapy from its origin, and use the benefits without accepting the cultural/human explanations which are given? Anderson and Jacobson suggest that separation is in fact possible but needs to be safeguarded by a careful scrutiny of all the aspects of any therapy.

> Separation can and does occur. Christians are like western medical practitioners and scientists who are atheists but still study God's creation, thereby discovering general revelation. They can separate a physical treatment in the natural realm, a false pagan interpretation from the treatment, and a practitioners false beliefs from the word of God in order to receive treatments without leaving themselves vulnerable to demonic forces.[15]

But they also warn that any use of such therapies which involves paying homage to their beliefs, or bowing to a divine master, or any procedures that by pass the conscious state of mind, should be avoided.

Another question which needs to be asked is: Is this a matter of fundamental importance and central to the very heart of the Christian faith? Or can it be seen as more of a *disputable* matter, which while important, does not impact on basic issues, such a salvation?

Anderson and Jacobson offer a helpful example:

> Suppose you were a missionary in China and came down
> with symptoms of a cold that you couldn't seem to get over.
> What if you went to a doctor who was highly recommended
> and was an expert in the area of herbs, and he prescribed a
> Chinese herbal concoction known as Ma Huang Tang. When
> you asked him how the remedy works, he explained that you
> had "encountered a wind cold evil" and were displaying a "Tai
> Yang stage pattern." The four substances in the concoction
> were designed to be acrid and warm and promote sweating,
> dispel cold, and "resolve the surface" (that is, bring harmony
> and balance rather than imbalance).

> Obviously as a Westerner, this explanation would not make
> much sense to you. Perhaps you recognize the explanation
> to be rooted in Taoism. As a Christian, you have at last two
> possible responses in this situation: leave the doctor's office
> and determine not to follow his advice, since the philosophy
> behind his practice and advice is obviously contrary to your
> Christian faith. Furthermore, you may feel the need to abstain
> from following his advice because you publicly represent the
> Christian faith, and you are concerned that your participation
> might be perceived as an endorsement of his pagan belief
> system.

> You could choose to believe that the Chinese people may have
> learned good things about herbs over the centuries and decide
> to follow the doctor's advice, but still reject his Taoist views.
> In this case, you accept the fact that God is the one who made
> the herbs for their medicinal value, but you do not accept the
> Taoist explanation as to why they work. With a little research
> you discover that Ma Huang Tang is a natural source for
> ephedra. Assuming that the herb helped your symptoms, you
> might attribute the benefits not to the balancing of yin and
> yang, but to the fact that ephedra stimulates beta receptors in

the smooth muscle of blood vessels, causing them to constrict and, thereby, act as a decongestant.

The authors then suggest that the direction you choose depends on your personal faith, your understanding of science, and the leading of the Holy Spirit, and add, "The issues addressed in (this) scenario are not uncommon, and you don't have to be missionaries in China to encounter them. They are happening with increasing frequency in the western hemisphere."

They suggest that these issues are "disputable matters" among Christians, similar to the issues of eating meat offered to idols, and whether Christians should continue the kosher traditions of the Jewish community, and conclude, "disputable matters are not fundamental to the Christian faith and are usually matters in which individual Christians may differ in opinion without impacting their salvation. Most, if not all, health care issues are disputable matters. They are matters of preference, and should never be allowed to divide our fellowship with other believers." Rather, they should be openly discussed in light of the principles given by Paul on such disputable matters, in Romans 14-15 and 1 Cor 8:1-13.[16]

Establishing guidelines for evaluation

Two valuable studies are provided by Anderson-Jacobson and Omathuna-Larimore:

Anderson and Jacobson suggest that what is needed in addressing these medical/health issues is a "reliable and enduring biblical model" that will stand the test of time. They offer a five-fold grid.[17]

- *the grid of history* — that is, what are the historical roots of any therapy — who invented it or discovered it? How was it developed?

- *the grid of faith* — how do the spiritual concepts underlying the founder and the medical system in question line up? Are they consistent with biblical teaching and the historical Christian faith?

- *the wholistic grid* — does the therapy address the whole person, or just one dimension, and disregards other important components of our humanity?

- *the scientific grid* — how does this approach relate to the scientific principles which are used to evaluate medical and health practices and philosophies? Does the method violate any proven scientific results derived from careful research?

- *the grid of spiritual discernment* — does the method and practice open the way for possible deception and control by spiritual powers opposed to God's purposes of health and wholeness, as in 1 John 4:1 and 1 Tim 4:1?

On this basis they offer valuable comments on some of the main medical systems and alternative therapies (in Chapters 9-20).

D. *Omathuna and W. Larimore* propose six areas for evaluation:[18]

- what spiritual beliefs underlie the therapy or are held by the practitioner?

- what financial and other resources are required to obtain and use the therapy?

- does the therapy have proven medical and health benefits, according to scientific evidence and research, or does it rely on anecdotal evidence only (for example, "it worked for me — so it must be O.K.")?

- does the therapy or the practitioner encourage reliance on your "inner guiding voice" or "spirit," or your "intuitive sense" rather than reason, scientific evidence and biblical principles?

• is there any evidence of medical fraud, where treatments are used and recommended (and charged for!) despite the lack of any proven benefit, and where desperate people are open to exploitation because of their desperate search for healing?

• will your involvement in the use of particular therapies have a negative impact on other Christians and possibly bring them into bondage to evil because of your example (as in 1 Cor 8:12)?

Omathuna and Larimore then examine six categories of therapies — conventional, complementary, scientifically unproven, scientifically questionable, energy medicine, quackery and fraud — and offer their conclusions as to the values, benefits, and possible dangers of many therapies, herbal remedies, vitamins, and dietary supplements (chapters 12, 13).

These modes are valuable in providing a framework or "evidential" foundation for a Christian understanding and response. It is important that Christians understand both the Christian and the New Age perspectives. The "thinking," or "intellectual" or "cognitive" aspects are essential — not just for "experts" or "professionals" in ministry, but for everyone involved in the healing ministry.

However, this understanding must also relate to the context in which people live their lives, and where they actually use or are attracted to particular therapies. It is like experts catching an endangered fish or animal, in order to check its health, mark or tag it in some way, in order to ensure its survival. But then it must be returned to its particular context, that is, the water, or the wilds, and so forth. Analyzing New Age and alternative health therapies from Christian perspectives is valuable and essential, but such evaluations must enable Christians to actually relate to those searching for health and meaning in the alternative scene. Having a sound evaluation framework is important — however, it should also facilitate dialogue and personal involvement with practitioners and seekers. Involvement in many New Age and alternative health festivals over the past decade has shown that one of the most important factors in relating to this scene is the starting point and attitudes which are adopted. Often Christians have excellent guidelines for evaluation which do not seem to get to first base because the impression is given that their main or only purpose is to show the weaknesses and flaws in a particular therapy or idea, and they don't really care about or want to understand how the practitioner understands it. Compare that with "People will not care about how much we know, until they know how much we care!" Many excellent Christian arguments, and valuable guidelines, often seem to be ineffective in promoting dialogue, because they are essentially argument-centered, not person-centered.

A common request for help is, "I work in an office where everyone is into some alternative therapy. When they ask me for my opinion as a Christian, I go through some of the guidelines and explain the Christian position. But what then? That is usually the end of the conversation, because I often seem to come across as "very dogmatic" and not ready to hear their perspective. I give my witness to the Christian understanding and also share my own testimony about the healing power of Jesus, but it doesn't seem to get very far. How can I relate to people so I can get past just "presenting the facts", which often seems to confirm their thinking that Christians really don't want to understand?

One of the essentials in any dialogue is a readiness and commitment to listen and learn in order to understand what the other is saying (not just the words but also the feelings involved), that is, to be as open and responsive as possible, accepting the fact that the other may not want to be involved at this level at all! This does not mean agreeing with their perspective — it simply means taking the risk and being ready to *start where they are* before instructing them as to the problems in their understanding and practice; for example, understanding why they have become involved in promoting this therapy, what they see as the benefits, and how the therapy impacts on their lives. If these issues are discussed before any examination of the therapy, then often the foundation is laid for mutual dialogue, because it shows that Christians are prepared to listen and learn before offering evaluations and critiques. This also allows Christians to share their understanding and questions about any therapy, and also their own experiences of healing, and to begin to work through some of the guidelines suggested.

Five issues have been useful in providing a framework for evaluation. These are similar to many points in the models presented, but they may be expressed differently. A series of questions are suggested which relate to the practitioner (as the starting point), origins, biblical teaching, scientific assessment, and personal involvement.

The Practitioner or Therapist

There are several questions which can be asked. For example, How did you become involved in the alternative scene? How do you understand the therapy works? Does the therapy help you? As a practitioner have you received any training and accreditation — courses, assessments, and so forth. What was the content of the courses? Were the courses helpful in gaining an understanding of the whole person? Would you share your spiritual journey and beliefs? How do these beliefs impact on the care you offer? Do you offer a particular world-view as an essential part of a particular treatment? — for example, when you teach yoga do you offer only skills of breathing, exercise and relaxation as aids to healing, or are these mixed with and dependent on the acceptance of Hindu philosophy and rituals ?

Origins

Ask: where the therapy come from? Who discovered or invented it? What is the underlying belief system on which it is based? If it comes from a non-Christian pagan background, and uses the language of universal energy — ki, prana, and so forth — ask whether this is essential to the effectiveness of the therapy, or can it be explained in other ways. For example, explain how the benefits of acupuncture and some other therapies have been reinterpreted in more orthodox medical terms. (This is the issue of separation/non-separation).

Acknowledge that various cultures have discovered the healing benefits of certain therapies, plants, herbs etc, which God has created for our well-being, and other non pagan explanations may be possible. If the therapy does offer health benefits, show that what you are questioning is not the benefits, but the way in which these have been described. However, be realistic! There ARE therapies where this separation and re-interpretation is not possible, and they should be rejected. Also, many therapists will reject this possibility and maintain the essential connection between the therapy and the belief system surrounding it.

Biblical teaching

Does the therapy recommend or include practices which contradict clear biblical teaching, for example, astrology, forms of divination, use of spirit mediums, and so forth? Is there encouragement to engage in practices which cause people to break a clear command from God, with the possibility of bringing them into bondage to evil? (see Deut 18:9-12; Isaiah 47:12-15).

Does the therapy *downgrade* Jesus — for example, as one of the ascended masters; as an example of Christ consciousness, who has mastered the "secrets" of the universe; as one conveyor of spiritual power, rather than the healing Lord, the promised Messiah, who was born among us, who died and rose again, and is worshipped as the ascended Lord of all. (See 1 John 4:1 and following.)

Does the therapy give an exalted place to spiritual beings (for example, angels) as agents of healing, rather than the healing power of Jesus Christ and the Holy Spirit?

Scientific assessment

Has the therapy been subjected to any reliable scientific and medical evaluation, or is it being recommended on the strength of personal reports as to its effectiveness? Do the claims made fit the facts? Ask for evidence of any assessments. If this request is ridiculed or rejected, politely suggest that this could be seen as a form of professional dishonesty, or even fraud (the discussion is likely to end at that point!)

Care must be taken not to completely reject a therapy because of the lack of substantial scientific or research evidence. This often happens slowly, and may only reflect the viewpoint and interpretations of a small part of the professional health establishment. Such evidence is not always foolproof. Compare that with medical treatments which work but cannot be explained through the available scientific data. Also note that some research conclusions have been shown to be inaccurate. However properly conducted research should not be discarded, but seen as a valuable component of any evaluation.

Personal questions are also important when you are evaluating or considering using any therapy.

Is the therapy worth the financial costs incurred, or am I (or others) throwing good money away on a doubtful benefit?

Will my use of such therapies cause problems for other Christians; for example, concern for the "weaker brother" (as in 1 Cor 8:1-13)? Am I prepared to discuss this with those who may be affected by my decision? If I feel that I should proceed with the therapy, can I stand firm against those who will criticize my decision?

Do I feel at ease in my mind, and at peace with the Lord, in tune with the Spirit in relation to this treatment? A good conclusion is: If in doubt, leave it out!

Am I prepared to discuss these issues of dispute and uncertainty with those I trust and respect, and, listen to their advice and comments?

There may be more questions which will come to mind. Such evaluation will take time and energy and careful thought, and is meant to be used in a flexible way. The purpose is to give a broad basis for consideration, and to equip the mind with information and ideas which will help to decide regarding the use of any therapy, and help create mutual relationships of respect and honesty.

Similarities and Differences

One problem in relation to the New Age and to some alternative therapies is the use of words and actions which are very similar to those commonly used by Christians, for example, words like love, spirit, God, Christ, and so forth, but which have particular alternative or New Age meanings. Also, certain actions or methods, for example, touch, breathing, meditation, visualizing, which are used by both alternative and Christian practitioners, may appear to be similar, but have very different meanings. It is therefore important to understand what words and methods (actions) mean for the practitioner and the particular therapy.

Two examples where there often appears to be similarities are therapeutic touch (similar to laying on of hands), and meditation, a common therapy or technique in both Christian and New Age practice. Further study of these practices reveal several important differences. This can be shown by thinking of <u>a picture</u> and <u>the frame</u> which surrounds, deepens and highlights the features of the picture. The picture represents the words, actions, symbols used, and the frame represents the larger world-view which surrounds and highlights the meaning of the picture.

Therapeutic touch and laying on of hands

Therapeutic touch (TT) is a very popular therapy, widely used in alternative healing, and the professional health service. It is based on the manipulation of non human energy forces, for example, prana, ki, and so forth which are regarded as the key to correcting any healing imbalances in the patient. The practitioner uses a form of meditation called "centering" to attune themselves to the patient, including mental peace, and "the intention to heal." Then hands are placed on or close to the patient, to sense the non-physical energies and assess the patient's energy field for imbalances and disturbances which are the indicators of illness. Any imbalance is corrected by "unruffling" where the hands are passed over the body to soothe out and stabilize the energy fields, or by directing energy to specific points in the body, all the time visualizing the healing effects of this balanced energy. The patient's energy field is then assessed.

Different explanations are given about the role of the practitioner. Many claim they are "enablers" only, in adjusting the energy flow. For others, the healer serves as a medium or conduit on behalf of the patient, that is, a channel through which spiritual energy and power (often described as "from the universe") is conveyed to the patient.

The laying on of hands may have similar actions and methods, like "centering" prayer, and varying methods of touch. Touch is an important aspect of all human relationships, including use by Christians. Following the example of Jesus, we lay hands on children and bless them and pray for them; we lay hands on people (or close to people) and pray for their healing and relaxation, blessing, freedom from stress, and so forth. We hold hands and extend our hands toward others when we pray, believing God's presence with us and among us. But what is the purpose of such actions (that is, the picture) and what is the frame surrounding these actions? It is not projecting or releasing any impersonal energy of the universe, but rather believing in God's presence with us and in us, and extending our hearts in **identification** with each other. There is an energy or power present, but it is the power of the Holy Spirit, who binds us together and responds to our healing needs. The other important aspect is that our actions and words affirm God's presence and action on our behalf, as God imparts his healing power to people lives. But the power is not ours — we cannot heal people. God is the source of healing — we affirm this in our actions and words. Any power present is from God, not from human origin (see 2 Cor 4:7). So laying on of hands involves both our **identification**, and God's **impartation**, but these are interpreted by the Christian "framework" or world-view (see Chapter 6).

Meditation is another popular therapy where there seems to be many similarities. It is practiced in most religions and has an important place in both New Age and Christian movements. It may involve a whole range of practices from relaxation exercises to a deep involvement in a particular religious philosophy. Does a common name and similar actions mean that the meaning and practice is the same? We will examine this using the picture-frame model.[19]

Similarities: The "Picture" = Outward Actions/Symbols

Name	Meditation is from a Greek word meaning "to measure out" and involves such ideas as "ponder," "reflect," "think on," "consider," "focus," "concentrate," "contemplate"
Posture	May involve kneeling, standing, lying prostrate
Means	Breathing exercises, use of prayer sentences, repetition of particular words, such as a "mantra," or the name of a "power" or "God" (in Christian spirituality, the use of the name Jesus)
Writings	As the basis, Christian scriptures or Hindu scriptures
Objects	As helps in reflection; a cross, crystals, a tree
Silence	In groups, or as individuals, and other similar "structures" to facilitate contact with the power or God

Differences: The "Frame" = World-view undergirding the Actions

	New Age	Christian
Purpose	To merge with God, to become one with universal energy	To worship God as revealed in Jesus Christ
Means	(a) Human intuition through an inward journey—to find the center of one's being (b) Various words and mantras (c) Often beyond use of reason	(a) By a divine revelation given in the Scriptures and a journey away from ourselves to God (b) Prayer in the Name of Jesus (c) Reason an essential aspect
Object	The ultimate reality— ourselves—as part of the universal energy, God, creation	God is the objective reality beyond ourselves
Experience	Subjective as we merge with the reality	Objective—based on the grace of God in Christ Jesus
Revelation, Insight, Illumination	When the inmost ultimate self is reached by journey into the soul	When God is encountered in revelation to which Scripture witnesses
Basis	The belief of Monism: everything is a manifestation of the same one consciousness, energy, power, immanence within	The belief in God the Creator, related to men & women, living among us but also beyond (immanent & transcendent)

Dr. C. J. Jung, the famous psychologist clarifies the basic difference between Christian and other forms of meditation in his book, *Psychology and Religion, East and West.*

> Between the Christian and Buddhist (method of meditation) there is a subtle but enormous difference. The Christian during contemplation would never say "I am Christ" but will confess with Paul: "Not I, but Christ liveth in me" (Gal. 2:20). The Buddhist form however says, "Thou wilt know that thou art the Buddha" . . . (whereas) . . . the Christian attains his end in Christ.[20]

The principles used in evaluating therapeutic touch and meditation can be adapted in considering other practices and words which appear to be similar in New Age and Christian usage, for example, love, spirit, Christ, transformation, and so forth.

The Future of NAM/Alternative Healing

Differences of evaluation and response will continue as Christians relate to these expressions of the new spirituality, from their particular biblical, theological, scientific, medical and pastoral perspectives. Where there are differences in understanding and approach, there needs to be dialogue and discussion, firstly with other Christians, to understand the various Christian attitudes; but there also needs to be a stronger effort among Christians to adopt a more open response to those involved in the New Age and alternative scenes.

Many Christians are satisfied to focus on the biblical and theological errors of the New Age, and the links between many alternative therapies and non-Christian world-views, that is, they use a "doctrinal/theological/origins" approach to invalidate the New Age world-view, and assume that this automatically invalidates any therapy which may be linked to that world-view. However, if this approach is used without any qualification, then we should not make use of any insights or therapies or discoveries which may arise from a pagan background. But our daily lives are permeated with many practices and ideas which were originally pagan in origin, but have been reinterpreted in more Christian terms, such as the "Christian" calendar and many aspects of the legal system, which are based on Roman, that is, pagan ideas, names and mythology. So, what about traditional healing treatments and insights which may have come from cultures which were (and some still are) pagan in origin, for example, Pacific island, Native American Indian, aboriginal, Maori, and are now used in western society, because of their proven healing benefits?

The doctrinal/theological approach has value in clarifying the significant weaknesses in the New Age world-view, and offers Christians a warning of possible danger areas, but it needs to be complemented by other evaluations as suggested.

Also, the way in which some Christian responses are given do not encourage any dialogue with those involved in the alternative scene. It is not difficult to show the differences between Christian and New Age and label the New Age as heretical, but it is much more challenging and risky for personal and respectful interaction with both alternative practitioners and seekers.

There is a growing desire among Christians to adopt a response with due regard to both positive and negative aspects, where dialogue and discussion are needed in examining the foundational ideas in the New Age, the medical and cultural backgrounds of many therapies, and the use or non-use of such therapies in both orthodox medicine and the Christian healing ministry.

Some issues which are receiving continuing study are:

The study of energy healing and its evaluation from biblical, theological, medical, and pastoral perspectives.

Continuing evaluation of particular therapies, for example, aromatherapy, reiki, reflexology, homeopathy, and so forth.

A more intentional "incarnational presence," that is, being there with practitioners and seekers at festivals, markets, celebrations, and so forth, that is, working on their turf rather than speaking at or to them from a "church" distance.

Development of creative ministries which try and bridge the gap between many involved in the New Age and the church.[21]

Conclusion

Wisdom is needed to avoid the extremes of being either completely positive and therefore taking on board some sub-Christian or non-Christian ideas and practices; or being completely negative and throwing out valuable insights which are not a threat to Christian understanding of God and the world. Any response needs to:

- realize the popularity and extent and use of such therapies

- recognize and respect the genuine desire of the majority of those offering these therapies — to help people experience healing (whilst also acknowledging that there will always be a minority who seek to exploit the vulnerable and gullible with extravagant claims)

- have courage to ask questions about each therapy — to non-Christian promoters, to Christians involved in the complementary scene, and to medical and health professionals who may have conflicting ideas in this whole area.

- encourage a desire to understand and help those involved in the alternative scene, rather than being satisfied just to condemn and often "demonize" it.

- see New Age and the alternative scene as a way to clarify and deepen our understanding of and involvement in a Christian healing ministry (that is, wrong ideas and practices can be used to " see the truth" more clearly, in the same way as heresies in the church have helped to clarify and affirm "sound doctrine").

Kevin Logan, Anglican minister and author/journalist, offers some practical advice.[22]

- **Do** be wary of "energy experts" who promise to manipulate invisible, unknown, unidentified, and unexplained fields or streams of power in the body.

- **Do** be wary of the god called One; the idea that God or the universal force or the cosmic energy is coursing through everything . . . All is not one. God, the ultimate in power and energy is within, but also remains apart and totally separate from His creation.

- **Do** avoid the psychic souls who delve into the depths of the occult and dredge up dubious spiritual solutions to cure your problems.

- **Do** ask questions and insist on comprehensive answers. Beware of the peddlers of gobbledygook.

- **Do** ignore testimonies of alleged success because people's feelings of wellness can be very fickle.

- **Do** consider the origins of the treatment being offered. If it comes from an occultic, spiritist, or Eastern mystical background, make further enquiries before accepting it as right.

- **Do** consider the roles of the world, the flesh, and the devil in your illness, whether physical, psychological, emotional or spiritual. The stress and pressure of the world, the demand and urges of the flesh, and the deception and deceit of the devil, may need more than a quivering acupuncture needle.

- *Do* examine your conscience when illness comes. Have you allowed yourself to be controlled by resentment and unforgiveness, and other attitudes which may be causing physical problems?

- *Do* remember that Christians have alternatives to the alternatives. We have a God who can repair life when it goes wrong. Often we don't give God a chance to bring his healing into our lives.

- *Do* beware of those who believe that there is no alternative but alternative medicine. Despite its many faults, orthodox medicine remains one of God's great gifts and should not be lightly discarded for what may be the latest fad which promises real life.

Sharing and Discussion

1. One writer describes the New Age as the "old lie"; man/woman putting themselves in God's place and wanting to be like God, as in Genesis 3:4-5. Do *you* think this is a good description of the New Age Movement?

2. How strong are New Age ideas and practices in people's lives from *your* point of view? Can *you* give some examples? (Check the magazines, tapes, and books in your local newsagent, bookstore, supermarket, library, and so forth — how many have a New Age flavor?)

3. Would *you* attend a Body, Mind, Spirit festival? If *yes,* what would *you* look for and hope to gain from it? If *you* feel *you* could not attend, why not?

4. Reflect on the four common responses to the NAM, that is, ignore, embrace, reject, examine. Do these describe the responses in your church or Christian group? If not, how would you describe the present responses?

5. Can we separate a particular method; acupuncture, meditation, and so on, from the philosophy or ideas on which it was originally, or may be presently built, which may be non-Christian and occultic?

6. Ask a Christian doctor to explain his or her attitude to alternative therapies, and then ask an alternative therapist for his or her views. Try and clarify the differences in their attitudes.

7. Does it really matter what therapy is used as long as the person receiving the treatment is restored to health? Is the end result of healing more important than the means by which it was experienced?

8. What has been your experience of the wholistic health movement, and your experience of the more traditional medical response to sickness? Are you satisfied with the help you have received from a particular source?

9. Should Christians concerned about healing regard the New Age Movement as an *enemy* to be exposed and opposed, or as an *unlikely source* which may be able to be used along with specifically Christian understandings of healing?

10. Choose one particular "alternative" therapy, for example, reiki, aromatherapy, crystal healing, channeling, and so forth and evaluate it some of the guidelines suggested in this chapter.

References for Further Reading

There is a very large range of books available on New Age and alternative healing. The following is a selection which address many issues relating to health and healing:

Ankerberg, J. and Weldon, J., *The Facts in the New Age Movement*, Harvest House, Oregon, 1988.

Ankerberg, J. and Weldon, J., *The Facts on Wholistic Health and the New Medicine,* Harvest House, Oregon, 1992.

Ankerberg, J. and Weldon, J., *Can You Trust Your Doctor?* Wolgemuth and Hyett, Tennessee, 1991.

Anderson, N., and Jacobson, M., *The Biblical Guide To Alternative Medicine.* Regal, CA, 2003.

Clifford, R. and Johnson, P., *Jesus and the Gods of the New Age,* Lion, Oxford, 2001.

Cole, M., (ed.), *What is the New Age?,* Hodder and Stoughton, London, 1990.

Coker, R., *Alternative Medicine, Helpful or Harmful,* Monarch, Crowborough, 1995.

Epperley, B., *Crystal and cross,* Twenty Third Publications, Mystic, CT, 1996.

Groothuis, D., *Confronting the New Age,* IVP, Illinois, 1988.

Huggett J., *Breath of Life,* Sovereign World, Tonbridge, England, 2004.

Lochhass, P., *How to Respond to the New Age Movement,* Concordia, St. Louis, 1988.

Logan, K., *Close Encounters with the New Age,* Kingsway, Eastbourne, 1991.

Miller, E., *A Crash Course on the New Age Movement,* Baker, Grand Rapids, 1989.

Millikan, D. and Drury, N., *Worlds Apart,* ABC Books, Melbourne, 1991.

Omathuna, D., and Larimore, W., *Alternative Medicine*, Zondervan, Grand Rapids, Michigan, 2001.

Pearson, M., *Christian Healing*, Chosen Books, Revell, Old Tappan NJ, 1990. Chapter 8.

Pfeifer, S., *Healing at any Price*, Word, Milton Keynes, UK, 1988.

Ray, D., *The Art of Christian Meditation*, Tyndale, Illinois, 1977.

Reisser, P. and Mabe, D., *Examining Alternative Medicine*, IVP, Downers Grove, Illinois. 2001.

Toon, P., *Meditating as a Christian*, Harper Collins, London, 1991.

12

THE MINISTRY OF DELIVERANCE—EXORCISM

Spectacular headlines and graphic pictures reported the death of a woman in an Australian country town. The woman had been sick for some time, and her friends were convinced that she was under the control of some evil power and that she needed the ministry of deliverance and exorcism. Her friends acted under their own authority because they believed that "the Lord had told them, in a word of knowledge," what was the problem, and how they should minister to her. The woman died as a result of injuries received during this ministry, and from the lack of professional medical care.

Death had apparently resulted from a crushed larynx which occurred as friends tried to rid her body of demons. Her friends believed that the woman was demon possessed and had been subject to attacks and control by demons since childhood. It appeared that this was the first attempt at exorcism for those involved. When the exorcism failed and death occurred, the friends sincerely believed that the deceased person would rise again from the dead, and be a powerful testimony for the gospel to all people. When this did not occur there was distress and confusion and a recognition that some mistakes had been made in understanding God's purpose, at least as far as the rising from the dead was concerned. But there was no denial of the exorcism attempt and those involved sincerely believed this is what God wanted them to do to help their friend.

Reactions to the tragic event included a genuine sympathy for those involved and a careful support for the idea of exorcism.

However, there was also a strong warning that such a ministry should only be given under the supervision of those experienced in this field and should be offered only after complete medical and psychiatric evaluation of a person's condition. Others ridiculed the whole idea, branding it as an alarming return to medieval superstition. Although the media helped to sensationalize the incident, it was quite clear that the question of deliverance is a very live issue and that many people, both Christian and non-Christian, accept the reality of demonic power in contemporary society.

- Someone says to you that they believe in the reality and power of demons to control people and to cause sickness and other problems. They ask you whether you share their belief. How would you respond?

- Does the church to which you belong (the denomination or the local church congregation) have any official policy on the ministry of deliverance? If so, briefly explain the policy. If not, do you think there should be a policy to offer guidelines for people interested or involved in or afraid of this particular ministry?

This chapter has been the hardest to write for several reasons: The Order of St. Luke has no *official* position on the ministry of deliverance. It recognizes the need for such a ministry and accepts the use of various methods within certain safeguards and guidelines.

- There is a lot of material written about this ministry reflecting various interpretations and practices, and it is therefore very difficult to offer a comprehensive overview of the subject.

- It is a volatile subject which produces strong reactions, either for or against. Often the responses given confirm the wisdom of the much quoted statement of C. S. Lewis:

There are two equal and opposite errors into which our race can fall, about the devils; one is to disbelieve in their existence, the other is to believe and to feel an excessive and unhealthy interest in them. They themselves are equally pleased by both errors and hail a materialist or magician with the same delight. (*The Screwtape Letters*).

- There is often a fascination with the subject, and people are eager to learn the latest techniques as to "how to do it" successfully, without bothering about any deeper issues involved.

In all probability this may be the chapter to which some readers will first turn in order to evaluate the soundness of approach — they may well judge the whole book by what they read!

It is important to note the purpose of the following material. It does not claim to offer *the* definitive statement or evaluation of this ministry, nor go into details as to techniques, nor retell experiences of exorcism. These aspects are available in other literature on the subject. Rather, it seeks to offer a broad overview of some of the main issues and principles relating to this ministry, which is a comparatively small but significant aspect of the total healing ministry.

This chapter aims to:

- Recognize the reality of evil and demonic powers and the need for a deliverance ministry within the larger ministry of healing;

- Outline the New Testament perspective on the reality of the battle between the kingdom of darkness and the kingdom of Jesus Christ;

- Clarify some different interpretations of key scripture verses about Satan and the evil powers;

- Examine when this ministry is required and the need for careful discernment in diagnosis;

- Outline some of the accepted methods used in this ministry;

- Consider some basic principles to guide people in the practice and evaluation of this ministry.

The Reality of Evil Powers — Need for Deliverance Ministry

There has been much study and discussion on this subject in recent years, and many reports have been completed to help the churches in their ongoing evaluation. One example of this is the Uniting Church in Australia which has issued several reports from its various State bodies, noting the interest, concern, and at times disagreement within the churches about this ministry. These reports referred to the following facts as an indication of this interest and concern:

- The Anglican Church both in Australia and England has commissioned several reports from committees of theologians, psychiatrists, educators, ministers and lay people.

- The recognition that the Roman Catholic, Orthodox and Anglican churches have officially accepted this ministry as a normal part of ministry to those who need it.

- Many churches and healing groups include this ministry as part of their understanding of healing. Some, especially Pentecostal churches, make it a major emphasis.

- Many hundreds of cases of deliverance/exorcism have been recorded and published in the ever-expanding literature on this subject. This includes several situations where an unwise use of this ministry has resulted in human tragedy, and indicated a need for a more informed understanding.

- The explosion of occult practices and the harm and bondage they cause in many people through either dabbling in occult phenomena, or deliberately exploring and affirming the use of the occult as a valid way to spiritual truth and understanding.[1]

In the healing ministry it is recognized that there are different types of sickness which require different types of ministry. Sickness may be physical, emotional, psychological, mental, spiritual, social, or a combination of these. Some would add a further dimension, that is, demonic sickness caused by the activity of evil powers. Others would not see the demonic as a separate category, but as a possible factor which can be present in any type of sickness.[2]

Many practitioners in the healing ministry refer to situations where a particular condition fails to respond to such ministries as counseling, prayer, laying on of hands and anointing, and it is only when the demonic factor is addressed that any progress occurs.

> In the healing ministry it is common to meet situations where the usual prayer seems quite ineffective. The person may be comforted and encouraged but their overall condition remains the same. Something more is called for . . . but what?[3]

After careful research of contemporary attitudes to the ministry of deliverance, another author finds that:

> A growing number of people including some who are qualified in the more scientific healing arts (medical, psychiatric and social science areas) now hold a place for the ministry of deliverance/exorcism. He suggests that there are some circumstances, although these are relatively rare, in which the ministry of exorcism is indicated.[4]

However, along with this recognition, there are many who are reluctant to become involved in any specific deliverance ministry because of such factors as:

- The danger of over-emphasis in seeing demons under every bush, and the cause of every sickness and problem.

- The fear of being seen as fanatical, unbalanced or too charismatic.

- The possible stigma of intellectual absurdity, "medieval hocus-pocus," and superstition, especially if suggested by peers in the professional health field and/or the ordained ministry of the church.

- The irresponsible use of this ministry by some healers.

- The sensationalism of the Hollywood treatment of this issue (for example, *The Exorcist 1* and *2*).

In the light of these deterrents, it is easy to understand why some people approach the subject of deliverance ministry either with extreme caution, or with complete rejection of all that is involved.

Because of these positive and negative responses, many churches acknowledge the need for continuing study and evaluation of deliverance ministry. At a seminar in Melbourne, Australia, representatives from seven churches and healing groups gathered for an interdenominational discussion of some of the issues confronting churches in relation to deliverance and exorcism. Amidst many different responses there was a unanimous affirmation of the urgent need for such ministries in the contemporary situation, the necessity for continuing in-depth study of the New Testament teaching, and the need for effective training and oversight of those involved in any form of deliverance ministry.[5]

For some who have long accepted the reality of this ministry, these recent developments may seem to be too little too late, because for many years some church leaders have refused to treat the subject seriously. However, the Melbourne discussion can also be seen as a significant development, a "breakthrough," because many churches in Australia are now tackling the issue on an official level, rather than leaving it as the concern of a small minority in the church.

One reason for this new awareness is the recognition that the ministry of deliverance is firmly based in the New Testament scriptures and that any honest evaluation must grapple with this solid biblical foundation.

Kingdoms in Conflict — The Battle Rages!

The New Testament clearly accepts the reality of evil in the world and attributes this reality to the work of Satan and to the evil powers under his control. The conflict between the rule of God and the power of Satan is depicted as a battle between the kingdom of light under the control of Jesus Christ and the kingdom of darkness under the control of Satan.[6]

The following are some of the main points in the New Testament understanding:

- There is a kingdom of light (John 12:35, 36), and a kingdom of darkness (Colossians 1:13).

- Each kingdom has its leader, the kingdom of light under Jesus Christ, and the kingdom of darkness under Satan (Matthew 12:25-28; 2 Corinthians 4:4; Ephesians 2:2; 1 John 5:19).

- These kingdoms have nothing in common and are in open conflict (2 Corinthians 6:14-17; Ephesians 5:8-11; Ephesians 6:10-12).

- Each person belongs to one or other of these warring kingdoms. When there is a response of repentance and faith in Jesus Christ, this is a rescue or deliverance from the dominion of darkness into the light (Acts 26:18; Colossians 1:13; 1 Peter 2:9-10).

- Both kingdoms have supernatural spiritual workers who seek to forward the purposes and plans of their leader, either for good or evil. The kingdom of light is served by the ministry of good angels (Hebrews 1:14), whereas the kingdom of darkness is served by demons and other evil powers, described as "the devil and his angels" (Matthew 25:41; Ephesians 6:12). One of the reasons for the coming of Jesus to the world was to destroy the works of the devil (Hebrews 2:14; 1 John 3:8).

- Jesus' ministry of healing and deliverance was a direct attack on the power of Satan and the kingdom of darkness (Matthew 10:7-8; 12:28-30). This attack culminated in the cross and resurrection where the evil powers and authorities under Satan's control were disarmed and their power broken (Colossians 2:15).

- Although mortally wounded and rendered ineffective, Satan continues to oppress and control people and situations (1 Peter 5:8-9).

- This conflict will continue until the final defeat of Satan and the complete destruction of the kingdom of darkness (Revelation 11:15; 20).

This broad overview is now explained in more detail. Although his teaching focused on the kingdom of God (Mark 1:15), Jesus did not give an exact definition of its meaning. However, the kingdom of God was clearly seen in his words and actions. It was the breaking into human life of a new dynamic in which the rule of God was experienced and the power of evil broken. Healing the sick, casting out of demons, and other acts of liberation were the signs that the kingdom was present (Matthew 10:7-8; 11:1-5; 12:28). Becoming a citizen of this kingdom was not a matter of natural birth, or of cultural and ethnic membership, or of living a meritorious life — rather, it was through repentance and faith in Jesus Christ and the work of the Holy Spirit (Mark 1:15; John 3:5).

As well as repentance and faith, the kingdom demanded a new and radical lifestyle which completely overturned the old values and traditions (Matthew 5, 6, 7). Unlike the people of his time who expected the kingdom of God to be a time of destruction and judgment on God's enemies, and the restoration of an ethnic and geographical territory centered on Israel (Acts 1:6), Jesus offered a kingdom of liberation, forgiveness and freedom to all people regardless of their ethnic and cultural background (Matthew 8:11-12). The kingdom of God was different from any earthly kingdom, both in character and purpose (John 18:36).

The kingdom of God was a reality to be experienced within the personal life of an individual (Luke 17:21), but it was also to be demonstrated and experienced in the wider spheres of community — in social, political, and family relationships. It was both a *present reality* demonstrated in the ministry of Jesus, and also a *future experience* when it would be established in its fullness. The citizen of the kingdom thus would experience its blessings in the present, but the citizen of the kingdom was also to pray for the kingdom to come (Matthew 6:10). The fullness of the kingdom would be revealed "at the end of the age." In the meantime, the citizens of the kingdom could experience its blessings while at the same time awaiting its fulfillment. Citizens of the kingdom live in the power of the kingdom while continuing to live in the world which belongs to the kingdom of darkness and is under the control of Satan.

Jesus came to destroy the works of the devil (Hebrews 2:14; 1 John 3:8), to break his control over human life, to bind the strong man, and to release those held in bondage (Mark 3:20-27; Luke 11:14-22). Casting out demons, healing the sick, and releasing people from the fear of death were signs of the breaking of Satan's control (Matthew 12:28; Hebrews 2:14). Jesus' ministry was a continuous battle against Satan and the evil forces under his command, from the victory of the temptations (Matthew 4:1-11) to the apparent defeat of the cross, where it seemed that the power of evil had prevailed and the darkness had overcome the light (Luke 22:53). The decisive battle in the conflict occurred at the cross and resurrection, where the forces of evil were dealt a death blow and their ultimate defeat was clearly demonstrated. Here Jesus broke the power of Satan and the evil forces controlling the world, and in the language of a military victory, "Having disarmed the powers and authorities, he made a public spectacle of them, triumphing over them by the cross" (Colossians 2:15). By his death and resurrection, Jesus crippled the forces of evil and destroyed Satan's power and control. So while the New Testament recognizes the reality of Satan, its main focus is not on *his* power, but on the victory by which he is defeated.

It is important to understand that while the cross and resurrection was the *decisive* battle in the conflict with evil, it was not the *final* battle; for the battle between good and evil still rages and Satan, the god of this age, continues to control vast areas of human life which have not responded to the freedom offered in Jesus Christ. He continues to control people and society by blinding their understanding of the true way (2 Corinthians 4:4). So great is the presence and power of evil that "the whole world is under the control of the evil one" (1 John 5:19).

How are we to understand the fact that Satan has been defeated yet he continues to cause havoc? The answer is in the meaning of the word "destroy" (Hebrews 2:14; 1 John 3:8). It does not mean to "wipe out completely" or to "obliterate" in the sense of complete and utter destruction; rather it means to "crush," "to render ineffective," "to bring to nought," "to rob of power," "to undo," "to render powerless or impotent." Through the cross and resurrection, Satan has been disarmed and his power broken, but he was not and is not completely destroyed. His complete and utter destruction will not come until the final victory of God (Revelation 20).

In the meantime, Satan continues to oppose the purposes of God and brings confusion, havoc, and misery on people and the world. Within the ultimate purposes of God, he continues to use his illegal power, but he is fighting a lost cause and his ultimate defeat is sure, because the decisive battle has been won — yet the war continues!

How a war already won can continue is illustrated by the end of World War II. In any war there are some crucial or decisive battles which determine the ultimate outcome. In the war in Europe, it was D-Day when allied troops secured a beach head at Normandy, an action which military experts saw as securing the final victory for the allied forces. There were still many battles to be fought before the V-E Day (Victory in Europe), when the final victory was achieved; but D-Day was the decisive turning point. In the Pacific war, a similar event occurred in two great battles, the Battle of Midway and the Battle of the Coral Sea. In these battles the power of the Japanese forces was broken and this marked the beginning of the end for the Japanese campaign. The V-P Day (Victory in Pacific) was still in the future but victory was assured.

So, to the eye of faith, the cross is the decisive battle where the power of Satan is broken, but the war continues and the fighting can be very heavy with many casualties. However, the ultimate victory is secure, because the decisive victory has already been won. So Satan is a defeated foe who continues to thrash about and must be confronted and opposed in the power of the victory of Jesus Christ. It is because he is a beaten foe that Satan seeks to do as much harm as possible before his ultimate destruction.

As the ruler of the kingdom of darkness, Satan controls a vast army of agents through whom he achieves his evil plans. He is "the ruler of the kingdom of the air," and under his authority are a vast group of hostile, supernatural forces, including rulers, authorities, angels, demons, unclean spirits, elemental spirits, the powers of this dark world, the spiritual forces of evil in the heavenly realms (Ephesians 2:2, 6:12). As the front-line troops, demons or evil spirits can harass, invade and control the body, mind, and spirit of a person or group. They are intelligent beings, often showing great physical strength and subtlety. In their desire to promote everything that is contrary to God's purpose for the world and the welfare of His people, these evil forces carry out every form of wickedness. They work on all levels of human activity, from influencing individuals to exerting control over the social order, even to the extent of exercising control over entire nations. For example, Daniel 10:13, 20 refers to the "Princes of Persia and Greece," and this is interpreted as being the "territorial spirits," responsible for controlling a particular city or country and keeping it under the evil influence of Satan. These influences may be felt in the social, economic, political, and religious systems, as well as in the disharmony in individual lives and family relationships. They also exert control through the use of natural phenomena and various occult practices which seek to use spiritual power to achieve particular ends.

However, despite his apparent power and control, the New Testament clearly affirms that Satan is a defeated tyrant, and that Christ has disarmed the powers of darkness. The reality of the conflict is clearly recognized, but it is always from the perspective of the victory which has been won through the death and resurrection of Jesus Christ. It is not a battle where the final outcome is in the balance; victory is sure because a decisive encounter has taken place. It is only in the light of this victory that the ministry of deliverance is possible.[7]

Before considering the outworking of Christ's victory in the ministry of deliverance, it may be helpful to understand some contemporary interpretations of the conflict between Christ and Satan; in particular the different interpretations given to key verses, such as Colossians 2:15 and Ephesians 6:12. What or who are the rulers, authorities, the powers of the dark world, and the evil forces against which we battle and which have been defeated through the cross and resurrection of Jesus Christ?

What Are Powers and Authorities?

Traditionally these powers have been understood as supernatural beings — demons, fallen angels, evil spirits operating under the control of Satan in the kingdom of darkness. This has formed the background for spiritual warfare and the reality of deliverance from these powers of evil. However, in recent years the powers and authorities have been interpreted, not as heavenly supernatural spiritual beings, but rather as earthly powers — such things as political institutions and economic entities, for example, multinational companies and the system of law and government which exercise control in every society. The powers are the spiritual dimensions of these structures which govern our lives, and are expressed in such things as the fixation on success, profit and greed, the arms race, environmental destruction, inequalities and injustice between rich and poor — these are the demons, the unclean spirits which must be confronted and cast out. These are the evil forces from which people and society need to be delivered. So the "supernatural" is replaced by "earthly" structures and systems which control people's lives and become the focus of our allegiance and bondage. For example, bondage to the claims of the nation or government above everything else, expressed in extreme nationalism, or to racial intolerance and hatred, expressed in ethnicism and ethnic cleansing, or to profit-making, expressed in the worship of the almighty dollar, and many other forms of control or idolatry.

This view re-interprets and removes some of the problems modem people may have with the belief in evil spiritual forces, Satan, and demons — which may seem to be out of place in contemporary scientific society. In this view, the warfare in which the church is involved is not so much against the invisible spiritual forces of evil, but against the very visible earthly powers and systems which imprison and destroy people. These need to be opposed so that people are delivered from their control, through such activities as political action for social justice and equality, solidarity with the poor, prevention of environmental destruction, opposition to economic exploitation, and peaceful opposition to war and militarism. So there is a need for deliverance and exorcism, but it is to be achieved through social and political action. In these ways people will be delivered from these powers which will be cast out or exorcised from society.

The contemporary problem of interpretation is clearly described by C. E. Arnold, who comments on the different interpretations of the relevance of Paul's teaching for today:

> Western society does not give credence to the notion of spirits, be they good or evil. To introduce the idea of evil spirits would be regarded by many as a reversion to primitive myths . . . traditional Christian interpretation has stressed the influence of the powers on individuals. The bulk of popular charismatic works on this topic have dealt primarily with ministering to people who are demonized. Both of these views assume that evil spirits really do exist. More recent interpretations of the powers, in contrast, have stressed the influence of the powers on a broad scale; that is, the powers work primarily through the structures of our existence. Such things as economic and political structures are most often cited (capitalism, socialism, nationalism) but also other factors enter in, such as social patterns, cultural norms, group habits (like the development of a mob spirit in a soccer match). These structures of existence are then viewed as the objects of our spiritual struggle and may be regarded as demonic. Many who hold to this view would regard the biblical references to the powers as symbols of non-personal realities . . . for most Christians the issue of the pervasive influence of the powers has not been a matter of careful reflection.[8]

The answer to this question will depend on attitudes to the authority of the scriptures; our evaluation of the world-view of the time when these words were written (is it real and true or mythical, according to current scientific understanding?); and to a large extent, by one's stance in relation to the church's involvement in society and the need for confrontation with all oppressive systems through the use of social and political action as legitimate expressions of the gospel. Many see these different interpretations as incompatible, whilst others who support one interpretation also acknowledge the need to be aware of other insights. Thus writers like M. Green and J. Stott, whilst acknowledging the need to recognize the influence of the demonic in all human structures in society, insist that the spiritual interpretation of the powers is the only valid way of interpreting the New Testament teaching, and that to identify the powers with the structures of earthly existence is to cause confusion. Green suggests that the recent tendency to regard the powers as the structures of earthly existence is attractive because it helps to get rid of unfashionable ideas like angels and evil spirits, and it also gives New Testament support to our very modern preoccupation with social structures. In commenting that the debate is often conducted on the basis of presupposition rather than on careful exegesis of the New Testament passage, Green concludes that:

> The truth of the matter is that words like principalities, powers, and thrones are used both of human rulers and of the spiritual forces which lie behind them. This is readily demonstrable: Luke 12:11 clearly refers to men . . . Acts 4:26 equally obviously indicates men . . . On the other hand it is perfectly manifest that the powers and thrones and authorities in Colossians 1:16, 2:15; Romans 8:38; Ephesians 6:12 are superhuman powers. There are some passages which could be taken either way, 1 Corinthians 2:8; Titus 3:1; Romans 13:1. Probably the ambiguity is deliberate. The main thrust of New Testament teaching is to see these powers as spiritual entities in the heavenlies, that is, the spiritual world. For example in Ephesians, they are described as being in the heavenlies, which makes it almost impossible to believe that earthly forces are in view. This does not for one moment mean that

the principalities and powers may not infect government, public opinion and the like. It simply avoids the confusion of identifying them.[9]

This chapter accepts the reality of deliverance from "the *spiritual forces of evil*" as a consequence of the conflict fought between Jesus Christ and Satan. However, whilst endorsing the reality of these spiritual enemies, there is also need to affirm demonic influence which may control and infect the structures and systems of any society. These spiritual powers subvert, control and destroy, often through human people and systems which are under their control, albeit without any realization or acknowledgment of this fact.

Having considered the contemporary interest in the deliverance ministry, its biblical foundations, and the different interpretations of some biblical verses, we are now able to focus more directly on the factors which indicate that such a ministry is needed, and the methods to be used. The following material deals with these aspects.

When is Ministry of Deliverance Needed?

There is no agreed definition of the words used to describe the work of Satan and the ministry of deliverance, and this can create confusion. The following words are commonly used:[10]

Oppression is the influence which is exerted on a person by one or more evil spiritual powers. Oppression is "the condition in which a person, while largely in control of his or her behavior, language and so on, cannot manage some area of his or her personality or life due to a demonic presence; for example, some form of compulsive behavior."

Many see oppression as a fairly common experience for Christians as Satan prowls about seeking people to devour and to cripple the effectiveness of Christian witnesses and service (1 Peter 5:8-9). It is the pervasive influence of evil in our lives and can be experienced in varying degrees of intensity.

Possession describes the condition in which a person or group is in a state of complete control by demonic powers; that is, their total life and behavior and various patterns of functioning. The New Testament describes this as being demonized.

Deliverance and Exorcism are sometimes used interchangeably, but many writers and practitioners make a distinction between them. For example, Brown suggests:

Deliverance is a ministry by which, in the name of Jesus and in the power of the Holy Spirit, people are set free from bondage to sin, guilt, demonic oppression or possession, destructive behavior, and ultimately alienation from God, who is the source of life and love.

Exorcism is a ritual action or actions, the purpose of which is to bind and cast out malevolent spiritual forces in the name of Jesus. It is one aspect of the ministry of deliverance.[11]

In this understanding, *deliverance* is a broader concept and refers both to the initial experience of exorcism, and also to the ongoing process of healing which flows from the casting out of the evil power.[12]

Other writers make a further distinction between deliverance and exorcism, the difference being in the extent or depth of the control being exerted by the evil spiritual power. Deliverance is a simple form of exorcism used for the relief of believing Christians suffering from some mild form of oppression; whereas exorcism is restricted to those who have been utterly taken over by Satan; that is, those under demonic possession.[13]

Some churches also distinguish between *major* and *minor* exorcism. *Minor* exorcisms are common and frequently used; for example, the petition "deliver us from evil" is a prayer to God and can be used by all Christians. It is a prayer for deliverance from all evil influences affecting a person or place. *Major* exorcism is a definite and specific command used in severe cases and only to be carried out after sufficient examination, and then only by authorized persons.[14]

In the following discussion the deliverance ministry includes the act of exorcism which involves release *from*, or out of, some control; but it also involves deliverance *to* something or someone; that is, to a fullness of life in God and the total experience of healing.

The Causes of Oppression and Possession[15]

This ministry is needed when any person, group, or place is oppressed by evil forces, but especially when *possession* is either suspected or dearly seen. These conditions can be caused by many factors; for example:

- Disobedience to spiritual truth and involvement in false beliefs and philosophies (Colossians 2:8-20).

- Unhealthy and irrational fears (Hebrews 2:14-15).

- Harboring of resentment, hate, revenge, anger and other attitudinal sins which foster a "root of bitterness" (Matthew 18:21-35; Ephesians 4:26-27, 30-32; Hebrews 12:14-15).

- Rejection of the principles of health and wholeness and engaging in excesses of conduct in relation to food, pleasure, sexual activity and so on (Ephesians 5:3-5; 1 Thessalonians 4:3-8; Hebrews 13:4).

- Involvement in false religion and idolatry (Exodus 20:2-3; Acts 15:20; 1 Corinthians 8:7; 1 John 5:21).

- Some physical sicknesses (Mark 1:21-28, 5:1-20, 9:14-29; Luke 13:10-17). Not all sickness and disease are caused by demonic control. Jesus did not cast out demons in several healing situations. (For example, John 5:8, 9:1-12.) There is a distinction made between the demonized and the sick (Matthew 8:16). Compare Matthew 8:28-34 (demon-possessed) and Matthew 9:2-8 (no mention of demonic activity).

By far the strongest cause is influence by, or involvement in, occult practices either by the person or by parents, relatives and friends. This ranges from attendances at séances involving astrology, necromancy, the use of ouija boards and tarot cards; to the use of divination, mediums, charms, amulets, fortune telling; to participation in various forms of spiritism, witchcraft, black magic and satanism.[16]

Indications when this Ministry may be Necessary[17]

The word "may" is important because it is possible to label situations and conditions as needing deliverance from the demonic when this may not be the real cause. It is easy to attribute things to the powers of evil when it may be a physical, emotional, or spiritual problem, which can be treated with some form of medication, counseling or spiritual therapy. Everyone is exposed to experiences, difficulties and misfortunes that may be influenced in some way by satanic powers, but which can be effectively handled through the means of repentance, faith, counseling, prayer and worship, and other forms of therapy and care. Usually these conditions do not require deliverance, but a more intentional use of the means of healing and help that are already available. In many of these difficult situations, the cause may stem from emotional disharmony or such attitudes as pride, rejection, disobedience, and so on, and may have little to do with evil spiritual forces.

A major error which many people make is to assume that the whole world is either under the control of God or Satan, and they therefore ignore the reality of natural human factors in problem situations.

> Some seem to assume that the whole world is either under the control of God or Satan; therefore everything that happens can be attributed either to a divine or satanic cause. With this kind of thinking, there can be no place for natural or human factors. This has led some Christians to grossly exaggerated views of the activities of evil spirits, so that all illnesses, including the psychological, and all temptations, are due to demonic forces. Even natural weaknesses and infirmities, and the temptations which, according to Paul are common to all men, are treated as cases in need of exorcism. Confusion and personal damage has been caused by such faulty diagnosis, for some people have been led to expect release from the disciplines, hardships and temptations of the Christian way of life.[18]

Harper notes that many of the problems faced by people have a natural explanation and are due to our selfishness, that is, our self-centered life lived in disobedience to God. What is needed is to "reckon ourselves dead to sin" through repentance and faith, not to seek for release through deliverance. Often what is needed is some form of discipline, or rest, or self-denial, or humility, or forgiveness, or a holiday!

> Often the real antidote is the basic Christian principle of repentance, without which a harmonious relationship with God and people is impossible. When this is neglected, people get themselves into impossible relationship tangles . . . We have to confess our faults to one another and seek forgiveness where necessary . . . Even if we can attribute a large measure of our problem to Satan's power and activity, we are still responsible before God and need to repent. The neglect of this basic principle is a cause of spiritual disorder in the church and amongst its individual members. Our warfare against Satan is no substitute for true repentance.[19]

A similar problem can arise from the belief that it is necessary to "name" particular demons as responsible for particular problems. So there are said to be demons of anger, lust, rejection, pride, jealousy, heaviness, fear, error, invalidity, treachery, slumber, confusion — the list is almost endless, and includes such suggestions as the demon of tooth decay! It is claimed that there are hundreds of particular demons waiting to afflict the human race, all of which can be, and need to be, named and identified.

Care needs to be taken with this method, because it is easy to blame a demon and try to cast it out, when what is needed is recognition of a physical or emotional problem, a careful study of the reasons for it, and a willingness to do something about it through appropriate means. That is not to say that there may not be demonic influence as part of the problem, but to ascribe all problems either totally or primarily to a demon, can or may mean denying the human factors involved. For example, if a person is controlled by anger, is this overcome by casting out the demon of anger; or by examining the cause of the problem, and understanding how anger can be truly expressed and used as one of the strong emotions given to us by God? Satan may indeed use our anger as a foothold to control us, but the answer is not in casting out the demon of anger, but in expressing anger in a positive way without sinning (Ephesians 4:26, 27). Or, if a person is controlled by lust, is the demon of lust to be exorcised, or should the addiction be confronted, confessed and then replaced by the stronger emotion of love? As for the demon of tooth decay, would a visit to the dentist, a good tooth brush, and cutting back sugar and sweets, be just as effective or more so than an attempt at exorcism?

The problem often comes from a wrong understanding of the word "spirit," where the meaning can refer to an independent spirit-being or to an attitude or disposition. Often these are confused. For example, 2 Timothy 1:7 speaks of a spirit of timidity or cowardly fear, so some assume that any deliverance from such fear or timidity must be by casting out the evil spirit or demon of fear; that is, an independent spirit-being. But the verse also speaks of the spirit of power, love and self-discipline. Are these also good spirits; that is, independent spirit-beings? If timidity or fear is a demon to be cast out; to be consistent, we would need to ask three good spirits to come in. However, love and self-discipline are not good spirits, but the fruit of the Holy Spirit. The spirit of power, love and self-discipline are the *attitudes* which result from the work of the Holy Spirit in us.

A wise comment from within the Pentecostal/Charismatic stream of church life is helpful:

> Much misunderstanding has arisen from a wrong interpretation of the word "spirit" as it is sometimes used in the Bible . . . The word spirit, in many cases, means an attitude or a disposition; for example, David spoke of a "broken" spirit (Psalm 51:17), Solomon, of a "lowly" spirit (Proverbs 16:19), Paul of a "gentle" or "meek" spirit (1 Corinthians 4:21), Peter of a "gentle and quiet" spirit (1 Peter 3:4), actually meaning a "quiet disposition" . . . Thus, unless the context shows that an independent spirit-being is meant, it seems best to take most phrases such as a "haughty" spirit, a spirit of "slumber," "jealousy" and many others, to be *sins of the dispositions* or *lusts of the flesh* and not demons. A serious danger in considering all these sins of the dispositions to be demons is that the individual may feel no responsibility for his or her actions and feel that the necessity for repentance is removed. The Bible calls men to repent of these things and put off these attitudes. The great conflict within us is not between the Holy Spirit and demons, but between the indwelling Holy Spirit and the flesh; that is, all the sensory apparatus that tends toward sin.[20]

So, whilst there is some validity in naming specific demons in order to clarify diagnosis, care must be taken not to cover up emotional, physical and spiritual conditions which should be addressed by repentance, confession, prayer and action!

When a person's condition, attitudes, or actions do not respond to all known treatments, disciplines and will power, a different type of ministry is needed. When a person is unable to control his or her conduct and displays addictive and sometimes bizarre behavior, then it is clear there is need for deliverance. Despite the dangers, we must accept the need to be ruthlessly honest in diagnosis of problem situations.

John Richards suggests four main areas which may indicate the need for deliverance. These relate to personality changes and physical/mental and spiritual changes.[21]

Personality changes include such things as physical appearance, outward changes in attitudes, behavior and moral character; and the lowering of normal levels of intelligence and speech.

Physical changes can be seen in violent and anti-social behavior, abnormal strength, changes in voice and facial expressions (trance-like, glassy or goggle-eyed), body convulsions, screaming, frothing at the mouth, body odor, insensitivity to pain, and physical conditions which do not respond to any treatment.

Mental/psychological changes may include unintelligible speech, abnormal reactions, seeing para-normal phenomena, seeking after occult power and knowledge, an overwhelming sense of depression, guilt, fear and anxiety, uncontrollable urges and addictions, fantasizing, and being out of touch with reality.

Spiritual changes, in blasphemy, rejection of Jesus Christ, hostile and fearful response to worship, prayer, and other actions and rituals relating to God; hostility to believers who seek to help; cursing in prayer; bitterness and unforgiveness which is allowed to grow and develop.

Along with all these, there may be indications from a person's background, for example, occult involvement or other forms of bondage and addiction from which the person cannot experience any freedom.

Many people respond to such a wide range of possible causes by giving up and leaving it to the "experts," or to those specifically trained and recognized as having this particular ministry. That response may be over-cautious, but it does emphasize the fact that careful diagnosis is essential before embarking on the deliverance journey. Many healing practitioners suggest that demonic oppression and especially demonic possession should be seen as the last possible cause of the problem and not the first; that is, examine all other possible causes before concluding that deliverance is necessary.

In such a complex area, it is important to understand and follow any guidelines offered by the church or healing group, and to always discuss situations with those experienced in this ministry. There must be a balance between boldness in affirming, claiming and applying the victory of Christ, and "rushing in where angels fear to tread."

Methods Used in this Ministry

Before any deliverance method is used, it is essential to be adequately prepared for such a ministry by understanding and being equipped in the area of spiritual warfare. Some ways in which we can prepare ourselves for spiritual warfare:

Our thinking: Not allowing our thoughts and minds to become an Achilles heel through which Satan can weaken our effectiveness, but be constantly renewed in our minds (Romans 12:1-2; Philippians 4:8).

Our Emotions: Not giving the devil a foothold by refusing to deal with emotions which have the power to wound ourselves and others (Ephesians 4:27).

Our Actions: Refusing involvement in anything which is going to give Satan an opportunity to oppress and control us.

Our Spiritual Understanding: Not becoming fascinated by the devil's power and subtlety. This can result in having a very big devil and a very small God, whereas the New Testament is clearly the other way round. Recognize and constantly affirm the reality of the victory of Jesus.

Being Realistic: John Richards notes that the main references to Satan in scripture refer to his power and position (for example, 2 Corinthians 4:4); his evil nature (for instance, John 8:44); and his defeat (for example, Romans 16:20). He then suggests that it is possible to over-emphasize any of these aspects:

If we overstress the devil's power, we will become defeatist. If we overstress his evil nature, we will become depressed. If we overstress his defeat, we will become unrealistic.[22]

What is needed is a realistic approach which recognizes the reality of Satan's power, but rests on the victory which has disarmed him and rendered him impotent. So Christians acknowledge the reality of evil, but do not "believe" in it, in the sense of entrusting themselves to it. The Christian believes in ***God***, and in **Satan's downfall**, because he is already defeated. (Compare that with M. Green: "I believe in Satan's downfall.")

Our Actual Involvement in the Fight

This involves understanding the principles of spiritual warfare, and actually living them out in daily life, not just talking about them. Richards points out that the concept of spiritual warfare can be a cover-up for selfish ambitions and weaknesses:

It is easy to assume that those who talk most about spiritual warfare are Christ's greatest soldiers; unfortunately, this is rarely if ever the case. The concept of spiritual warfare provides the situations and the terminology in which the rejected can find meaning, the insecure can find status, and the bored can find drama. There are those who positively feed on these things in order to bolster their own egos, to give them status in the Christian community, and/or to wield power over others.[23]

With this warning Richards affirms that the first item to consider in our spiritual warfare is not the armor as depicted in Ephesians 6:10-17, rather it is all the spiritual conditions which are given in Ephesians 1-5.[24]

Unless we read Ephesians backwards, the armor is the last thing that will concern us. Military equipment is of no use whatever to a soldier who is not disciplined, trained and obedient . . . for the Christian soldier, there is no point considering the weaponry available in Chapter 6, unless he or she first has been thoroughly trained according to Chapters 1-5.

Accordingly, any preparation must include:

• A relationship with Jesus Christ (Ephesians 1:3, 2:6).

• Receiving the Holy Spirit for our enlightenment (Ephesians 1:17).

• Working together as a team, not as individual commandos (Ephesians 2:19).

• Living worthily, as our special calling (Ephesians 4:2-3, 22-23, 25-32).

• Not giving the devil any foothold through compromising in moral behavior (Ephesians 4:27, 5:7-14).

- Being constantly filled with the Holy Spirit (Ephesians 5:15-20).

- Harmonious and loving relationships (Ephesians 5:21, 6:9).

On this foundation the armor for warfare will be effective, but without this preparation it will be of little or no use.

This preparation then becomes the foundation on which the following methods can be used.

The Methods to be Used

There are many variations in methods, but the following are usually included in any act of deliverance or exorcism of persons or places (where appropriate).[25]

- The powers of Satan are verbally bound in the name of Jesus Christ in order to silence and pacify the demons present.

- The demons are commanded to leave the afflicted person, to do no harm to the sufferer or to others present, not to re-enter the person, and to go away into a state of subjection to Jesus Christ.

- The afflicted person is asked to confess and repent of past sins, to disown the power of darkness, to receive Christ or affirm faith in Christ. This may be followed by anointing, laying on of hands, and prayer for the infilling of the Holy Spirit.

- The person is asked to renounce any involvement with possible causes of demonic control, especially occult practices. This is a challenge to choose freedom in Christ as well as a commitment to change the pattern of behavior and destroy the networks of bondage associated with it. It is a refusal to allow demonic forces any further hold over his or her life.

- After this release the person needs to be helped to keep moving on in the experience of renewal. While not an essential part of the actual exorcism, it is important that future growth into wholeness is adequately addressed. Deliverance is to be an ongoing experience in the overall process of healing.

One writer suggests a helpful fivefold procedure which includes most of the points made, but expresses them in a different order.

- Recognition — discerning the problem.
- Repentance — of unconfessed sin and turning to Jesus Christ.
- Renunciation — of any involvement in evil practices.
- Release — through authoritative prayer.
- Renewal — after-care for continuing growth in grace.[26]

Having noted the various aspects of this ministry, we can now summarize some of the important principles which need to be followed in any practice and evaluation of this ministry.

Principles of Deliverance Ministry[27]

Whether we are actually involved in deliverance ministry or not, the following principles will assist in our approach and understanding:

The deliverance ministry is a valid ministry and is one aspect of the total healing ministry of Jesus Christ. Do not be afraid to recognize it as one of the resources for healing the whole person.

This ministry is based on the authority of the victory of Jesus Christ and not on any technique or human authority. Jesus Christ through his death and resurrection has conquered the forces of evil, and salvation and freedom is through him alone.

Christian people will be affected by the power of evil, because of failure to live constantly in the victory of Christ through the power of the Holy Spirit. Therefore confession of sin, repentance, and acceptance of God's pardoning grace remain as daily essentials, in order to prevent any control or oppression by any evil power.

Avoid the assumption that the world is either under the control of God or Satan, and thus ignore human responsibility in problem situations. Do not blame everything either on God or Satan, but recognize the fact of human involvement.

Recognize that the powers of evil gain access to human lives in many ways. It is important to exhort people to keep away from any activity or philosophy which opens the way for demonic influence and control. This is especially so in relation to involvement in occult practices and ideas.

Give a greater place in thinking to the love and power of God than to the activities of Satan. Do not believe in Satan — rather believe in his downfall! Being more God-conscious will prevent us from giving Satan too high a place in our thinking. Do not develop a "Satan Syndrome," except in the sense of rejoicing in his defeat by Jesus Christ. Some writers refer to Satan as "it" and only acknowledge him as one who is already defeated and who will soon be crushed underfoot! (Romans 16:20).

Any involvement in this ministry must be preceded by adequate preparation and must involve genuine Christian faith and living, and knowledge of how to effectively use the soldier's armor in spiritual warfare.

Do not rush into this ministry without careful thought, and do not attempt it on your own. Work within the guidelines and regulations laid down by the church, and do not act as a lone ranger; rather be subject to the fellowship of the church, and work in cooperation with others.

Do not attempt this ministry as a quick-fix to a difficult problem, but only minister after careful diagnosis and preparation. This may involve a multi-disciplinary team approach, seeking to be involved with others who have special gifts in this area. Draw upon the experience and advice available from trained and experienced practitioners.

Ensure that any person who receives this ministry is adequately cared for after any act of deliverance, to ensure effective spiritual and personal growth.

Do not look for success in this ministry — rather serve and minister after the manner of Jesus Christ (Mark 10:45). Note carefully Jesus' words to his disciples, and rejoice in the heavenly rewards (Luke 10:20).

Do not be taken in by the lure of the spectacular and sensational, but try to be biblical and balanced. Refuse to be either a materialist or a magician.

Conclusion

Despite the many variations of interpretation and practice, and the need for caution and discernment, it is important that we keep a balanced perspective. We acknowledge the complex issues, and yet also realize the need to de-mystify the subject as much as possible. Satan and his evil forces are in reality "tiresome intruders," who can be, and need to be, put in their place. The victory has been won, and we move forward in the power of Jesus Christ, alert and aware of the enemy, but not frightened nor fascinated by it.

The words of two famous Christians help to give the needed focus:

> The best way to drive out the devil, if he will not yield to the text of scripture, is to jeer and flout him, for he cannot bear scorn. — *Martin Luther*

One does not gain much ground against the devil with a lengthy disputation, but with brief words and replies such as "I am a Christian, of the same flesh and blood as is my Lord Christ the Son of God; settle your accounts with him." Then the devil does not stay long. — *Martin Luther*

Soldiers of Christ arise and put your armor on,
Strong in the strength that God supplies through His Eternal Son,
Strong in the Lord of Hosts and in His mighty power,
Who in the strength of Jesus trusts is more than conqueror.
— *Charles Wesley*

From strength to strength go on,
Wrestle and fight and pray,
Tread all the powers of darkness down
And win the well fought day. — *Charles Wesley*

Sharing and Discussion

1. How would you respond to someone who says that it is impossible for modern people to believe in Satan, and that the idea of demons attacking people is a reversion to old superstitions?

2. Is it realistic to talk about the victory of Jesus Christ when "Satan is alive and well on planet earth" — in fact it seems he is doing pretty well if you care to look at the world's chaotic situation! In what sense has the decisive battle been won?

3. "Spiritual beings" *or* "earthly political and social structures" -- what do you think is the best way to interpret Ephesians 6: 12?

4. A friend asks you to explain the difference between oppression and possession and to give an example of each. How would you respond?

5. Are deliverance and exorcism the same? What are some of the ways these words are defined? What is the meaning which your church gives to these words?

6. Read the section on the causes of demonic oppression and possession. Which are the most significant causes? What causes have you experienced or read about in your understanding of the deliverance ministry?

7. List the possible signs which could indicate the need for deliverance.

8. Michael Harper says that "Our warfare against Satan is no substitute for true repentance." What does he mean? Why is this important?

9. What does "spiritual warfare" involve if we are going to be effective against the wiles of Satan?

10. Read the section on naming the demons. What are the strong and weak points of this method?

11. A friend asks you to explain what actually happens in a deliverance; that is, how is it done? Explain your response by using the 5 "R's" suggested by Parker (recognition, repentance, renunciation, release, renewal).

12. Read again the guiding principles for deliverance ministry. Which of these principles need to be emphasized today? Why?

References for Further Reading

Amid the very wide range of available material, the following are recommended:

Arnold, C. E., *Powers of Darkness,* IVP, Leicester, 1992.

Brown, B., *The Uniting Church and the Ministry of Deliverance,* Consultative Committee on Healing, Synod of Victoria, Uniting Church in Australia, Melbourne, 1992.

Green, M., *I Believe In Satan's Downfall,* Eerdmans, Grand Rapids, 1981.

Harper, M., *Spiritual Warfare,* Logos International, New Jersey, 1970.

Horrobin, P., *Healing Through Deliverance,* Sovereign World, Chichester, 1991.

Kraft, C., *Defeating Dark Angels,* Sovereign World, Kent. 1993.

Kraft, C., *Confronting Powerless Christianity.* Baker, 2002.

McNutt, F., *Deliverance From Evil Spirits,* Chosen Books, Baker, Grand Rapids, Michigan, 1996.

Murphy, E., *The Handbook for Spiritual Warfare,* Thomas Nelson, Nashville, Tennessee, 1992.

Pearson, M., *Christian Healing,* Chosen Books, Revell, Old Tappan NJ, 1990, Chapter 7.

Perry, M., *Deliverance,* SPCK, London. 1987.

Parker, R., *The Occult,* IVP, Leicester, 1989.

Richards, J., *But Deliver Us From Evil,* Darton, Longman & Todd, London, 1974.

Richards, J., *Spiritual Warfare,* Network, No. 5, Floreat Flame Books, Mirrabooka, undated.

Sherlock, C., *Overcoming Satan*, Grove Spirituality Series No. 17, Grove Books, Bramcote, Nottingham, 1986.

Twelftree, G., *Christ Triumphant*, Hodder and Stoughton, London, 1985.

Uniting Church in Australia, *Study Documents and Reports on the Deliverance Ministry*, Department for Mission and Parish Services, Queensland Synod, Brisbane, 1989.

Wagner, C. P., & Pennoyer, F. P., *Wrestling with Dark Angels*, Regal, California, 1990.

Woolmer, J., *Healing and Deliverance*, Monarch, Crowborough, 1999.

13
WHAT ABOUT THOSE WHO ARE NOT HEALED?

Selwyn Hughes is the Director of Crusade for World Revival, and has presented counseling and encouragement seminars in many different countries. He is also involved in the healing ministry and has written a book, *God Wants You Whole*. In the book's preface, Hughes speaks of the fact that his own wife has not received healing.

> I set out to write this book five years ago, but when my wife Enid was taken ill with what is known as Simmons disease, I abandoned it. I said to myself, `I can hardly write a book on the subject of healing when my own wife is sick. I'll wait until she is better, and then write it.'"

> Enid did not get better. And now, five years later, there is little evidence of healing. In fact, her doctors have diagnosed that in addition to Simmons disease she also has pernicious anemia and pancreatitis.

> A good deal of prayer has been offered for Enid, yet she is unhealed. Her sickness is not being healed, but it is certainly being used. Although I have prayed and exercised as much faith as I have in relation to Enid's condition, I am not able to explain why, up to this moment, my wife has not been healed. Over the 34 years I have been a minister, I have seen God work countless physical miracles in the lives of people. I have prayed for hundreds of people and seen them restored to health. But my prayers for my wife seem to be unavailing.

> Quite frankly, I do not know all the reasons why some are

healed and some are not. Some of the reasons are clear to me, while others are still unrevealed. Doubtless we will have to wait until eternity to fully comprehend the reasons why healing does not come for some people. One preacher summed up the problem by saying that the subject of healing is one of the greatest mysteries in the universe. We are big enough to ask the questions, but not big enough to understand all the answers.[1]

Reflect on Hughes' comments. Would his wife's lack of healing weaken the arguments contained in the book? Would it affect your reading of the book?

This chapter aims to:

- Clarify some of the issues involved when people are not healed.

- Consider some of the explanations given to explain non-healing.

- Suggest ways to respond to the reality of non-healing.

The experience of Selwyn Hughes opens up the problem of the un-healed, or those for whom prayer is offered; who receive the various ministries of healing; such as laying on of hands, anointing, and Holy Communion, but who are not healed from their sickness in any discernible way. It is a problem which causes confusion in the minds of many people. Some people give up any involvement in the healing ministry because healing does not come to those for whom they have prayed, some cease to pray for themselves and others because healing does not come, and others don't really see any problem at all as they explain the lack of healing by declaring that it is all due to insufficient faith. The problem of those who are unhealed is acknowledged by all involved in the healing ministry and several writers have attempted to give various reasons.[2]

In considering the different explanations, it is helpful to think of possible hindrance areas which block healing. There are at least four broad hindrance areas under which the various reasons can be placed.[3]

Hindrances to healing can occur in the society in which we live, in the church, in the person needing healing, and within the healing ministry itself — in those who are praying for and believing for another person's healing. Before these various hindrance areas are considered, two important facts need to be stated in relation to this issue of the lack of healing.

Firstly, we should accept that it is God's normal will that people be healed. In the teaching and practice of Jesus it is clear that sickness was seen as an evil to be confronted and healed. Jesus never gave the impression that sickness was to be accepted as a blessing, or a "cross to be borne," or a means of deeper spiritual growth and commitment. Jesus clearly distinguished between the suffering which results from persecution (which all Christians are to accept), and the sickness which has its source in Satan's opposition to God and in human disobedience and sin. Jesus taught that opposition and persecution was to be expected, and therefore suffering would be part of true discipleship. But sickness was to be healed. Healing the sick was an essential part of the commission given to his disciples, and this remains the commission for his followers today (Luke 9:1-2, 10:9).

It is true that in some situations God may use the experience of sickness to achieve His particular purposes, but our starting point is that sickness is contrary to His will and purpose and that God's normal will is that people will be healed. (See Chapter 5, Sickness, Suffering and the Will of God.)

Secondly, healing must be defined as wholeness and not only physical cure. It may be possible for a person to remain unhealed in some aspect of physical health, and yet to be whole within themselves. Physical cure therefore should not be seen as the total meaning of healing. It is a significant aspect, but not the total experience of wholeness.

Hindrances Blocking Healing

Attitudes and Influence of Society

Each person is strongly influenced by the society in which he or she lives. Social norms, attitudes, values, and accepted responses are absorbed and reflected in our thinking and behavior. Often this process is unnoticed, and unless we take steps to prevent this influence, we are shaped and molded by the social setting in which we participate. In Western society, three aspects are very significant in relation to our understanding of healing and the healing ministry.

We live in a very secular world, which is dominated by a scientific and technological approach which seeks to explain everything in analytical, logical, material and scientific ways. We distrust or reject anything that cannot be explained in these terms, and this can lead to a lack of recognition of spiritual values and realities. Prayer and other spiritual therapies and resources do not fit into these secular categories, and are therefore rejected as unscientific and of little or no value in the real world.

General social attitudes toward sickness can have a negative influence. Often sickness brings out negative emotions like fear, anger, depression, withdrawal, and others. These attitudes can quickly extinguish hope and are easily passed on to others, for example, through words and actions of discouragement. This will prevent people from seeing any positives in a threatening situation, especially if the illness is severe and possibly terminal. Negative attitudes may be in the sick person, or in family or friends surrounding the sick person. Sometimes people will not seek healing because they fear they may not be healed, and they may end up worse off. (Why have your hopes raised, only to have them dashed again?)

A third negative influence may be in relation to the high place of medical science and the belief that the only valid way of healing is through accepted medical practices. Some medical workers act as if there is no other way, no room for healing apart from rigid adherence to the prescribed treatment from medical doctors. The medical profession and health services are rightly given an important place in modern society. Their contribution to the health of any community is acknowledged and gratefully appreciated. However, the over-emphasis on physical health which dominates many societies can give the medical profession an almost God-like character, so that any other alternative therapy or approach to healing which is outside the accepted medical procedure is suspect. Fortunately, many medical workers are acknowledging the limitations of orthodox medical treatment and are open to new possibilities and treatments for healing. (See Chapter 9, Healing and Medical Science — Pills or Prayer or Both?)

Hindrances Within the Church

There can be a lack of corporate faith in the church as to the validity and effectiveness of the healing ministry. This lack of faith may stem from a particular theological and biblical interpretation that healing and the healing miracles belong to the past, and are something which belonged to the early stage of church history and are not meant for the present time. Or, it can be the belief that the gift of healing has ceased, and that any healing today is therefore invalid. Such interpretations can lock the healing ministry into a particular time in history; such as the age of the apostles and the establishment of the church, with no contemporary relevance. Where this interpretation is constantly taught, then there is a general weakening of expectation in relation to healing, and the whole ministry can become suspect. These negative interpretations can be strengthened by any exaggerated and unproven claims by healers within the healing ministry, and the fact that some of the biblical and theological interpretations used by healers display a lack of sound knowledge of the scriptures.[4]

Some leaders within the church fear the loss of professional and theological credibility and the respect of their colleagues in ministry if they openly support the healing ministry. Often the genuine theological questions raised by the ministry of healing are not treated seriously either by those who support such a ministry or by those who oppose it. As stated in the preface, there are few substantial courses in most theological schools and Bible colleges which treat the subject of healing seriously, and if it is considered at all, it is often relegated to the "Cinderella" department in theological studies. It will be difficult for any renewed understanding and practice of the healing ministry to be a reality while it remains on the theological fringes.

Many within the church, both clergy and laity, do not really accept the teachings of scripture as relevant and valid for today. For example, the healing stories in the gospels are often seen as stories from the first century, from which we gain some spiritual and moral insight, but not meant to be taken literally and applied to today's situation. If they are treated seriously, they are often interpreted in spiritual terms; for example, healing of the sick is often interpreted as healing of the sin-sick soul, and there is very little attempt to treat the healing stories as significant for the church today in relation to actual physical, mental and psychological healing.

In the church as in society, particularly Western society, there is a general acceptance of a secular world-view which interprets and confines the supernatural in terms that can be understood and explained in scientific and technological categories and language. Where these attitudes exist, they lead to diminished emphasis on the healing ministry and make it difficult for healing to become a reality in the church.

Hindrances Within the Person Needing Healing

Many people are unable to receive healing, or be open to the possibility, because of the thoughts and ideas they carry in their minds.

This especially relates to many common conceptions of God, who is often seen as one who inflicts pain, suffering and sickness on people as a just punishment for their sins. There is little understanding of God as the compassionate father, and this often results in a blocking off of any expectation of God bringing healing to their lives. Francis MacNutt deals with this problem when he writes:

> We desperately need to return to the vision of the God revealed in and by Jesus Christ; a tender, loving and compassionate God who raises us up and makes us whole wherever we have been cast down by the world of evil — whether we have sinned and need forgiveness, or are sick and need physical healing. Even now the kingdom of God is among us, saving and healing and destroying the kingdom of evil. In short, the nature of God as manifested visibly in Jesus Christ, is love.[5]

It is this inability to relate to and trust in a loving father which can form a strong barrier to healing in our lives. Sometimes God has to heal a person's theology before He can heal his or her life. Where our theology remains unhealed, then often healing and wholeness cannot occur.

One particular belief which can hinder healing is that when sickness comes to us, it should be accepted as God's will, so we should become resigned to it. Sometimes people refer to sickness as "their cross" which God has given to them. But in the New Testament, the cross is never seen as sickness. A cross is something which we take up ourselves (Matthew 10:38). It relates to commitment and may involve persecution and suffering, but it is not to be equated with sickness.

The person may not receive healing because they have not sought the appropriate medical help. The healing ministry does not set itself over against the work of doctors and others in the healing profession. Rather, the healing ministry believes that the work of the doctor and medical science is one of the gifts which God has given, and part of the healing process.

Sometimes the person's motivation for healing is not strong, and some may even wish to hold on to their illness because they have an emotional investment in it. For some, sickness is a means of gaining attention, sympathy, or the concern of other people. Healing could mean that they must start a new way of life, accept new responsibility, and this would be too demanding for them. So, the word which Jesus addressed to the man by the pool, "Do you want to be healed?" (John 5:6) is something that must be faced by each sick person.

Within a person's life there may be sinful attitudes or habits, particularly in the area of resentment and lack of forgiveness toward others.

For example, the lifestyle of the person may be preventing healing, in that the person is not using either body or mind in the way that God intended, but is misusing his or her body and ignoring the plain laws of health in relation to such matters as diet, thought patterns and physical exercise.

There can be an over-emphasis on the problem so that the person is not able to develop any expectation of healing. All the person's thoughts and words relate to the problem. They talk about it all the time, worry about it all the time, and so the focus of their attention is on the problem rather than the possible solution.

There can be a lack of faith and expectation in relation to healing. The person may feel their situation is hopeless or, out of fear, they may over-emphasize the problem or they may feel their faith is inadequate or that only a particular special healer will be able to help them. Some people go from healer to healer seeking this special help. Often their faith is misplaced. Their faith is in the healer, or sometimes in faith itself, rather than in God.

Hindrances Within the Healing Ministry Itself

There can be a lack of genuine compassion for the sick person. There is great strength in a loving community, and when many people in the community of faith share together, this releases a great volume of compassion and love, and love is the climate in which healing can take place.

Within the healing ministry there can be a misplaced faith in a special healer, or guru, who is thought to possess special gifts of healing. Others from within the fellowship of the church, who should be involved, feel that they do not have the necessary gift, and so they do not pray for the person, but they leave it to the special up-front healer. This then means that there is a reduced prayer being offered for that person because people feel inadequate in their praying.

Sometimes the wrong type of ministry is being offered, because there has not been a correct diagnosis or evaluation of the person's need. Sometimes there may be a need for counseling, or for a word of forgiveness, or occasionally for confrontation. Francis MacNutt suggests that there can be faulty diagnosis, and he points out three common failures. Prayer is offered for physical healing when inner healing is the basic need. Prayer is offered for deliverance when inner healing is the actual need. Prayer is offered for inner healing when deliverance is the primary need.[6] So it is essential to rely on the Holy Spirit and to seek discernment in understanding the real need. If the real need is not addressed, healing will not take place.

Often within the healing ministry there is a lack of time given to the sick person. Sometimes there is an attempt to do too much in too little time. Many people think that a sick person must get well quickly, and that healing must be instantaneous. Most healings however do not happen instantaneously, and quite often healing occurs as the result of a long process.

Some situations of sickness require what has been called "soaking prayer" when a person is surrounded by prayer over a long period of time. Often those involved in the healing ministry are not prepared to give long periods of time to one person. However, some situations are so serious that healing will only come as the person is surrounded by soaking prayer over an extended period of time.

Sometimes those involved in the situation work on a very limited understanding of healing. There may be such a concentration on physical healing that other aspects are ignored. Healing is wholeness, and is expressed in healthy relationships as well as in a healthy body. If relationships with God and others are broken, then these also need healing. Healing may not be given for a physical malfunction while these other aspects are ignored. There may need to be repentance, obedience, and a change of perspective before physical healing is possible. Wholeness is the goal, not only one aspect of it.

Also, it must be remembered that in one sense all healing is partial, especially physical healing. The human body will wear out and we all must die at some time. So, while it is true that we may experience *substantial* healing in this life, we are subject to groaning and weakness as a normal part of our human existence (Romans 8:22-23). We should seek healing, so that we may glorify God in all aspects of our being — body, mind, spirit, and in all our relationships. In doing this, we need to keep in tension the possibilities of true health and wholeness, and the fact that human life is limited. We should seek to be whole, and live life to the fullest while God continues to grant us daily life and strength, remembering that our lives are in His hands.

Sometimes within the healing ministry, there is a refusal to accept the reality of death as the ultimate healing. Often death is seen as defeat, whereas it should be recognized that, sometimes, healing in its fullest sense is only possible through death. Death is therefore the ultimate healing, and not necessarily a defeat. For the

Christian, death is not the great enemy, but can be seen as a great victory, because it opens up to us the more abundant life in the presence of Christ. Rev. Andrew Pearce, former Warden of OSL, Australia, affirmed that "the greatest healing of all takes place at death. This is quite opposite to the commonly accepted idea that death is the great enemy which is to be avoided at all costs."[7]

All these reasons may throw light on perplexing questions which arise when people are not healed. The issue of non-healing or failure in the healing ministry is one of the mysteries of the gospel which we cannot fully understand. The gospel declares that God has revealed Himself in Jesus Christ as the compassionate God whose will is to heal. But also in His wisdom, this same God keeps His own counsel so that there are some things we will never fully understand. In our present lives we see through a dark glass, or we see a poor blurred reflection (I Cor. 13:12). The Living Bible helpfully translates this verse as "We can see and understand only a little about God now, as if we were peering at his reflection in a poor mirror." The Good News Bible translates the verse "Like a dim image in a mirror." We are faced with the fact that the secret things belong to God, and His ways and judgments cannot be completely understood (Romans 11:33; Deuteronomy 29:29). God pleases to make Himself known in Jesus Christ, and yet He is also the God who in some ways chooses to remain hidden. He is both the hidden God and the revealed God. Martin Luther, the great reformer, spoke of God as both "deus absconditus" (God hidden), and "deus revelatus" (God revealed). We need to keep a balance between our understanding of God's will and our ignorance of His will. God's ways and thoughts are not ours (Isaiah 55:8), and despite the many insights that God gives in relation to healing, ultimately there is much that we do not understand.

The subject of failure in healing needs to be acknowledged, for whenever this is denied, an element of phoniness can creep into the ministry and many people will distance themselves from this ministry, because their honest questions have been dismissed or answered in a simplistic way. To assert that the final answer is with God is not a refusal to face the issues, rather it is an honest response that after much thought and prayer has been given, and some possible answers have been suggested, ultimately the answer is with God. God is the One who can be trusted to work out His good will and purpose for each person.

How then can we respond when healing does not seem to come? Bishop Owen Dowling suggests that there are *four* things we can do.[8]

- We can accept the situation as a stretching or testing of our faith, which presents the challenge to persevere in prayer and compassion for the sick person.

- If we feel we do not have enough faith, we should ask others to add their faith to ours, and to exercise faith for us and with us, so that faith is added to faith. We need to accept and depend upon the faith of others, and not try to do it all ourselves. We have to allow others to believe for us, if we feel that our faith is unable to function properly in relation to this particular sickness. We need help with our unbelief, and we need others to assist us.

- We need to keep on trusting God as we reach out and receive help from others. This recognizes that we do not have all the answers, and we share our sense of need, and perhaps also our confusion and puzzlement. We accept the mystery and acknowledge that we simply do not know why some people get better and some do not. Our role is to continue to cooperate with what we believe is God's purpose for wholeness, health and salvation. This will mean continuing to pray faithfully and expectantly; it will mean trying to think through and research some of the reasons for non-healing; it will mean sharing our thoughts and insights with others, and through all this to keep on trusting God, even if we do not have all the answers to the problem.

- We need to accept that, in each situation, something is happening, even though it may be different from what we desire and what the sick person also desires. Whenever people are prayed for and that person comes to Christ with a receptive mind and spirit, then we can be assured that Christ blesses and helps that person in some way. Many involved in the healing ministry affirm that there are few who, having properly understood spiritual healing, then turn from God because they are not healed.

Emily Gardiner Neal cites the experience of a rector of an Episcopal Church:

> In my years of work in the healing ministry . . . I have yet to see anyone who has lost faith because physical healing was not received, and this obtains also for the members of any family which has lost a loved one. I have never known such a family to be bitter because we prayed and built up false hopes. Instead the loved ones tell me gratefully how the patient was without pain; how he grew discernibly closer to the Lord, and how the family was strengthened and comforted.[9]

Neal then affirms that "all who are physically sick, whether or not their bodies are cured, can received spiritual healing, which dwarfs by comparison any healing of the body."[10]

This would be supported by many involved in the healing ministry. Whilst it may be thought, and is often said, that people's faith and trust will be destroyed if they are not healed, the evidence suggests that this does not occur in most situations. Of course there will be exceptions to this, but there are many testimonies that people who have been ministered to, have entered into a deeper experience of God's grace and have come to a richer understanding of life, even though a particular form of healing was not experienced. Where the meaning of healing has been adequately explained, few people seem to be shattered by a lack of healing. It is often those who look on as spectators who experience the problem most acutely.[11]

In conclusion, the mystery of non-healing remains and many answers can be suggested. Some of them will be valid in some situations, others will be invalid. But the mystery remains. Therefore, each person is challenged to continue to reflect on this issue and continue to share and discuss the many reasons why people may not be healed.[12]

Sharing and Discussion

1. Share your own experiences and understanding of non-healing. Have you ever prayed for others, or been prayed for yourself, without any apparent healing resulting? How did you feel about this, and how did you resolve the issue?

2. After your initial personal reflection, discuss the following question with others. Do you think Selwyn Hughes was right in continuing to write a book on healing even though his own wife was not healed? Would it be more honest to refrain from writing? Would the fact of his wife's sickness weaken his presentation of the healing ministry?

3. Which of the four hindrances have you seen in situations where there has been no healing?

4. Discuss the idea of death as the "ultimate healing." How can you convey this understanding to people who live in a society which generally ignores the reality of death and which sees "living a healthy life in the here and now" as all important.

5. Discuss the suggestion by Owen Dowling that there are "four things we can do" when we are faced with non-healing, either for ourselves, or for others. Which of these have you found helpful? Have you also found other ways to help in this situation? Share your experiences with others.

6. Read the extracts from Emily Gardiner Neal. How do you respond

to the claim that something always happens, even though we may not understand or see it in ways we expect or desire? Is this a cop-out, which ignores the truth, and is simply covering the problem by using spiritual clichés, or is this a profound truth? Can you share any experience which supports her words, or throws some doubt on her claims?

References for Further Reading

Althouse, L., *Rediscovering the Gift of Healing*, Abingdon, Nashville, 1977, pp. 83-86.

Cosslett, N., *His Healing Hands*, Hodder and Stoughton, London, 1985, Chapter 10.

Hillman, R., *There is Hope, Anzea*, Homebush West, Sydney, 1992.

MacNutt, F., *Healing*, Hodder and Stoughton, London, 1988, Chapter 18.

Moonie, P., "The Problem of the Unhealed," *For His Love's Sake*, OSL, Australia, undated, Chapter 8.

Pearson, M., *Christian Healing*, Chosen Books, Baker, 1990. Chapter 4.

Wagner, J. K., *Blessed to be a Blessing*, The Upper Room, Nashville, 1980, Chapter 5.

Wimber, L., *Power Healing*, Hodder and Stoughton, London, 1987, Chapter 8.

Wright, F., *The Pastoral Nature of Healing*, SCM-Canterbury Press, London, 1985, Chapter 3.

14
HEALTH AND HEALING — THE WIDER SOCIAL DIMENSIONS

One of the definitions of health in Chapter 1 focused on the wider aspects which must be included in any understanding and practice of healing. The definition proposed by the Christian Medical Commission of the World Council of Churches defines health as:

A dynamic state of well-being of the individual and society, of physical, mental, spiritual, economic, political and social well-being; of being in harmony with each other, with the material environment and with God.[1]

In our consideration of healing up to this point, we have mainly focused on individual sickness and healing, and have attempted to understand the significance of the healing ministry largely in relation to personal needs. It is now important to balance this individual emphasis with a focus on some of the social aspects of healing and reflect on their meaning for a comprehensive understanding of Christian healing. This may be unfamiliar territory for some, because overall, the emphasis in the healing ministry has not been focused on the broader social aspects of healing. However, it is an important issue and deserves careful consideration, even though it may raise questions for which there are not yet clear answers.

In recent years this concern about the wider meaning of health and healing has been carefully examined.[2] For example, since 1980, the Christian Medical Commission of the World Council of Churches has conducted several regional consultations on this theme in Africa, Europe, Asia, Latin America, Australia and the Pacific. Reports of these consultations have focused on the meaning of health and healing in particular situations, many of which are in the "third undeveloped world" or what is now called the non-Western/developing world. In most of these situations people do not have the same technological infrastructure that Western countries take for granted, and their standard of living is often much lower than what Western nations expect as a right. Some reports from these consultations will be used in this chapter to assist in our reflection on the wider aspects of healing.

Respond to the following three situations:

You are working in one of the crowded shantytowns of a large seaside city in a developing country in Asia. The squatter village, as it is known by the locals, is situated close to the busy port and factory areas. Many thousands of people cram into this area; living in very crowded conditions, in houses made of materials scrounged from garbage dumps or bought cheaply from manufacturers' castoffs. The water supply is inadequate, with two taps serving several hundred people who have to spend hours each day waiting to fill their buckets. There is no effective sanitation in the settlement and the people who live close to the sea use it as their toilet. There are two small medical centers which try to help the sick, but the supply of drugs and medicine is never sufficient to meet all the needs. Most of the men in the village are port and factory workers, and their wages go entirely to purchase necessities of food and clothing for their families. Wages are very low, and many workers feel they are exploited by the wealthy business leaders. As you look at their living conditions, you begin to see how all these are connected: poverty, disease, sickness, overcrowding, wall-to-wall people, economic exploitation, and need!

Yet some of the residents of the shantytown are cheerful and show strong courage in difficult circumstances. They attend a small church in the village, and the worship times are full of joy and encouragement. The gifts of the Holy Spirit are thankfully accepted and used, including the gift of healing. Many in the church regularly pray for people to be healed, and ask for prayer themselves.

This joyful worship is in contrast to most of the people of the shantytown, who believe that they are in this bad situation because the spirits are punishing them for evil things they have done, both in the past and present.

One of the church elders, Alphonso (a factory worker living with his wife and large family in two small rooms with no heating and poor facilities), comes to you and asks this question: "My friend, we have been talking about healing and wholeness and this idea of *shalom*. My wife and I are really keen on this, and we constantly pray for ourselves and our children to be whole. But alas, we are often sick, and no matter how hard we try, we can't seem to stay well. Is something wrong with our prayers? Are the other people right when they say the spirits are attacking us? Is this healing and wholeness you talk about possible in this situation? Why are we so often sick?"

How would you respond to Alphonso? Is "wholeness" possible in this situation? What could be done to make healing and wholeness more of a reality?

In Liberia, in northern Africa, the Christian Health Association organizes special health workshops for church evangelists and teachers. As they go from village to village they pass on this knowledge to the people. In the village of Ndambo, the evangelists (the regular preachers of the gospel) worked with the people to try and overcome some of the health problems. They explained how people could make special home-made solutions to help when their children became sick with diarrhea dehydration. They also helped to dig wells to provide safe drinking water and to reduce the incidence of diarrhea among the people.

Through proper education about immunization and nutrition, the Christian Health Association was able to reduce the infant mortality rate in the village. So the people of Ndambo learned that health is not just a medical matter, but that the community could gain control over diseases that formerly struck fear in their hearts. Gradually the people of Ndambo began to understand and experience the down-to-earth message of God's love because their children were not dying as they had before.[3]

Is this health message an essential part of the Good News which the evangelists should be offering to the people, or really just an optional extra to the gospel of God's love in Jesus Christ? What does "wholeness" mean in this situation?

In the Marshall Islands, where sixty-six atomic bombs were tested many years ago, people still suffer from long term effects of radiation, such as thyroid cancer, leukemia, and congenital birth defects. Many residents relocated to safer but much less fruitful habitations as their islands became contaminated. Thus, they have become dependent for their survival on outside help, exchanging sovereignty for money. Healthy eating habits have been replaced by the unhealthy consumption of canned and junk food, resulting in a higher incidence of obesity, diabetes and hypertension.

The testing site at Kwajalein Atoll, which originally supported a large and generally healthy community, is now a prohibited "wasteland" as far as the people are concerned. Eight thousand former inhabitants of that atoll crowd on to a much smaller island a few miles away, creating an ugly slum in the vast expanse of the Pacific.[4]

What are the wider dimensions of healing and wholeness in this situation? What practical actions are needed to make "shalom" possible?

This chapter aims to:

* Consider three models of health and sickness and understand the perspectives on which they are based.

* Understand the wider social aspects of healing, and the relationship between healing and issues such as justice and peace.

- Evaluate the Western emphasis on individualism in relation to health and healing, and consider the possibilities for and challenges to the church in becoming a truly healed and truly healing community.

Our understanding of the dimensions of healing and wholeness are determined by what we think about people, what we think about the meaning and cause of sickness and disease, and what we think is the most effective way to bring healing and health to those who are sick. Put simply, the answers we give to three basic questions strongly influence our overall understanding and practice of healing:

- Who is this person who is sick? What is our understanding of the person?

- Why is this person sick? What is our understanding of the causes of sickness and disease?

- What is the best treatment or help to overcome this sickness? What is our understanding of the solution?

In contemporary Western society, there are three main models for understanding sickness and healing. They are the *medical, psychological,* and *social* models. Although there is some overlap, each of these models has a particular perspective which gives different answers to the above questions, and results in different emphases in practice.[5]

Models of Sickness and Health

The Medical Model

People in Western and developed countries are familiar with this model because it underlies our thinking about sickness and health. It is the main working model for the major health agencies and institutions in our society. The medical model includes the following:[6]

- There is a concentration on the physical body which is seen as an integrated machine needing to be fixed or repaired if it breaks down or is damaged.

- Illness is described in terms of biology, chemistry and physics (often unintelligible to the non-professional!).

- Illness is a deviation from the normal working of the machine and is caused by germs or other "nasties," which are independent entities attacking the body from outside (and thus gaining access to the machine).

- Illness is something which attacks and affects each individual machine, causing it to malfunction.

- Treatment consists in a skilled person "intervening" to repair the damage usually through the use of drugs, surgery and medication.

- If there are no effective treatments available to cure or repair the particular damage, then we look forward in hope because scientific research will eventually (preferably sooner rather than later) produce the necessary drug or procedure.

- There is no blame or shame attached to any sickness, because it is something which happens from outside the sick person.

The medical model is very influential in contemporary society, as it provides a vast range of intervention possibilities for almost every disease. Most people trust the model, and also trust those who represent the model to the public — doctors, specialists, nurses and other health care workers. Over the last two centuries this model has become the common and dominant understanding of illness and its treatment in most technologically developed societies.

Some of the problems of this model have already been mentioned (see Chapter 9). There are three main problem areas arising out of the model, in relation to the wider dimensions of healing:

- The model tends to be individualistic in its evaluation of people, illness and treatment. The focus is on the individual person, as a "malfunctioning machine" which needs to be repaired, so that it can function effectively.

- The medical model can show more interest in obtaining a cure than in actually caring for the person. So, in order to show the benefits of technological and scientific discovery, treatments can be prescribed which may be of very little help in giving quality of life and care to the patient. It may even seem as though the sick person becomes a means to an end: the use of the latest scientific breakthrough!

- The model tends to isolate disease from the wider social factors which can be very important in the cause and treatment of disease. It also often ignores the fact that we do not live and move as individuals, but as part of a social community.

The Psychological Model

Whilst accepting the fact that physical and organic factors are important in understanding any illness, this model believes that by themselves such perspectives are inadequate in understanding the person and his or her needs. People are not satisfactorily explained in terms of biology and chemistry, but other mental, emotional, and spiritual perspectives must be recognized. The use of the word "psychosomatic," literally soul/mind/body, explains the fact that the type of illnesses people get, the way they describe them, how it affects them, and the way they try and deal with it are all strongly affected by their mental perceptions and reactions. Pattison comments that:

There is no shortage of evidence to show how psychological factors, such as perception, emotional life, events, and character, impinge upon illness. Although the precise mechanisms of psychological and physical interaction are often obscure, *prima facie*, one would expect this kind of relationship to exist. All human life is based on physiology.[7]

Such illnesses as coronary disease and cancer have been linked to certain character types, and conditions of stress, tension, bereavement, and changed circumstances are known to contribute to problems like asthma, peptic ulcers and ulcerative colitis. Again, diseases associated with bad eating habits, smoking, and alcohol use can be largely psychological in their cause and treatment.

This model broadens the medical model, and when taken together these two models probably constitute the generally accepted understanding of sickness and disease, as most people now realize the significance of both factors. However, in correcting the narrow perspective of the medical model, the psychological model likewise tends to be very individualistic in its evaluation of people and illness; the difference being that the emphasis is not on their physical and biological make-up, but rather on their character and behavior patterns. But there is often an inadequate recognition of the wider social aspects of healing and sickness.

The Social Model

This model accepts many of the insights from the medical and psychological models but moves beyond them by stressing the importance of social factors in relation to health and sickness. The sick person is never just an individual, but always a person in a community. So, in answering the question: "Why is this person sick?" this model is not satisfied with just a biological answer, or with a character/behavior answer. Rather, it asks whether there are also social reasons why particular diseases occur.

Any investigation of societal factors affecting health show there is a close connection between a person's health and his or her living conditions, economic and social status, and belief patterns.

Living conditions have a profound effect on the quality of health. Facilities such as water supply, sanitation, housing, and air quality, are of crucial importance to community health. It is well known that many diseases are transmitted through polluted air, impure drinking water, and poor sanitation. Other factors like hygiene and nutrition are equally significant. Doctor E. Ram, Director of International Health at World Vision International and previously Director of the Christian Medical Commission, Geneva, comments:

> Throughout the world the problems of ill health are strongly related to and dependent on such factors as poverty, poor housing, poor environment, lack of safe drinking water, lack of food, malnutrition, under-nutrition, high fertility rate, illiteracy, unemployment and low income, land tenure, and inaccessibility of social services. Despite the "magic" of modern medicine and daily pronouncements of major breakthroughs in medical technology, the most basic health needs of the majority of the world's population are not met in even a rudimentary manner.[8]

Another writer, Thomas McKeown, argues that the growth of public health over the last two hundred years owes more to the recognition of, and attention to these factors, than to any developments in medicine.

> Medicine has contributed very little to the aggregate growth of public health in the last two centuries. The great epidemics of infectious diseases which used to carry off so many citizens have been eliminated more by better hygiene, nutrition, sanitation, and living conditions than by new therapeutic methods whose beneficial effects are confined to fairly narrow areas such as surgical advances.[9]

Social status can also be an important factor, because those in the lower social groups usually have less resources and opportunity for adequate health care. Inequalities of income and facilities deprive many people of a healthy lifestyle. For example, a poor family can only buy poor quality food which in turn affects their overall health. Many families cannot afford medical care and rely on outside assistance from Governments and other agencies. Factors such as war, terrorism, environmental pollution and destruction, can also be very significant in relation to health and healing.

The important thing to note is that these factors involve social and political organizations and decisions, if there is to be any real change. Improvements in water supply, housing, sanitation, wages, availability of and access to adequate medical resources are issues which must be addressed by social and political authorities. It is at this point that factors like social inequality and injustice become relevant to an understanding of health and healing.

Beliefs and cultural patterns are also very significant in understanding perspectives on health and healing. For example, many non-Western societies focus more on the cause of sickness than how to treat it. They are concerned about why a person is sick, rather than how a person became sick. Did the person act wrongly toward others? Has he or she offended some spiritual power? Has he or she obeyed the accepted patterns of behavior?

These are some of the questions which will be asked, and these will give completely different answers compared to the scientific understanding of modern Western biomedicine.

So a person's world-view is of crucial importance, that is, how the person understands the world in which he or she lives, and how each will relate to it and make sense of it. A person's attitude to sickness and health flows directly from this understanding which itself is formed by his or her involvement in particular social and cultural situations.[10]

How does a Christian understanding of health and healing respond to these three models? It accepts the valid insights from each model, but also recognizes the inadequacy of any model which ignores other legitimate perspectives. In practice, it means that any evaluation of health and healing must take note of the complex nature of sickness, and be prepared to examine all the relevant factors involved when a person becomes sick. This is especially so in relation to social factors which are often ignored by many Christians, especially those who live in Western developed countries.

It is important to note that this broadening of the "healing map" worries some Christians, who think that this stretching of the factors involved in healing is invalid from a biblical perspective. They believe that the biblical emphasis is directed to the individual, especially in the healing work of Jesus, which usually involves the sick person and Jesus as the healer. They maintain that there is very little explicit social content in the many stories of healing in both Old Testament and New Testament. Rather, some feel that this "broadening" emphasis is just a contemporary push of social-minded liberal thinkers, who are "into" the latest ideas about equality and environmental issues, and the catch-all bag of social justice! Some believe there is little if any connection between this wider social dimension, and the essential healing offered in the gospel and experienced through the power of the Holy Spirit. These criticisms need to be evaluated in order to appreciate the significance of these wider issues for our understanding and practice of the healing ministry.

The Social Dimension of Healing

The Biblical Witness to Healing

In much popular thinking it is accepted that the biblical promises of healing are directed to individual people, and this is how many Bible verses and stories are interpreted. For example, Exodus 15:26 "I am the Lord who heals you" is usually applied to individuals, even though the original statement was given to the community as a whole. Also, the healing incidents in the ministry of Jesus are given an individual emphasis. For example, "I tell *you*, take up *your* mat and go home" (Mark 2:11); "*Your* faith has healed *you*" (Luke 8:48); "Do *you* want to get well?" (John 5:6). It is true that the promises of healing are to be applied to personal lives and that the healing work of Jesus had profound meaning for the individual. This must be clearly emphasized, or the meaning of the promises and the stories are distorted. However, it is also true that each individual and personal healing had profound social implications which affected the community around the solitary individual. An example will show this. When Jesus healed the leper (Luke 5:12-16), this involved at least four different aspects of healing.

- *Physical healing* as the person's body was restored.

- *Psychological healing* as the person's self-image was re-made, possibly after years of rejection.

- *Spiritual healing* as the person was now able to be part of the community's religious practices and worship God as part of the people of faith.

- *Social healing* as the person was restored to family and community relationships which before had been barred.

For healing or wholeness to be experienced, each of these aspects needed to be addressed.

The same dimensions can be seen in the story of the woman with the flow of blood (Mark 5:21-34; Luke 8:40-48) and many other healing incidents in the ministry of Jesus. If we approach these stories with a wider perspective, new aspects of healing are discovered, even though they may not be mentioned in the actual text itself. If we approach the stories from a purely individualistic angle, then that is all we will see, but in doing so we will have separated the healing event from its wider personal, social and religious significance.

In his healings, Jesus impacted upon all levels of society, but especially the poor, blind, lame, deaf, the lepers and the demon-possessed. These chronically ill people were at the bottom of the social scale and were discriminated against socially as well as religiously (especially when their condition was attributed to sin: John 9:2). So when Jesus brought healing; he gave life, hope and salvation; he also empowered the helpless and hopeless in a new way. This was an essential part of the person's restoration to "wholeness" and "shalom." Luke portrays Jesus as:

> The one who refuses to recognize any social, ethnic, political or religious barriers. In his boundary-breaking ministry, Jesus embraces all. In doing so, he affirms them; more importantly, he empowers them. The insignificant and oppressed people of Israel, the poor, the bonded slaves, the leper, the women, the children, the enemies of Israel, Gentiles and Samaritans, those regarded as "sell-outs", the tax collectors; all of those who were accustomed to cringing in the presence of the social and religious establishment, are empowered to lift up their heads and hold them high, to recognize their own dignity, and to begin to see themselves in a new light. After their encounter with Jesus they are transformed into people who know themselves to be God's children.[11]

So while healing was an intensely personal experience, it also had profound social implications, as healed people were restored to community with others. Healing and community are thus closely linked. As previously stated, Jesus responded to people in community, and not just as abstract individuals. He came to transform the whole of human experience, and in that process he challenged everything that was oppressive and demeaning.

This link between healing and community can also be seen from another perspective; not only did the healing affect the community, but the community social factors were in themselves one of the causes of the problem; that is, they often created the need for healing. As with many developing countries today, social conditions in biblical times were often a potent factor in the sicknesses which people experienced. Poverty, oppression, exploitation, social injustice, occupation by a controlling power, lack of medical knowledge and resources; these were part of the total situation and would have had similar effects then, as these factors do today.

But did Jesus actually address these social factors in his healing ministry? A surface reading of Jesus words and actions could suggest that Jesus did not directly address these wider issues, and therefore was more focused on the individual person and their healing and salvation. However, that is to read the gospel stories from a western individual perspective, rather than from the perspective of what was actually happening in the cultural and social situation of the New Testament. The healings Jesus offered touched all aspects of a person's life and so laid the foundation for new social and community relationships as well as individual relationships with God. In his statement of his mission, Jesus applied the words of the prophet Isaiah to his own ministry, and spoke of a deliverance which involved the broken hearted, the poor, the captives, the oppressed — all social as well as individual conditions (Luke 4:18-19, 7: 21-23). Jesus' approach was the outworking of the "shalom" principle of the Old Testament which related to all aspects of personal and community life.

The scriptures of the Old Testament are socially aware as well, and address both individuals and the nation as a whole. The strong health regulations given to Israel, for example, in Leviticus chapters 11-19, reflect the desire of God for each individual and the whole community to be healthy in all respects: physically, psychologically, socially and spiritually. Individual health and social health were intertwined together and could not be separated.

The Old Testament prophets declared God's will to the people and they castigated the rich upper classes for their failure to apply their worship to social situations. Social inequalities and injustice were rampant as the wealthy classes of society exploited and misused the poorer classes. By these actions "shalom" was destroyed because people lived as selfish individuals and deliberately ignored their social responsibility to care for each other (Isaiah 58:1-10; Micah 6:6-8; Amos 2:6-7, 5:21-24). As a result of such selfishness and irresponsibility, the people of Israel as a whole became sick and unhealthy — socially, politically, morally, spiritually, and, especially in the underprivileged and depressed lower classes, often physically.

The contemporary situation

The close connection between social factors and health and healing can be clearly seen in many contemporary situations. In speaking of the need for social justice in health care, Dr. E. A. Allen, the Director of Services in Bethel Baptist Church in Kingston, Jamaica, reports that:

> The person is a social being as much as he is a psychological and physical being . . . In my medical and psychiatric experience, social alienation or loneliness on the one hand and social oppression on the other, are extremely common aspects of most psychological illness and problems. They also contribute to several physical disorders as well.[12]

In relation to the general state of health services in the world, Dr. David Morley, an authority in international community health, believes that poverty and lack of education due to injustice are the greatest causes of disease in today's world, despite the amazing advances in medical technology. Dr. Morley compares the health budgets in developed and undeveloped countries:

> Whereas US $400 is spent per person on health in the

developed countries, only US $4 is spent on the average individual in the Third World. This trend is reflected in the fact that most people in the world today do not have access to adequate health care. Nevertheless, within most countries, even the poorest countries, those of good means can enjoy almost first-rate medical care. Medical care is increasingly the domain of the drug companies, private hospital corporations, and medical technology manufacturers — not of the people.[13]

A recent headline in a report from the World Bank underscored the connection between poverty and poor health:

"POOR MISS OUT ON A HEALTHIER WORLD"

While health care around the world has improved dramatically in recent years, the poor are still ravaged by destructive diseases. The high cost of treatment and the increasing use of drugs like tobacco are reaping a grim harvest as tobacco and other companies turn to developing countries for their customers, thus setting the stage for added illness. The World Bank report notes that tobacco-related deaths from heart disease and cancer are likely to double by 2010 to two million a year; and if present smoking patterns continue, they will grow to more than twelve million a year by 2050. This highlights an area of exploitation by affluent, profit-seeking Western companies, which is a direct cause of ill health for millions of people. This pattern of abuse must be addressed along with the basic flaw of inequality.

. . Basic flaws in the global health system include a mis-allocation of public funds on health strategies . . . a disproportionate amount of government spending benefited the affluent, while the poor lacked access to basic health services and received low quality care . . . Nearly two million children died each year of such diseases as measles, tetanus and whooping cough that could be prevented by inexpensive vaccines . . . if developing countries, governments and donors could adopt policies that more effectively reach the poor, the potential for health improvement is enormous.[14]

Recent surveys which analyze issues of world health, poverty and injustice have found that there have been few improvements in the health situation; rather the situation has become much worse. Beginning from the World Health Organization (WHO) Declaration of 1978 (the Alma-Ata Declaration), and surveying efforts since 1980, it has been reported:

> Sadly, the aims of the WHO initiative have not been fulfilled. Poverty is increasing in most developing countries and is having a devastating impact on the physical and mental health of the majority of the worlds population, a quarter of whom, around 1.3 billion people, live in extreme poverty, and earn less than one US dollar each day. Over half of those living in sub-Saharan Africa lack a safe water supply and two thirds lack proper sanitation facilities. The mortality statistics for the poorest quarter of the human race are appalling. These people are ten times more likely to die under the age of 15 years than are those from the richest quarter of the human population. They are nine times more likely to die of infectious diseases; women are more likely to suffer early death from all causes, and, in addition, are between 10 and 100 times more likely to die in childbirth than their counterparts in affluent countries. Even the most basic requisites for healthy living are unaffordable and an estimated 190 million children under five years in age suffer from chronic malnutrition, and one million are forced into becoming street orphans each year. Millions more die of starvation that is preventable by adequate sanitation, clean water supplies and immunization programs.[15]

The stark realities of such health issues can easily become lost in statistical quagmires and erudite discussions among health experts, and often have little or no impact on many people in more developed countries. The enormity of the problem often acts as a deterrent to effective action, and the problem of "aid fatigue" or "compassion fatigue" lessens effective responses, except for special situations such as the response to the Christmas 2004 tsunami, and so forth.

So, while it is comparatively easy to multiply examples of the connection between social factors and health in developing countries, these facts appear far removed from familiar situations in highly technological and progressive Western societies like Australia, Great Britain, Canada, and the U.S.A., among other places.

Are the same issues relevant to contemporary western societies? The answer is, "Yes," it is clear that similar realities of social inequality and injustice have a very negative effect on health in our own society. For example, in a pastoral statement on the distribution of wealth in Australia, the Australian Catholic Bishops' Conference emphasized the close connection between economic disadvantage and inadequate health care.

The care of the sick is a demand of the gospel. The church has always encouraged, and now rejoices in, the progress made in modern medical science, making it possible in ways and to an extent never previously imagined, to carry out Christ's injunction to heal and care for the sick . . . **Health is one of the key structures affecting and affected by wealth distribution.**[16]

The statement refers to a national study which finds a high correlation between health and wealth. The worst health problems are found in working class people in remote areas and those without good housing, heating and adequate income. The survey concludes that:

> Good health is dependent on adequate income for food and housing much more than on medical and hospital services . . . health has little to do with the health system; there is no correlation between the use of hospitals and the health system

... there are serious problems about the just distribution of medical services despite the efforts by governments to ensure that adequate and equitable provision exists for the health needs of the population . . . In justice, those who cannot afford to pay for services have the right to necessary health, medical and hospital services . . . everyone has the right to basic health services.[17]

These realities show that health and healing cannot be divorced from issues of justice, exploitation, peace, and so on. This growing awareness is reflected in statements arising from the world regional conferences on health and healing organized by the Medical Commission of the World Council of Churches since 1980. In response to the question: "What is health?" the conclusions are:

Health is a Justice Issue

The number one cause of disease in the world is poverty, which is ultimately the result of oppression, exploitation and war. Providing immunization, medicine, and health education by standard methods cannot significantly ameliorate illness due to poverty. The churches are called on to see this as a justice issue, to be raised in the centers of power — local, national, regional, and global . . . There is a call for commitment to more just distribution of available resources for health.[18]

Health is a Peace Issue

Deaths due to armed conflict and other forms of political violence have continued to be a reality of health . . . for thousands in the world; state terrorism through low intensity conflict, torture, imprisonment, and other forms of human rights violations, has made wellness of body, mind and spirit/wholeness an impossibility. The threat of nuclear annihilation hangs over the entire globe, often suppressing life-giving hope. No medications can remedy the personal and social illness arising out of the world climate of militarism. Churches are reminded of the blessedness of being peacemakers.[19]

Health is an Issue of the Integrity of Creation

A significant proportion of illness in the world is self-inflicted. What we impose upon ourselves individually and collectively, whether out of ignorance, greed or lack of self-control, causes physical, mental, spiritual, and ecological damage which is not addressed by medical technology.

This is seen in factors like:

- Lifestyles and values which breed individualism and disrupt community life.

- Lifestyles which are destructive to health through wrong eating habits and drug use.

- The struggle for military and technological supremacy which endangers the health of the planet.

- Materialism which replaces community as a significant value.

In these situations, the church is called to advocate and protect the integrity of creation with a genuine concern for the human body and the conditions which are necessary to sustain life.[20]

Health is a Spiritual Issue

Despite the glaring social inequalities, it is true that:

Even in the midst of poverty, some people stay well, while among the world's affluent many are chronically ill. Why? Medical science is beginning to affirm the biblical emphasis on beliefs and feelings as the ultimate tools and powers for healing. Unresolved guilt, anger and resentment, and meaninglessness, are found to be very potent suppressors of the body's powerful health controlling immune system, while loving relationships in community are among its strongest augmenters. Those in loving harmony with God and neighbor, not only survive tragedy or suffering best, but grow stronger in the process. When we choose the spiritual dimension of life, we opt for the abundant life, which is wholeness-life, a gift of God.[21]

This fourfold understanding of health as relating to issues of justice, peace, environmental care, and spirituality, gives a sound foundation for tackling some of the realities relating to health and healing today. Each aspect is important and cannot be neglected. To emphasize one at the expense of the other, leads to imbalance and division in the church's use of resources. Those who opt for radical social justice, peace, and environmental issues — but ignore the spiritual realities — present a diluted understanding. At the same time, those who proclaim healing as a spiritual issue only, also offer a distorted biblical understanding of health and healing. The amount of zeal which often accompanies both of these emphases does not make up for the imbalances in these respective perspectives. The precarious situation requires a united approach, based on recognition of the validity of all of these issues.

However, this emphasis on the wider dimensions of healing, presents real difficulties for many Christians, especially those in developed Western countries. There are at least two problem areas: the fact that individualism is regarded as a sacred right, and the lack of effective ways to respond to these issues. These two aspects are considered in the remainder of this chapter.

The Problem of Individualism

In any attempt to understand illness and its treatment, it is important to realize that this is closely related to cultural values and meaning. In considering typical Western approaches, Pattison notes:

> Western biomedicine, with its scientific language and its focus on individual pathology, fits in with a generally secular view of the universe and a strong emphasis on the supreme importance of the individual as the basic unit of social discourse.[22]

This emphasis on individualism prevents many Christians from thinking about and trying to tackle some of the wider social dimensions of healing. It includes the way the Bible is interpreted almost entirely in personal, individualistic ways; the emphasis of so much contemporary worship which focuses on **God and Me**, and the abundance of literature which offers personal liberation and freedom. It is a focus on "Me-ism" which has little or no place for the idea of community and the social factors which promote community. The gospel, as the answer to individual needs only, is a product of a capitalist market, consumer economy, where the individual is supremely important both as a producer and consumer of goods. It is often reflected in the way some of the healing incidents in the ministry of Jesus are interpreted, without any attention to wider social and community factors. Thus it is common for many of the healing incidents to be re-interpreted in personal, "spiritual" terms; so that a particular sickness is seen as a type of sin or spiritual blindness or spiritual deformity, with Jesus as the healer, in the sense of spiritual healing and salvation. It may be legitimate to point out some of the spiritual lessons to be learnt from these healing incidents, but not at the expense of grappling with the actual physical, emotional and social healings which are involved. This "personalizing" and "spiritualizing" approach has resulted in the tendency of much contemporary theology and preaching to "shun man's concrete physical side in favor of more abstract theological principles and allegorical sermons about spiritual blindness and the like."[23]

An example of spiritualizing the meaning of the healing miracles

is given by R. Kent Hughes. In a sermon on the Healing of the
Leper (Mark 1:40-45), he suggests that Christ's healing miracles
were parables which portray the effect of the Holy Spirit's work in
people's lives. So when Jesus healed the blind, this was a portrayal
of his illumination of darkened hearts . . . In relation to the leper
story, Hughes comments:

> Realizing that Christ's miracles were parables, we must note
> that leprosy was especially symbolic of sin, and the healing
> of it especially of deliverance from sin. Though the leper
> was not worse or guiltier than his fellow countrymen, he
> was nevertheless a parable of sin, an outward visible sign of
> innermost spiritual corruption . . . the spiritual reality for all
> of us is that we are spiritual lepers. This is what the image is
> meant to teach us.[24]

Pattison indicates how this emphasis on individualism affects both
the understanding and practice of the healing ministry.

> This basic attitude pervades the whole of life, including
> religious life, where personal piety and individual religious
> experience are exalted over the need to develop corporate
> identity and a sense of social justice. While religious healing
> methods may take place in a corporate context, they raise
> no awkward questions about the fundamental shape of the
> social order, for they see illness as no more than personal
> sin, individual misfortune, or spiritual oppression. Religious
> healing stays strictly in the realm of the personal and private,
> offering personalized help to needy individuals. As such,
> like most medical practice, it is deeply congruent with the
> dominant social philosophy of our time, in a way that social
> action for justice on the part of Christians is not.[25]

Another writer offers a similar critique:

> Healing is an integral part of the church's ministry.

Nevertheless the Western church is deeply implicated in the very institutions, systems and lifestyles that are in question today. Theology also participates in the global crisis, to the extent that it provides support for these systems and structures.

In popular Christianity, much of the present day revival in faith healing is linked with excessive individualism and a "theology of success" that glorifies abundance, holds suffering as evidence of poor faith, and looks askance at Christians committed to a lifestyle of simplicity, self-denial and solidarity with the poor.[26]

It is true that the whole area of social analysis has often been ignored in the healing ministry. There is a very strong emphasis on the value of ministry, prayer, laying on of hands, anointing, and so on; but often very little on the actual prevention of illness, especially in relation to some of the social factors involved. So, for example, if a person who has been a smoker or moderate-to-heavy drinker genuinely seeks healing, he or she will be encouraged to be open to God in repentance and faith, and will be offered various forms of ministry. But will there be anything said or done about the industries which manufacture the disease producing substances — that is, the tobacco and liquor companies? Pattison gives a generalized and challenging critique when he asserts:

Christian healing, like much medical healing, makes the sick individual its object and concern. Illness is divorced from social structures. It can only be cured, not prevented. It is a personal misfortune, and has nothing to do with principles of justice. In taking this general line, Christianity actually reinforces the idea that illness is a personal matter, which cannot be prevented, and so passively supports the prevailing social order, whatever its cost in terms of widespread suffering throughout society.[27]

It is important to note that there are some benefits from this individualism which should not be ignored, and a spiritual emphasis helps many people cope in a society where alienation abounds and where people feel confused in an impersonal, materialistic and increasingly technological world. It affirms the importance of the individual in an increasingly complex world, and it gives meaning to situations where the secular emphasis tries to drive out the reality of God and the supernatural dimensions of life. In these ways it is a helpful emphasis, but it can become twisted into a subjective preoccupation with personal, spiritual, and healing issues, to the neglect of the wider dimensions of healing.

Therefore, anyone realistically involved in healing has to grapple with the need to balance the individual and the social aspects of this ministry. To emphasize the social issues at the expense of the individual, or to ignore the social aspects in order to promote individual health and healing — both of these responses lack credibility and fail to do justice to the biblical idea of "shalom." By themselves they are incomplete and need to be seen as belonging together. Social justice, peace, environmental concern, and a deeply personal experience of the Holy Spirit, all come together to produce the wholeness or "shalom" which is the meaning of true healing.

However, it is one thing to recognize the significance of the wider social dimensions of the healing ministry, but quite another to respond to the actual situations which are often dominated by social, political, and religious attitudes and structures, which may resist any change to familiar patterns and ideas. Can this challenge be adequately addressed?

The Church as a Healing Community

The challenge for the church and any other groups involved in the healing ministry — for example, the Order of St. Luke — is to create a genuine healing community which encourages wholeness in all its activities, and tries to move beyond its own doors into the surrounding society. The church is called to be a community of practical love, for love is the greatest motivator for healing. God heals because He loves. Love motivates concern for others and demands action where there is sickness and suffering (1 John 3:14, 16, 18). It involves a concern for justice and peace, a concern for the creation, and compassion and encouragement for people affected by illness and disease. But can such a challenge ever be more than mere rhetoric?

The various regional conferences conducted by the World Council of Churches grappled with the practical realities of these issues. There was a strong realization that nothing would happen if this issue was left in the hands of church leaders and official church bodies like synods, conferences, and assemblies. These gatherings may be able to offer impressive statements, exhorting the church to action, but nothing will really happen unless it begins at the level of the local congregation. Out of all the discussions, the following challenges were presented to each local congregation to consider:[28]

The Congregation as a Healing Community

Do not abdicate healing to the medical professionals but become involved through:

- Praying for the sick.

- Providing opportunities for confession and forgiveness.

- Laying on of hands.

- Anointing with oil.

- Sharing in Holy Communion.

- Using creative healing services.

- Supporting those involved in healing.

- Using the charismatic gifts for healing.

- Training people to be involved in a healing ministry.

The Congregation as a Caring Community

Attempting to "do good to all people, especially to those who belong to the family of believers" (Galatians 6:10) involves caring for the sick, lonely, handicapped, oppressed, and those grappling with problems like divorce, unemployment, broken family relationships, and so on.

The Congregation as a Health/Healing/Teaching Center

By encouraging Bible studies on health, healing and wholeness.

- By discovering the causes of ill health and asking important questions about biomedical ethics.

- By encouraging people to take responsibility for their health.

The Congregation as an Advocate for Justice, Peace, and the Integrity of Creation

- By encouraging public opinion (starting in the church) in support of the struggle for justice and equality in health matters.

- By working with others of goodwill and growing together in social awareness.

- By supporting the elimination of oppression, racism, class inequalities and lack of opportunities.

The Congregation as a Supporting Group

- By offering support for those involved in providing adequate health services.

This is particularly relevant for developing countries where health facilities are often very inadequate. This could mean support for aid organizations and church programs providing the basic resources which facilitate good health.

The Congregation as a Co-operating Group

- By supporting all those involved in the healing process, including health professionals, family care groups, and social welfare groups, as well as other church groups.

Some of these issues may already be addressed by local congregations, but they do provide a continuing challenge. An example is given of a congregation which tries to do this:

> The Bethel Baptist Healing Ministry in Kingston, Jamaica, is a congregation-sponsored, holistic, community-based service. It offers a setting where care is provided (in the church) by Christian medical personnel, who work together with pastors and psychologists to provide prayer and spiritual counseling as well as medicines. When the word "healing" is used, it refers to healing of the whole person by means of counseling, medicine, faith and prayer, as well as by community. Hence, the motto of Bethel's ministry "Total Healing to the Whole Person.[29]

Where does a group like the Order of St. Luke fit into this picture? It can be one of the groups God uses to encourage the church to become a truly human community. This is part of what it means to help restore the healing ministry to the normal stream of church life. As a group committed to healing and wholeness, it has an opportunity to encourage an understanding of healing which refuses to accept any one-sided approaches and seeks to promote a true understanding of wholeness. It works and prays to help people to be whole in body, mind and spirit and to work for a community where "shalom" may be experienced at least in some measure. Many may respond that this is quite impossible and is a vague pipe dream. It is true that such a goal may never be achieved, but is it worth working toward? That is the question which the healing ministry must consider as it grapples with the wider dimensions of healing.

Sharing and Discussion

1. What do you think are the strong and weak points of each of the three models of sickness and its treatment — the medical, psychological, and social models?

2. Think of your own sickness or the sickness of someone you know. What social aspects were involved for you and others in that situation — for example, family, friends, work, hospital, finance and so on?

3. Is all this talk about health being a justice, peace, environmental and spiritual issue, over-stretching the idea of healing too broadly for you, and thus weakening the biblical emphasis on individual healing and salvation?

4. Discuss how you see issues of justice, peace, poverty, equality, to be factors in health care and healing in your own community situation, and in the country as a whole.

5. How important are world-views in affecting how we think about sickness and health? Write down the main ingredients of your own world-view, that is, your basic assumptions about God, people, the world, and what sickness is. Why is it important to understand other people's world-view when we try and help them?

6. Reflect on the six points about the congregation being a healing community. Is it practical and realistic to think of a "normal" congregation being a "healing community" in the sense suggested; or is this far beyond the understanding and available resources of most congregations? What is the understanding of your own congregation?

7. Why is "individualism" so strong in our thinking and practice? How is this demonstrated in our lives and communities? Is it possible to change this way of thinking and acting?

8. Is it possible to tackle some of the BIG political, social, and economic issues relating to health and healing, or are they too complex and should be left to the "experts" to solve? Is there any way for the churches to make a significant contribution?

9. Choose some of the healing stories in the New Testament and discuss the personal, social and religious factors involved. Some suggested stories are Mark 1:40-45, Mark 2:1-12, Mark 5:21-34; John 5:1-16. After reflecting on these stories, reflect on other healing stories with "a wider" perspective.

References for Further Reading

Australian Catholic Bishops' Conference, *Common Wealth for the Common Good*, Collins Dove, Blackburn, 1992.

Allen, E. L., *et al.*, *Health, Healing and Transformation*, MARC, World Vision International, Monrovia, 1991.

Christian Medical Commission, *Healing and Wholeness*, WCC, Geneva, 1990.

Epperley, B., *God's Touch*, Westminster John Knox Press, Louisville, KY, 2001.

Heath, Faith and Healing, International Review of Mission, WCC, Geneva, Vol. 90, Nos. 356-357, Jan-April 2001, p, 87-160

Pattison, S., *Alive and Kicking* SCM-Canterbury Press, London, 1989.

Pilch, J., *Healing in the New Testament,* Fortress, Minneapolis, 2000.

Wellock, P., *In Search of Wholeness,* OSL Australia, 2005.

Epilogue

We have come to the end of our consideration of various topics relating to the healing ministry. Not all important issues in this ministry have been considered, and there is a continuing need for other issues to be addressed. In the healing ministry, different issues will continue to arise, because the problems of sickness and disease will always be part of our human life.

There will be continuing questions asked about such conditions as AIDS, Alzheimer's disease, birth defects, disabilities, and many others. Ethical and moral questions arise as new technologies and scientific breakthroughs become part of many societies. The stark problems of poverty and racial and social inequalities continue to haunt the world and point to the desperate need for wholeness and healing for all people. We shall continue to experience difficulties, both in trying to understand these situations in the light of faith, and then seeking to offer a healing ministry to those involved.

Participation in this ministry offers the privilege of being involved with people at the point of their need; being committed to be channels of divine healing; and the challenge of grappling with the puzzling questions which are part of sickness, disease and human weakness. This book has offered a foundation for a balanced, biblical approach, and you are encouraged to keep on growing in your understanding and practice of this ministry, which is at the heart of the gospel.

APPENDIX 1
THE HEALING STORIES IN THE GOSPELS

From: J. Wilkinson, *Health and Healing*, Handsel Press, Chapters 4 & 5; see also J. Wilkinson, *The Bible and Healing*, Chapter 6.

Wilkinson divides the healing events into two main categories — the healing of individuals, and the healing of groups. He also gives outlines of the type of diseases healed, the initiative for healing, and the motives for healing.

Accounts Of Healing Of Individuals

The accounts of the healing of sick or possessed individuals in which some clinical detail of the disease and its healing is given may be further classified into three distinct groups according to the nature of the healing. These groups include examples of physical healing, the exorcism of demons, and the raising of the dead. These groups may be classified as follows in accordance with their occurrence in the four gospels:

Accounts of Physical Healing

In one Gospel only

	Matthew	Mark	Luke	John
1. The two blind men	9.27-31			
2. The deaf mute		7.31-37		
3. The blind man of Bethsaida		8.22-26		

	Matthew	Mark	Luke	John
4. The woman with a spirit of infirmity			13.11-17	
5. The man with dropsy			14.1-6	
6. The ten leprosy patients			17.11-19	
7. The ear of Malchus			22.50-51	
8. The nobleman's son				4.46-54
9. The impotent man				5.1-16
10. The man born blind				9.1-41

B. *In two gospels only*

	Matthew	Mark	Luke	John
11. The centurion's servant	8.5-13		7.1-10	

C. In three gospels (In the order of Mark)

	Matthew	Mark	Luke	John
12. Peter's mother-in-law	8.14-15	1.30-31	4.38-39	

13. The man full of leprosy	8.1-4	1.40-45	5.12-15
14. The paralytic	9.1-8	2.1-12	5.18-26
15. The man with the withered hand	12.10-13	3.1-6	6.6-11
16. The woman with the flow of blood	9.20-22	5.25-34	8.43-48
17. Blind Bartimaeus	20.29-34	10.46-52	18.35-43

Accounts of the Exorcism of Demons

In one Gospel only

	Matthew	Mark	Luke	John
1. The dumb demoniac	9.32-34			

In two Gospels only

	Matthew	Mark	Luke	John
2. The blind and dumb demoniac	12.22-24		11.14-16	
3. The synagogue demoniac		1.21-28	4.31-37	
4. The Syro-phonecian girl	15.22-28	7.24-30		

In three Gospels

	Matthew	Mark	Luke	John
5. The Gadarene demoniac	8.28-34	5.1-20	8.26-39	
6. The epileptic boy	17.14-21	9.14-29	9.37-43	

Accounts of the Raising of the Dead

In one Gospel only

	Matthew	Mark	Luke	John
1. The widow's son at Nain			7.11-16	
2. Lazarus				11.1-46

In three Gospels

	Matthew	Mark	Luke	John
3. Jairus' daughter	9.18-19, 23-26	5.22-24, 35-43	8.41-42, 49-56	

Healing of Individuals

Now that we have identified the twenty-six accounts of the healing of individuals by Jesus in which details are given of the sick and their sickness, it is possible to classify them according to the nature of the disease from which they suffered. In most cases the diagnosis cannot be any more than a general or symptomatic one, but in a few cases sufficient significant details have been recorded which allow a more specific diagnosis to be made. In the following classification of the diseases healed by Jesus the references given are those of the verses which contain the relevant information about the diagnosis.

Physical disease:

A. Acute disease

1. Fever:
The nobleman's son (John 4.52).
Peter's mother-in-law (Matthew 8.14; Mark 1.30; Luke 4.38).

2. Acute anterior poliomyelitis:
The centurion's servant (Matthew 8.6; Luke 7.2).

3. Incised wound:
Malchus' ear (Luke 22.50).

4. Unknown fatal diseases:
Widow's son at Nain (Luke 7.12).
Jairus' daughter (Matthew 9.18; Mark 5.23; Luke 8.42).
Lazarus (John 11.3 and 13).

B. Chronic disease:

1. Nervous disease
a. Paraplegia or paralysis of the lower limbs:
The paralytic (Matthew 9.2; Mark 2.3; Luke 5.18).
The impotent man (John 5.5-7).

b. Paralysis of the hand:
The man with the withered hand (Matthew 12.10; Mark 3.1; Luke 6.6).

c. Blindness:
The two blind men (Matthew 9.27).
The blind man of Bethsaida (Mark 8.22).
The man born blind (John 9.1).
Blind Bartimaeus (Matthew 20.30; Mark 10.46; Luke 18.35).

d. Deafness and defective speech:
The deaf mute (Mark 7.32).

2. Rheumatic disease of the spine (spondylitis ankylopoietica)
The woman with a spirit of infirmity (Luke 13.11).

3. Chronic heart failure:
The man with dropsy (Luke 14.2).

4. Gynecological disease: Fibroid tumors of the uterus.
The woman with the flow of blood (Matthew 9.20; Mark 5.25; Luke 8.43).

5. Skin disease:
The ten leprosy patients (Luke 17.12).
The man full of leprosy (Matthew 8.2; Mark 1.40; Luke 5.12).

A close examination of the references in these cases will reveal how often it is Luke who records the significant detail. It is he who tells us that Peter's mother-in-law had a high fever (Luke 4.38); that the leprosy patient was covered with leprosy (Luke 5.12) NEB; that the withered hand was the man's right hand (Luke 6.6); and that the young man of Nain was the only son of his mother, and she was a widow (Luke 7.12). This awareness of the significance of detail is a reflection and confirmation of Luke's medical training.

Demon possession:

A. With specific physical manifestations described

1. Major epilepsy:
The synagogue demoniac (Mark 1.26; Luke 4.35).
The epileptic boy (Matthew 17.15; Mark 9.17-27; Luke 9.39).

2. Acute mania:
The Gadarene demoniac (Matthew 8.28; Mark 5.2-7; Luke 8.29).

3. Mutism or an inability to speak:
The dumb demoniac (Matthew 9.32-33).

4. Mutism accompanied by blindness:
The blind and dumb demoniac (Matthew 12.22; Luke 11.14).

B. With no specific physical manifestations described
The Syrophoenician girl (Matthew 15.22; Mark 7.25).

Healing of Groups

In addition to the twenty-six accounts of the healing of individuals which occur in the gospels, there are twelve other references to occasions when Jesus healed sick people. In these we are given few details and simply told that he healed an unspecified number of sick people in a group.

A. References in on gospel only

	Matthew	Mark	Luke	John
1. In an unnamed city			5.15	
2. In the Temple	21.14			

B. In two gospels only

	Matthew	Mark	Luke	John
3. On a tour in Galilee	9.35	(6.5)		
4. In answer to John the Baptist	11.1-6		7.18-23	
5. At Genneseret	14.35-36	6.54-56		
6. In the hills	15.30-31	7.31-37		

7. In Judaea   19.2   (10.1)

C. *In three gospels*

	Matthew	Mark	Luke	John
8. At Caper-naum	8.16-17	1.32-34	4.40-41	
9. On an-other tour in Galilee	4.23-25	1.39	(4.44)	
10. By the seaside	12.15-16	3.10-12	6.17-19	
11. At Nazareth	13.58	6.5	(4.24)	
12. After the return of the Twelve	14.14	(6.34)	9.11	

Incident	Reference	English	Greek
1. In an un-named city	Luke 5.15	infirmity	astheneia
2. In the Temple	Mathew 21.14	blindness	tuphlos
		lameness	chlos
3. On a tour in Galilee	Matthew 9.35	disease	nosos
		illness	malakia
4. In answer to John the Baptist	Luke 7.21	disease	nosos
		plague	mastix
		evil spirits	pneumata ponera
		blindness	tuphlos

Incident	Reference	English	Greek
5. At Genneseret	Matthew 14.35	sickness	kakos echo
6. In the hills	Matthew 15.30	lameness	cholos
		lameness	kullos
		blindness	tuphlos
		mutism	kophos
7. In Judaea	Matthew 19.2	no description given	
8. At Capernaum	Matthew 8.16	demon possession	dimonizomai
		sickness	kakos echo
	Luke 4.40	sick with various diseases	astheneo nosois poikilais
9. On another tour in Galilee	Matthew 4.23-24	disease	nosos
		illness	malakia
		sickness	kakos echo
		suffering from torture/torment	basanois echo
		demon possession	daimonizomai
		epilepsy	seleniazomai
		paralysis	paralutikos
10. By the seaside	Mark 3.10	plague	mastix
		unclean spirits	pneumata akatharta
	Luke 6.17	disease	nosos

| 11. At Nazareth | Mark 6.5 | sickness | arrostos |
| 12. After the return of the twelve | Matthew 14.14 | sickness | arrostos |

The Initiative In Healing

The identity of the person who took the initiative which resulted in a miracle of healing performed by Jesus is not always clearly indicated in the gospel record. The writers of the gospels do not appear to have been particularly interested in this detail of the miracles. The result is that in some cases we are left in doubt about whom it was who made the first move in bringing the sick to the attention of Jesus. The following list is an attempt to classify the narratives of the miracles of healing according to who it was who took the initiative in each case. In some cases the identification can only be regarded as possible.

Those in which Jesus himself took the initiative:

1. The woman with a spirit of infirmity (Luke 13.12).
2. The impotent man (John 5.6)
3. The ear of Malchus (Luke 22.51).
4. The widow's son at Nain (Luke 7.14).

Those in which the sick took the initiative:

1. The two blind men (Matthew 9.27).
2. The ten leprosy patients (Luke 17.13).
3. The man full of leprosy (Mark 1.40).
4. The woman with the flow of blood (Mark 5.27).
5. Blind Bartimaeus (Mark 10.47).
6. The synagogue demoniac (Mark 1.24).
7. The Gadarene demoniac (Mark 5.6).

Those in which others took the initiative:

1. The deaf mute (Mark 7.32). Persons not identified.
2. The blind man of Bethsaida (Mark 8.22). Persons not identified.
3. The nobleman's son (John 4.47). His father took the initiative.
4. The man born blind (John 9.2). The disciples took the initiative.
5. The centurion's servant (Matthew 8.5). His master took the initiative.
6. Peter's mother-in-law (Mark 1.30). The disciples took the initiative.
7. The paralytic man (Mark 2.3). His friends brought him.
8. The dumb demoniac (Matthew 9.32). Persons not identified.
9. The blind & dumb demoniac (Matthew 12.22). Persons not identified.
10. The Syrophoenician girl (Mark 7.26). Her mother came to Jesus.
11. The epileptic boy (Mark 9.17). His father brought him to Jesus.
12. Lazarus (John 11.3). His sisters sent for Jesus.
13. Jairus' daughter (Mark 5.23). Her father came to Jesus.

Those in which Jesus' enemies appear to take the initiative:

1. The man with dropsy (Luke 14.1-3).
2. The man with the withered hand (Luke 6.6-7).

The Motive For Healing

In fewer than half the accounts of the miracles of healing performed by Jesus is any indication of his motive given. In most cases it is implicit rather than explicit, and the following list is an attempt to identify and classify the motives which appear to underlie most of the healing incidents whether individual or multiple which are recorded in the gospels.

1. An expression of compassion

a. The man full of leprosy (Mark 1.41).
b. The dead son of the widow of Nain (Luke 7.13).
c. Blind Bartimaeus and his friend (Matthew 20.34).
d. Healing after the return of the Twelve (Matthew 14.14).

2. A response to a cry for mercy

a. The two blind men (Matthew 9.27).

b. Blind Bartimaeus (Mark 10.47 and parallels).

c. The epileptic boy (Matthew 17.15 and Mark 9.22).

d. The Syrophoenician girl (Matthew 15.22).

e. The ten leprosy patients (Luke 17.13).

3. In answer to faith

a. The centurion's servant (Matthew 8.10 and Luke 7.9).

b. The paralyzed man (Mark 2.5 and parallels).

c. The two blind men (Matthew 9.28-29).

d. The Syrophoenician girl (Matthew 15.28).

e. The epileptic boy (Mark 9.24).

f. Blind Bartimaeus (Mark 10.52 and Luke 18.42).

4. A manifestation of glory

a. The nobleman's son (John 4.54, d. 2.11).

b. The man born blind (John 9.3).

c. The raising of Lazarus (John 11.4).

5. A fulfillment of scripture

a. The evening healings at Capernaum (Matthew 8.16-17).

b. The demonstration to the Baptist's disciples (Matthew 11.2-6 and Luke 7.18-23).

c. The healings by the seaside (Matthew 12.15-21).

Appendix 2
The Healing Stories In The Acts Of The Apostles

From: J. Wilkinson, *Health and Healing*, Handsel Press, Edinburgh, 1980; see also J. Wilkinson, The Bible and Healing, Chapter 13.

The Healing Of Individuals

Accounts of physical healing:

1. The lame man at the gate of the Temple	By Peter	Acts 3.1-10
2. Paul's recovery of sight	By Ananias	Acts 9.17-19
3. Aeneas healed of paralysis	By Peter	Acts 9.32-35
4. Cripple healed at Lystra	By Paul	Acts 14.8-11
5. Cure of father of Publius	By Paul	Acts 28.8

Accounts of the exorcism of demons:

6. The Philippian slave girl	By Paul	Acts 16.16-18

Accounts of the raising of the dead:

7. Tabitha (Dorcas) at Joppa	By Peter	Acts 9.36-41
8. Eutychus at Troas	By Paul	Acts 20.9-12

The Healing of Groups

1. The sick in the streets of Jerusalem	By Peter	Acts 5.15-16
2. The sick in Samaria	By Philip	Acts 8.6-7
3. The sick at Ephesus	By Paul	Acts 19.11-12
4. The sick at Malta	By Paul	Acts 28.9

Other Possible References

1. Wonders and signs in Jerusalem	By all the apostles	Acts 2.43
2. More wonders and signs in Jerusalem	By all the apostles	Acts 5.12
3. More wonders and signs in Jerusalem	By Stephen	Acts 6.8
4. Signs and wonders in Iconium	By Paul and Barnabas	Acts 14.3

The Diseases Healed

It is possible to classify the narratives of healing miracles on the basis of the diseases whose healing they describe. Insofar as the diseases can be identified we may classify them as follows:

Physical Disease

Acute diseases:
1. Acute blindness: Paul in Acts 9.8
2. Acute fatal head injury: Eutychus in Acts 20.9
3. Acute bacillary dysentery: Father of Publius in Acts 28.8
4. Acute fatal disease of unknown nature: Tabitha in Acts 9.37

Chronic diseases:

1. Lameness of locomotor disability:
a. The man at the gate of the Temple in Acts 3.2
b. The cripple at Lystra in Acts 14.8

2. Paralysis due to neurological disorder:
Aeneas in Acts 9.33
In Acts 8.7 there is a reference to "many who were paralyzed or lame" who were healed by Philip.

Demon Possession

1. The Philippian slave-girl of Acts 16.16

ENDNOTES

Chapter 1

1. Christian Medical Commission, *Healing and Wholeness,* WCC, Geneva, 1990, p. 6.

The expanded WHO definition is cited in E. Lucas, "What is health? Towards a Christian understanding" in *Christian Healing — What Can We Believe?* SPCK, London, 1997, p. 60.

See also *Health, Faith and Healing,* International Review of Mission, WCC, Geneva, Vol. 90, Nos. 356-357, Jan-April 2001, p. 21.

2. Issues relating to the wider social aspects of health and healing are considered in Chapter 14.

3. J. A. Sanford, cited in J. K. Wagner, *Blessed to be a Blessing,* The Upper Room, Nashville, 1980, p. 29.

4. For helpful insights in relation to the understanding of health and healing in the scriptures, including words used in Old Testament and New Testament to describe healing, see:

M. Brown, *Israel's Divine Healer,* Zondervan, Grand Rapids, Michigan, 1995.

J. Wilkinson, *Health and Healing,* Handsel Press, Edinburgh, 1980.

J. Wilkinson, *The Bible and Healing,* Handsel Press, Edinburgh, and Eerdmans, Grand Rapids, Michigan, 1998.

5. For helpful comments on the significance of "*sozo,*" "*therapeuo*" "*iaomai,*" see M. Maddocks, *Twenty Questions About Healing,* SPCK London, 1981, p. 5.

6. L. Weatherhead, *Psychology, Religion, and Healing*, Hodder & Stoughton, London, 1952, p. 466.

7. J. K. Wagner, *Blessed to be a Blessing*, The Upper Room, Nashville, 1980, p. 29.

8. W. Clebsch & C. Jaekle, *Pastoral Care in Historical Perspective*, HarperCollins, New York, 1967, p. 33.

9. Christian Medical Commission, p. 6.

10. N. Jackson. *The Ministry of Healing*, Anglican Diocese of Ballarat, Victoria, Australia, 1990.

11. M. Maddocks, *Twenty Questions about Healing*, SPCK, London, 1981, p. 5.

Chapter 2

1. There has always been debate about the significance of Jesus. One writer comments, "No other name has inspired greater devotion, evoked greater aversion, or ignited greater controversy." Two helpful discussions on contemporary responses to Jesus are:

D. Groothuis. *Jesus in an Age of Controversy*, Harvest House, Oregon, 1996.

M. Wilken and P. Moreland. *Jesus Under Fire*, Zondervan, Grand Rapids, Michigan, 1995.

2. G. Bennett, *Commissioned to Heal*, Divine Healing Mission, London, undated, p. 2. The questions of authority and truth are important in contemporary society and church. The Christian claim that the scriptures are the source of truth for everyone is rejected by many people who believe that truth is personal and each person has their own truth which is real for them, and that there is

no one truth that applies to everyone. There are many different truths which are formed by culture and social situation, and these can be discovered and embraced by human reason. So there is no over-arching revelation or authority for everyone — no one "story" which applies to everyone (often called a "meta-narrative") — there is only my truth and your truth, or our truth, and all these truths have equal authority. This way of thinking is one aspect of "post modernity".

The issues of authority and the significance of the scriptures are discussed in many books on Christian theology. Three helpful studies are:

M. Erickson, *Christian Theology*, one volume edition, Baker, Grand Rapids, Michigan, 1990.

A. E. McGrath, *Christian Theology*, Blackwell, Oxford, 1994, Chapter 6.

B. Milne, *Know The Truth — A Handbook of Christian Belief*, IVP, Leicester, Rev Edition, 1998, Chapter 3.

For discussion on the significance of "post modern" thinking for the Christian faith, see

P. Copan, *True For You, But Not For Me*, Bethany, Minneapolis, Minnesota, 1998.

D. Dockery (ed.), *The Challenge of Post Modernism — An Evangelical Assessment*. Victor, Wheaton, Illinois. 1995.

C. Loscalzo, *Apologetic Preaching — Proclaiming Christ to a Post Modern World*. IVP. Downers Grove, Illinois, 2000.

T. R. Philips & D. L. Okholm, *Christian Apologetics in the Postmodern World*, IVP, Downers Grove, Illinois. 1995.

3. M. Kelsey, *Psychology, Medicine and Christian Healing.* HarperCollins, New York, 1988. Chapters 3-5 offer helpful analyses of both Old Testament and New Testament understanding of healing, especially the healing ministry of Jesus.

For comments on the wider dimensions of Jesus ministry, see further references in endnote 4; see also Chapter 14 of this book; also see:

R. Kydd, *Healing Through the Centuries — Models for Understanding,* Hendriksen, Peabody, Mass, 1998, pp. xvi-xx.

4. For a discussion of the healing miracles of Jesus, and the significance of the wider cultural and social backgrounds in understanding healing, see:

B. Epperley, *God's Touch,* Westminster John Knox Press, Louisville, Ky. 2001.

M. Harper, *The Healings of Jesus,* Hodder & Stoughton, London, 1986.

J. Pilch. Healing in the New Testament — Insights from Medical and Mediterranean Anthropology, Augsburg Fortress, Minneapolis 2000.

5. J. Wilkinson offers detailed studies of the healings, types of diseases, and motives for healing, in *Health and Healing,* Handsel Press, Edinburgh, 1980, Chapters 4-6, see also J. Wilkinson, *The Bible and Healing.* Handsel Press, Edinburgh and Eerdmans, Grand Rapids, Michigan. 1998.

6. One understanding of the healing ministry of Jesus emphasizes that his death on the cross is the source of all healing. Based on such verses as Isaiah 53:4-5, Matthew 8:17, and 1 Peter 2:24, this interpretation sees healing as included in salvation through

the cross or Atonement of Jesus Christ to be received by faith in the same way as forgiveness of sin, acceptance by God, and other blessings. For helpful discussions on the concept that "healing is in the Atonement," see:

B. Barron, *The Health and Wealth Gospel*, IVP, Illinois, 1987, Chapters 3-5.

J. S. Baxter, *Divine Healing of the Body*, Zondervan, Grand Rapids, 1979.

G. D. Fee, *The Disease of the Health and Wealth Gospels*, Concerned Christian Growth Ministries, North Perth, 1985.

L. Morris, *The cross of Jesus*, Eerdmans, Grand Rapids, 1988, Chapter 6.

7. M. Kelsey. p. 78.

8. *Ibid.*, pp. 32, 33.

9. W. Barclay's commentaries on the gospels offer detailed explanations of prevalent beliefs and customs. See also:

B. Epperley, *God's Touch*. Westminster John Knox Press, Louisville, KY 2001.

M. Harper, *The Healings of Jesus*. Hodder & Stoughton, London, 1986.

J. Pilch, *Healing in the New Testament*. Augsburg Fortress, Minneapolis 2000.

Chapter 3

1. J. Wilkinson provides an excellent outline of the healings and

types of disease in the Acts of the Apostles. See *Health and Healing*, Handsel Press, Edinburgh, 1980, pp. 85-86. See also *The Bible and Healing*, Chapter 13-14.

2. For a helpful discussion on these issues, see J. Glennon, *Your Healing is Within You*, Hodder & Stoughton, London, 1978, pp. 154-165.

3. For a detailed examination of "the thorn in the flesh" see J. Wilkinson, *Health and Healing*, Chapter 11, and *The Bible and Healing*, Chapters 16-19.

4. The following six arguments are explained in: "The Gift of Healing has Ceased: Six Biblical Reasons Why," in *Evangelical Action*, Bible Union of Australia, Volume 13, No. 5, April-May 1989.

5. P. Hacking, "A ministry easily over-emphasized," in J. Goldingay (Ed.), *Signs, Wonders and Healing*, IVP, Leicester, 1989, pp. 160-162.

6. P. Hacking, p. 163.

7. D. Huggett, "A ministry to be encouraged," in J. Goldingay, pp. 139-140.

8. M. Maddocks, *The Christian Healing Ministry*, SPCK, London, 1990, p. 104.

9. *Ibid.*, p. 107

10. For comments on the global and ecumenical expression of the healing ministry, see:

A Time To Heal, House of Bishops, London, 2000. Chapter 4.

Health Faith and Healing. International Review of Mission, WCC,

Geneva, Vol. 90, Nos. 356-357, Jan-April 2001.

Chapter 4

1. This historical development has been researched by several authors. Four valuable studies are:

B. Brown, *Liturgy, Ritual, and Healing*, Unpub. D.Min Thesis, Melbourne, 1991.

R. Kydd provides a Pentecostal-charismatic perspective, offering six models for understanding the diversities of method, theology, and social application that have characterized the healing ministry over the centuries. See R. Kydd, *Healing through the Centuries — Models for Understanding*, Hendriksen, Peabody, Mass., 1998.

M. Kelsey, *Psychology, Medicine and Christian Healing*, HarperCollins, NY, 1988, Chapters 7-10.

F. MacNutt. *The Nearly Perfect Crime — How the Church Almost Killed the Healing Ministry*, Chosen Books, Baker, Grand Rapids, Michigan, 2005.

2. M. Kelsey p. 123.

3. *Ibid.*, p. 155.

4. *Ibid.*, p. 169.

5. *Ibid.*, p. 17.

6. *Ibid.*, p. 17. For an evaluation of the influence of Martin Luther's and John Calvin's teaching on healing, for the church from the Reformation to the present day, see B. Brown, Chapter 4. See also F. MacNutt. *The Nearly Perfect Crime*, Chapter 17.

7. F. MacNutt gives a valuable overview of developments in the 20ᵗʰ century, focusing on the charismatic-renewal, and third wave movements, especially in the American scene. He briefly refers to the amazing growth of the church and healing ministries "throughout the world" (pp. 201-4), but apart from a brief reference to the work of OSL, gives little attention to the renewal of healing ministries in the so called "established churches" (especially in U.K., Australia, and New Zealand).

8. A helpful discussion of the different approaches outlined in this section is given by D. Duncan, *Health and Healing: A Ministry to Wholeness,* St. Andrew Press, Edinburgh, 1988, Chapter 10. Duncan discusses some of the differences especially in relation to the healing of the memories, but his words have wider application to the healing ministry as a whole.

9. *Ibid.,* pp. 111-112

10. *Health, Faith and Healing,* International Review of Mission, p. 4.

11. A forthcoming study in Australia offers an introduction to various perspectives and practices in this ministry, and points to the need to recognize the value of different perspectives. See *From Where I Stand – Christian Perspectives on the Ministry of Healing.* OSL Australia.

Chapter 5

1. The author acknowledges his indebtedness to G. Collins for his insights on the significance of sickness in counseling and healing. See G. Collins, *Christian Counseling,* Word, Milton Keynes, UK, 1989, Chapter 22.

2. For more detailed explanations of these responses see Collins, p. 332.

3. See Collins, p. 334.

4. This historical development is outlined in M. Kelsey, *Psychology, Medicine and Healing*, HarperCollins, N.Y., 1988, Chapters 8 and 9.

5. *Ibid.*, p. 12.

6. Examples are:

K. Blue, *Authority to Heal*, IVP, Leicester, 1987.

J. Glennon, *Your Healing is Within You*, Hodder & Stoughton, London, 1978.

F. MacNutt, *Healing*, Hodder & Stoughton, London, 1988.

7. Arguments for a clear distinction between sickness and suffering are presented by K. Blue, J. Glennon, and F. MacNutt. Arguments opposing any such distinction are presented by P. Masters, *The Healing Epidemic*, The Wakeman Trust, London, 1988; C. S. Storms, *Healing and Holiness*, Presbyterian and Reformed, New Jersey, 1990.

8. Differing interpretations as to the nature of Paul's "thorn in the flesh" are given by the above-mentioned writers. See also J. Wilkinson, *The Bible and Healing*, Handsel Press, Edinburgh & Eerdmans, Grand Rapids, Michigan, 1998, Chapters 16-19.

9. Two contemporary examples of this response are Joni Eareckson and Jennifer Rees Larcombe. See *Healing and Wholeness*, Crowborough, East Sussex, No. 1, Jan/March, 1991, and No. 5, Jan/March, 1992. Each of these authors tell their stories in their books: J. Eareckson, *Glorious Intruder*, Scripture Press; J. R. Larcombe, *Unexpected Healing*, Hodder & Stoughton.

10. P. Yancey, *Where is God When It Hurts?*, Zondervan, Grand

Rapids, 1977. An excellent discussion on the subject of suffering, evil, and the character and purpose of God is given in D. Carson, *How Long, O Lord?*, Baker, Grand Rapids, 1990.

11. J. Glennon, *Your Healing is Within You*, Hodder & Stoughton, London, 1978, p. 164.

Chapter 6

1. H. Frost, *Miraculous Healing*, Marshall Morgan and Scott, London, 1981, p. 5.

2. F. MacNutt, *Healing*, Hodder and Stoughton, London, 1988, pp. 162 ff.

3. P. Tillich, *Systematic Theology*, Vol. 3, James Nisbet, Digswell Place, Herts, UK, 1964, p. 298.

4. F. Wright, *The Pastoral Nature of Healing*, SCM-Canterbury Press, London, 1985, p. 33.

5. Cited in F. MacNutt, *Healing*, p. 204.

6. *Ibid.*

7. See J. Gunstone, *Prayers for Healing*, Highland Books, Crowborough, East Sussex, 1987, for many examples of prayer.

8. A. Arbuthnot, *Healing and Wholeness*, Crowborough, East Sussex, No. 1 January/March 1991, p. 14.

9. A. Sanford, *The Healing Light*, Arthur James/Daystar, Fortitude Valley, Australia, 1986, p. 36.

10. B. Green, *Healing and Wholeness*, No. 1, January/March, 1991, p. 15.

11. OSL Service of Ministry to the Sick, OSL Australia, undated, p. 26.

12. J. Richards, *The Question of Healing Services,* Daybreak/D.L.T., London, 1989, p. 96.

13. *Ibid.,* p. 97.

14. J. Glennon, "Guidelines for Healing Today," *Sermon Notes,* St. Andrew's Healing Ministry, Sydney, June 11, 1990.

Chapter 7

1. F. MacNutt, *Healing,* Hodder and Stoughton, London, 1988, pp. 119-120.

2. J. Richards, *Faith and Healing,* Network No. 6, Floreat Flame Books, Mirrabooka, undated, p. 31.

3. Canon J. Glennon was the founder of St. Andrew's Healing Ministry in Sydney. His description of the prayer of faith is contained in *Your Healing is Within You; How Can I Find Healing?; Sermon Notes From St. Andrew's Healing Ministry, Sydney;* and an article: *The Theology of Healing.*

4. J. Glennon, *How Can I Find Healing?* Hodder and Stoughton, London, 1984, pp. 21-23; J. Glennon, *Your Healing is Within You,* Hodder and Stoughton, London, 1978, pp. 166-167. J. Glennon, *The Theology of Healing,* OSL, Australia, undated.

5. *Ibid.,* p. 3.

6. *Ibid.,* p. 5.

7. J. Glennon, *How Can I Find Healing?* p. 80.

8. *Ibid.*, p. 53.

9. F. MacNutt *Healing*, Chapters 8 and 9.

10. F. MacNutt, *Healing*, p. 124.

11. *Ibid.*, pp. 125-126.

12. *Ibid.*, pp. 128-129.

13. *Ibid.*, p. 134.

14. *Ibid.*, pp. 147-148.

15. *Ibid.*, p. 134.

16. C. S. Storms, *Healing and Holiness*, Presbyterian and Reformed Publishing, New Jersey, 1990, p. 113.

17. P. Masters, *The Healing Epidemic*. The Wakeman Trust, London, 1988, p. 151.

18. *Ibid.*, p. 153.

19. *Ibid.*, p. 154.

20. J. A. Motyer, *The Message of James, The Bible Speaks Today*, IVP, Leicester, 1985, p. 200.

21. *Ibid.*, pp. 199-200.

22. Cited in K. Blue, *Authority to Heal*, p. 49.

23. J. Richards, *Faith and Healing*, p. 30

24. Helpful insights on "abuses of faith", "name it and claim it",

and other harmful ideas are given by K. Blue, *Healing Spiritual Abuse*, IVP. Downers Grove, Illinois, 1993; and C. Kraft, *Confronting Powerless Christianity*, Baker, Grand Rapids, Michigan, 2002, Chapter 5.

Chapter 8

1. A. Pearce, "Healing of the Memories," *Basic Booklet No. 7*, Order of St. Luke, Australia, 1982.

2. D. Turner, "Is Inner Healing A Valid Ministry," J. Yutaka Amano and N. L. Geisler, *The Infiltration of the New Age*, Tyndale, Wheaton, Illinois, 1989, p. 64.

3. H. N. Maloney, "Inner Healing," *Baker Encyclopedia of Psychology*, Baker, Grand Rapids, 1985, p. 579.

4. D. A. Seamands, *Healing of Memories*, Victor Books, Illinois, 1985, p. 24.

5. *Ibid.*, p. 12.

6. S. Hughes, "The Healing of Memories — is it a Valid Biblical Ministry?," *The Christian Counselor*, C.W.R., Farnham, Surrey, Volume 1, No. 1, Winter 1991, pp. 16-17.

7. This point outlines the process in a general way, and does not attempt to apply to any actual situation. For helpful guidelines as to the content of prayer and a more detailed "how-to" approach, see suggestions in F. MacNutt, *Healing*, Chapter 13, and D. A. Seamands, *Healing of Memories*, Chapters 9, 10, 12. For helpful guidelines in applying this healing to our personal lives, see O. Dowling, "Healing of the Past" *Healing Contact*, OSL-Australia, No. 128, June 1991.

8. A helpful description of the methods of three leading practitioners

(F. MacNutt, Betty and Ed. Tapscott, and Ruth Carter Stapleton) are given by H. N. Maloney, pp. 581-582.

9. R. Green, *God's Catalyst,* Hodder & Stoughton, London, 1991. p. 138.

10. F. MacNutt, *Healing,* Hodder & Stoughton, London, 1988. p. 190.

11. D. A. Seamands, p. 27.

12. Cited in H. N. Maloney, p. 581.

13. D. A. Seamands, pp. 150-151.

14. *Ibid.,* p. 152.

15. D. Augsburger, *The Freedom of Forgiveness,* Moody Press, 1970, pp. 39-40.

16. D. A. Seamands, p. 188.

17. F. MacNutt, p. 186.

18. For further comment on possible indications for the healing of memories, see D. A. Seamands, Chapters 6 and 7; S. Hughes, Volume 1, Nos. 1-4.

19. S. Hughes, Volume 1, No. 2, p. 7.

20. D. Matzat, *Inner Healing — Deliverance or Deception?,* Harvest House, Oregon, 1987, p. 35.

21. *Ibid.,* p. 42.

22. S. Hughes, Volume 1, No. 3, p. 16. See also D. Hunt and T.

A. McMahon, *The Seduction of Christianity,* Harvest House, Oregon, 1985.

23. R. Green, p. 142.

24. D. A. Seamands, cited in Amano and Geisler, p. 73.

25. D. A. Seamands, pp. 61-62; the principles are outlined pp. 62-78.

26. S. Hughes, Volume 1, No. 3, pp. 15-18.

27. There is a lot of material written on this topic from a Christian perspective, both for and against. For a negative critique refer to D. Matzat, Chapters 5-7; for a positive affirmation within certain guidelines, refer to D. A. Seamands; and M. A. Pearson, *Christian Healing,* Chosen Books, F. H. Revell, New Jersey, 1990, Chapter 6.

28. Adapted from M. A. Pearson, *Christian Healing,* Chosen Books, F. H. Revell, New Jersey, 1990, pp. 116-118.

29. R. Wise, "Church Divided," cited in Matzat, pp. 81 and 85

30. M. A. Pearson, p. 118.

31. H. N. Maloney, pp. 583-584.

32. D. A. Seamands, p. 189.

Chapter 9

1. E. H. Cobb, "Christ Healing," *Sharing,* OSL, San Antonio, March 1988, pp. 10-13.

2. *Ibid.,* p. 14.

3. S. Pattison, *Alive and Kicking,* SCM-Canterbury Press, London, 1989, p. 49.

4. M. Kelsey, *Psychology, Medicine and Christian Healing,* HarperCollins, New York, 1988, p. 166.

5. The author acknowledges the insights of S. Pattison in this section.

6. J. Gunstone, *The Lord is our Healer,* Hodder and Stoughton, London, 1986, p. 144.

7. Cited in F. Wright, *The Pastoral Nature of Healing,* SCM-Canterbury Press, London, 1985, p. 8.

8. M. Maddocks, *The Christian Healing Ministry,* SPCK, London, 1990, p. 164.

9. *Ibid.,* p. 165.

10. Questions about the validity of claims to healing by non-physical or spiritual methods are examined and evaluated by:

D. Lewis, *Healing — Fiction, Fantasy, or Fact?,* Hodder and Stoughton, London, 1989.

R. Gardner, *Healing Miracles, A Doctor Investigates,* Darton, Longman and Todd, London, 1986.

11. Cited in M. Maddocks, *A Healing House of Prayer,* Hodder and Stoughton, London, 1987, p. 77.

12. M. Maddocks, *Journey to Wholeness,* SPCK/Triangle, London, 1986, p. 41.

13. J. Richards, *Gospel and Medicine,* Network No. 6, Floreat Flame Books, Mirrabooka, undated, pp. 32 ff.

14. *Ibid.,* p. 32.

15. J. Gunstone, p. 158.

16. Based on J. Richards, p. 37.

17. Cited in J. Richards, p. 38.

18. *Ibid.,* p. 38.

19. M. Scheel, "Missionary Work and Healing," *International Review of Missions,* WCC, Geneva, Vol. 53, No. 211, July 1964, p. 265.

20. Based on M. Maddocks, *A Healing House of Prayer,* p. 77.

21. *Ibid.,* pp. 77-78.

Chapter 10

1. For fascinating insights into the wonders of the body, see: P. Brand and P. Yancey: *Fearfully and Wonderfully Made,* Zondervan, Grand Rapids, 1980, and *In His Image,* Hodder and Stoughton, London, 1982.

2. Cited in *Healing and Wholeness,* Crowborough, East Sussex, No. 3, July/September, 1991, p. 24.

3. For a detailed study of the human mind, refer to: G. Collins, *Your Magnificent Mind,* Baker, Grand Rapids, 1988. The author acknowledges the insights of Dr. Collins in the section on The Healthy Mind.

4. *Ibid.,* p. 16.

5. *Ibid.,* pp. 31-32.

6. *Ibid.,* p. 35.

7. N. Cousins, *Human Options,* Norton, New York, 1981, cited in Collins, p. 58.

8. Collins, p. 62.

9. The recognition and acceptance of the reality of our emotional life is often neglected by Christians who may see it as "secular psychology." It is a very important component in true healing. For more in-depth treatments of emotions, refer to:

R. Baldwin, *Healing and Wholeness,* Word, Milton Keynes, 1986.

L. Crabb, *Understanding People,* S. J. Bacon, Melbourne, 1987.

D. Seamands, *Healing for Damaged Emotions,* Victor/Scripture Press, Illinois, 1981.

H. N. Wright, *The Christian Use of Emotional Power,* F. H. Revell, New Jersey, 1974.

10. Based on the definition of worship given by William Temple, *Readings in St. John's Gospel,* Macmillan, London, 1955, p. 68.

11. O. Dowling, "The Eucharist, Healing, and Living in Communion," in *Healing Contact,* OSL, Melbourne, Issue 129, September 1991. A helpful overview of the use of the seven historic sacraments as vehicles of healing, is given in: M. Pearson, *Christian Healing,* Chosen Books, 2002, Chapter 9.

12. Australian Hymn Book 446.

Chapter 11

1. M. Raiter. *Stirrings of the Soul,* Matthias Media, Kingsford, 2003.

2. For information on new religious movements, see:

A. Brockway & J. Rajashekar, *New Religious Movements and the Churches*, WCC, Geneva, 1987.

J. Saliba, *Perspectives on New Religious Movements.* Geoffrey Chapman, London, 1995

For material on the rise of the NAM and new spirituality in western societies, and the problem of definition, see:

J. Drane. *What is the New Age Still Saying to the Church?* Harper Collins, London, 1999.

J. Herrick, *The Making of the New Spirituality.* IVP. Downers Grove, Illinois, 2003.

I. Hexham, *Encountering New Religious Movements.* Kregel, Grand Rapids, Michigan, 2004.

J. Newport, *The New Age Movement and the Biblical Worldview.* Eerdmans, Grand Rapids, Michigan, 1998.

D. Tacey, *Re-enchantment.* Harper Collins, Sydney, 2000.

D. Tacey, *The Spirituality Revolution*, Harper Collins, Sydney, 2003

M. Raiter, *Stirrings of the Soul*, Mathias Media. Kingsford, 2003.

P. Johnson (ed.), *Religious and Non-Religious Spirituality in the Western World*, Lausanne Committee for World Evangelisation, Morling Press. 2004

3. D. Groothuis, cited in *What is the New Age?*, in M. Cole (ed.), Hodder & Stoughton, London, 1990, p. 6.

4. E. Miller. *A Crash Course on the New Age Movement*, Baker, Grand Rapids, Michigan, 1989, p. 15

5. Most writers on the New Age give a similar outline of beliefs, although with some different emphases. This outline from:

P. Lochhass. *How to Respond to the New Age Movement*, Concordia, St. Louis, 1998, p. 3-4.

6. Many Christian writers on the New Age offer responses and evaluation. An excellent overview of various Christian responses, that is, Evangelical and fundamentalist, mainline Protestant, Orthodox, and Catholic, is given by:

J. Saliba. *Christian Responses to the New Age Movement*. Geoffrey Chapman, London, 1999.

7. For the influence of New Age in contemporary society, see:

J. Newport. *The New Age Movement and the Biblical Worldview*, Eerdmans, Grand Rapids, Michigan, 1998.

E. Winker, *The New Age is Lying to You*, Concordia, St. Louis, 1994.

For New Age influence in health care, see:

P. Reisser & D. Mabe, *Examining Alternative Medicine*, IVP, Downers Grove, Illinois, 2001, Chapter 1. "A nation takes notice".

8. For discussion on the use of these terms, see:

D. Omathuna & W. Larimore, *Alternative Medicine*, IVP, Downers Grove, Illinois, 2001, Chapter 1.

P. Reisser & D. Mabe, Chapter 2.

9. See Chapter 9. Healing and medical science — pills or prayer or both?

10. S. Pfeifer. *Healing at any Price*, Milton Keynes, 1988, p. 3.

11. Quoted in "Alternative therapies and the New Age," by G. Tuckwell & D. Flagg, in *Healing and Wholeness*, Crowborough, No. 9. Oct-Dec 1992, p.10.

12. D. Millikan & N. Drury, *Worlds Apart*, ABC Enterprises, Melbourne 1991, p. 33.

13. R. Foster, *Celebration of Discipline*, Hodder & Stoughton, London, 1989 Chapter 2; and *Prayer*, Hodder & Stoughton, London, 1992, Chapter 13, and D. Seamands, *Healing of Memories*, Victor, Illinois, 1985.

See also "Under Fire," Christianity Today, Vol. 30, Sept. 18, 1987.

14. Many authors offer analyses and evaluation of alternative therapies, including the issue of background and origin. See:

N. Anderson & M. Jacobson, *The Biblical Guide to Alternative Medicine*, Regal, CA, 2003.

A Time To Heal, Church House, London, 2000, Chapter 10

J. Ankerberg & J. Weldon, *Encyclopedia of New Beliefs*, Harvest, Oregon, 1996.

R. Coker, *Alternative Medicine — Helpful or Harmful*, Monarch, Crowborough, 1995.
D. Omathuna & W. Larimore, *ibid*.

P. Reisser & D. Mabe, *ibid*.

J. Watt. *The Church, Medicine, and The New Age*, Churches Council for health and healing. London, 1995.

For generally positive responses to the use of certain therapies, see:

R. Clifford & P. Johnson, *Jesus and the gods of the New Age*, Lion, Oxford, 2001, Chapter 6.

J. Huggett, *Breath of Life*, Sovereign World, Tonbridge, England, 2004.

B. Epperley, *Crystal and cross*, Twenty Third Publications, Mystic, CT, 1996, Chapter 4.

B. Epperley, *God's Touch*, Westminster John Knox Press, KY, 2001.

S. Parsons, *Searching for Healing*, Lion, Oxford, 1995.

R. Pollard, "Jesus among the alternative healers — sacred oils, aromatherapists and the gospel," in I. Hexham. *Encountering New Religious Movements*, Kregel, Grand Rapids, Michigan, 2004, Chapter 13.

15. N. Anderson & M. Jacobson, p. 191

16. *Ibid.*, pp. 111-112.

17. *Ibid.*, Chapter 3-7.

18. D. Omathuna & W. Larimore, Chapters 12, 13.
19. For material on meditation, see:

R. Foster, *The Celebration of Discipline*, Chapter 13;

J. Glennon, *Christian Meditation*, Healing Ministry Centre, Newtown, 1986.

D. Ray, *The Art of Christian Meditation*, Tyndale, Illinois, 1977.

P. Toon, *Meditating as a Christian*, Harper Collins, London, 1991, part 1.

20. Cited in D. Ray, p. 17.

21. For examples of some creative responses to these issues, see:

I. Hexham, *Encountering New Religious Movements*.

P. Johnson, *Religious and Non-Religious Spirituality in the Western World*.

For a person centered approach in explaining the Christian faith, see:

D. Clark. *Dialogical Apologetics*, Baker, Grand Rapids, Michigan, 1993.

22. K. Logan, *Close Encounters with the New Age*, Kingsway, London, 1991, pp. 174-178

Chapter 12

1. Report of the Committee on Healing, Synod of Victoria, Uniting Church in Australia, Melbourne, 1979, p. 19. For Anglican (UK) reports see details in J. Richards, *Exorcism, Deliverance and Healing*, Grove Worship Series, No. 44, Grove Books, Bramcote, Nottingham, 1976. For recent development, see *A Time to Heal*, Church House, 2000, Chapter 9.

2. An example of the influence of the demonic in sickness is

outlined in F. MacNutt, *Healing*, Ave Maria Press, Notre Dame, Indiana, 1974, Chapter 11.

3. F. Rigg, *Healing the Oppressed*, Order of St. Luke, New Zealand, November, 1989.

4. B. Brown, *The Uniting Church and the Ministry of Deliverance*, Consultative Committee on Healing, Synod of Victoria, Uniting Church in Australia, 1992, p. 4.

For a qualified psychologist's perspectives and experiences on the reality of demonic influence, and the need for exorcism in particular situations, see:

J. Roodenburg, "The drama of the Demonic" and "Salvation, Psychotherapy, or Exorcism," in *On Being*, Hawthorn, Melbourne, Vol. 20, No. 7, August 1993, pp. 4-9.

5. Consultation on the deliverance ministry sponsored by the Victorian Council of Churches, Melbourne, June 24, 1993. Examples of this continuing evaluation are the reports of two State Synods in the Uniting Church in Australia:

— Department for Mission and Parish Services, *Study Documents and Reports on the Deliverance Ministry*, Queensland Synod, Uniting Church in Australia, Brisbane, 1989.

— B. Brown, *The Uniting Church and the Ministry of Deliverance*, Consultative Committee on Healing, Synod of Victoria, Uniting Church in Australia, Melbourne, 1992.

Other churches have produced similar reports. Enquiries should be made to each church as to their status and availability.

6. The New Testament accepts the reality of Satan and does not seek to prove this. For the relevance of this belief for contemporary

society, see M. Green, *I Believe in Satan's Downfall,* Eerdmans, Grand Rapids, 1981, Chapter 1, and J. Woolmer, *Healing and Deliverance,* Monarch, Crowborough, 1999.

7. There are many books which describe the plans and activities of the kingdom of evil and its defeat by Jesus Christ.

— G. Dow, *Those Tiresome Intruders,* Grove Pastoral Series, No. 41, Grove Books, Bramcote, Nottingham, 1990.

— M. Green, *I Believe in Satan's Downfall,* Eerdmans, Grand Rapids, 1981.

— P. Horrobin, *Healing through Deliverance,* Sovereign World, Chichester, 199

— C. Kraft, *Confronting Powerless Christianity,* Baker, Grand Rapids, Michigan, 2002

— C. Kraft, *Defeating Dark Angels,* Sovereign World, Kent, 1993.

— F. H. Leahy, *Satan Cast Out,* The Banner of Truth Trust, Edinburgh, 1990.

— C. Sherlock, *Overcoming Satan,* Grove Spirituality Series, No. 17, Grove Books, Bramcote, Nottingham, 1986.

— G. H. Twelftree, *Christ Triumphant,* Hodder & Stoughton, London, 1985.

— C. P. Wagner and F. D. Tennoyer (Eds.), *Wrestling with Dark Angels,* Regal, California, 1990.

— C. P. Wagner, *Territorial Spirits,* Sovereign World, Chichester, 1991.

— W. Wink, The Powers — Volume 2, *Unmasking the Powers,* Fortress Press, Minneapolis, 1984.

8. C. E. Arnold, *Powers of Darkness,* IVP, Leicester, 1992, p. 167. For further discussion on the meaning of the powers see:

— M. Green, *I Believe in Satan's Downfall,* Eerdmans, 1981.

— T. H. McAlpine, *Facing the Powers,* MARC, World Vision International, Monrovia, 1991.

— J. W. R. Stott, *God's New Society — The Message of Ephesians,* The Bible Speaks Today, IVP, Illinois, 1979, Chapter 12.

— W. Wink, Trilogy on The Powers — Volume 1, *Naming the Powers,* Fortress, Minneapolis, 1984; Volume 2, *Unmasking the Powers,* Fortress, 1986; Volume 3, *Engaging the Powers,* Fortress 1992. (This is a very valuable treatment of the theme and is the most detailed and comprehensive available. It is solid reading and very worthwhile.)

9. M. Green, *I Believe in Satan's Downfall,* Eerdmans, Grand Rapids, 1981, p. 85.

10. Based on *Uniting Church Synod of Victoria Report,* 1979, p. 19. Other helpful definitions of these terms are given by B. Brown, *The Uniting Church and The Ministry of Deliverance,* p. 2; J. Wimber and K. Springer, *Power Healing,* Hodder and Stoughton, London, 1986, Chapter 6.

11. Brown, p. 2.

12. This difference is also emphasized by J Richards, *But Deliver Us from Evil,* Darton, Longman and Todd, London, 1974, Chapters 6 and 7.

13. See Green, p. 132.

14. M. Perry, *Deliverance*, SPCK, London, 1987, Chapter 10. For a discussion see J. Richards, *But Deliver Us from Evil, pp.* 164, 179-184.

15. It is impossible to list all possible causes. Most writers on this subject suggest various causes especially occult involvement. See the following for helpful comments:

— N. & P. Gibson, *Evicting Demonic Squatters and Breaking Bondages,* Freedom in Christ Ministries, Drummoyne, Sydney, 1987, Chapters 8-17 (especially p. 63).

— M. Green, Chapter 5.

— R. Parker, *The Occult,* IVP. Leicester, 1989, Chapters 7 and 8.

— Uniting Church Synod of Victoria, 1979 Report, p. 22.

— T. Marshall, *Foundations for a Healing Ministry,* Sovereign World, Chichester, 1988.

16. The extent and dangers of occult practice are described in the following:

— E. G. Frederickson, *How to Respond to Satanism,* Concordia, St. Louis, 1988.

— N. & P. Gibson, Chapter 16.

— M. Green, Chapter 5.

— D. W. Hoover, *How to Respond to the Occult,* Concordia, St. Louis, 1977.

— R. Parker, *The Occult*, Chapters 7 and 8.

— M. Perry, *Deliverance*, SPCK, London, 1987.

— J. Richards, *But Deliver us from Evil*, Darton, Longman and Todd, 1974.

17. Most writers and practitioners in this ministry offer lists of possible indications. The following give helpful suggestions:

— N. & P. Gibson, Part II.

— M. Harper, *Spiritual Warfare*, Logos International, New Jersey, 1971, Chapter 10.

— R. Parker, *The Occult*, Chapters 7 & 8, and pp. 124-126 (based on J. Richards).

— J. Richards, *But Deliver us from Evil*, pp. 156-157.

More detailed discussion on the need to carefully evaluate possible indications is given in:

— J. W. Montgomery (Ed.), *Demon Possession*, Bethany Fellowship, Minnesota, 1976, Chapters 14, 18, 22 and 23.

18. M. Harper, *Spiritual Warfare*, Logos International, New Jersey, 1971, p. 93.

19. *Ibid.*, p. 94.

20. From an official statement of the General Assembly of the Assemblies of God, Gospel Publishing House, Springfield, Missouri, 1972, cited in G. P. Duffield & N. M. van Cleave, *Foundations of Pentecostal Theology*, Life Bible College, Los Angeles, California, 1983, pp. 495-496.

21. J. Richards, *But Deliver us from Evil,* pp. 156-157.

22. J. Richards, *Spiritual Warfare,* Network No. 5, Floreat Flame Books, Mirrabooka, W. A., undated, pp. 6-7.

23. *Ibid.,* p. 8.

24. *Ibid.,* p. 9.

Many books contain helpful material on the armor to be used in Spiritual Warfare, for example:

— M. Green, Chapters 7 & 8.

— M. Harper, *Spiritual Warfare,* Chapters 8 & 9.

— G. Mallone, *Arming for Spiritual Warfare,* IVP, Illinois, 1991.

— E. Murphy, *The Handbook for Spiritual Warfare,* Thomas Nelson, Nashville, Tennessee, 1992. Murphy offers a detailed biblical, theological, world-view, and practical examination of many of the issues involved in the deliverance ministry, including spiritual warfare.

— R. Stedman, *Spiritual Warfare,* Multnomah Press, Oregon, 1975.

— C. P. Wagner and F. D. Pennoyer, *Wrestling with Dark Angels,* Chapter 2

25. Uniting Church 1979 Synod Report, p. 21.

26. Based on R. Parker, *The Occult,* pp. 126-144, cited in "Deliverance and Healing, *Healing and Wholeness,* Crowborough, East Sussex, Number 11, July/September, 1993, p. 28.

27. Helpful guidelines are outlined in, *Study Documents and Reports*

on the Deliverance Ministry, Queensland Synod, Uniting Church in Australia, Brisbane, 1989, Appendix 1, p. 1.

Chapter 13

1. S. Hughes, *God Wants You Whole,* Kingsway, London, 1984, p. 9.

2. See appropriate chapters in references at the conclusion of this chapter.

3. The idea of hindrances was suggested by Dr. B. Brown in a series of sermons on the Healing Ministry given in Wesley Church, Melbourne, 1980. The author acknowledges his debt to Dr. Brown for his seminal thoughts on this issue.

4. Refer to Chapters 3 and 4 for examples of these attitudes.

5. F. MacNutt, *Healing,* Hodder and Stoughton, London, 1988, p. 109.

6. *Ibid.,* p. 261.

7. A helpful discussion on death as the ultimate healing is given by A. Pearce, "Ultimate Healing: *For His Love's Sake,* OSL, Australia, undated, pp. 73-80. For helpful material on ministering to people in situations of terminal illness and approaching death, see O. Dowling, "Healing Ministry and Dying," *Healing Contact,* Issue 131, March 1992, pp. 2-3.

8. Suggested by O. Dowling, *"When Healing Doesn't Seem to Come,"* undated seminar material.

9. E. G. Neal, *The Lord is Our Healer,* Prentice Hall, London, 1961, p. 184.

10. *Ibid.,* p. 184. Chapters 18 and 20 deal with difficulties in the

healing ministry including the issue of non-healing and death.

11. An example of honest reflection and response to non-healing is given by: R. J. Hillman, *There is Hope, Anzea*, Homebush West, Sydney, 1992. Dr. Hillman, a Uniting Church minister, struggled with non-curable cancer for many years. He writes as an involved "wounded healer," and not as a detached observer. He accepted with gratitude various forms of help and support, involving medical, physical, and spiritual therapies, recognizing these as good gifts from God. His book is a realistic and moving account of his journey in sickness, faith and hope, and is highly recommended "for those who are ill and those who care for them." Dr. Hillman died in April 1992.

12. An excellent overview of some of the issues relating to suffering, failure, death, care of the uncured, and the church's theology of creation and healing, is given in a 1989 report of an interdenominational working party of medical professionals and clergy. Although dealing specifically with hospice care, the report offers excellent guidelines and help in thinking about the healing ministry as a whole. See: *Mud and Star, A report of a working party on the impact of hospice experience in the church's ministry of healing*, Sobell Publications, Oxford, 1991, especially Sections 1 and 2.

Chapter 14

1. Christian Medical Commission, *Healing and Wholeness*, WCC, Geneva, 1990, p. 6.

2. See S. Pattison, *Alive and Kicking*, SCM-Canterbury Press, London, 1989; and Christian Medical Commission, *Healing and Wholeness*, WCC, Geneva, 1990. A recent study is offered by P. Wellock, *The Search For Wholeness — A Christian Perspective*, OSL Australia, 2005.

3. From an African consultation on Health and Healing; Christian

Medical Commission, *Healing and Wholeness,* WCC, Geneva, 1990, p. 8.

4. From a Pacific consultation on Health and Healing; WCC, Geneva, 1990, p. 25.

5. I am indebted to S. Pattison for a description of these models, and acknowledge the value of his analysis. S. Pattison, *Alive and Kicking,* SCM-Canterbury Press, London, 1989, Chapter 2.

6. Based on Pattison, p. 23.

7. *Ibid.,* p. 25.

8. E. R. Ram (et. al), *Health, Healing and Transformation,* MARC, World Vision International, Monrovia, 1991 pp. 101, 102.

9. T. McKeown, *The Role of Medicine* (1979), cited in Pattison, p. 27.

10. For the importance of a person's world-view and how it affects all aspects of life, see: D. Burnett, *Clash of Worlds,* MARC, Eastbourne, 1990; J. Sire, *The Universe Next Door,* IVP, Leicester, 1988; M. Jones, *The Universe Upstairs — A Cartoon Guide to World Views,* Frameworks/IVP, Leicester, 1991. Most textbooks on anthropology discuss these aspects in detail. For a Christian perspective see: P. Hiebert, *Cultural Anthropology,* Baker, Grand Rapids, 1983; S. Grunlan and K. Mayers, *Cultural Anthropology,* Zondervan, Grand Rapids, 1979; C. Kraft, *Christianity in Culture,* Orbis, MaryKnoll, New York, 1979.

11. D. J. Bosch, "Mission in Jesus' Way; A Perspective from Luke's Gospel," *Missionalia,* Volume 17, Number 1, April 1989, p. 8.
For the wider social/community dimensions of health and healing, as demonstrated in the healing stories of the gospels, see B. Epperley, *God's Touch,* and J. Pilch, *Healing in the N.T.*

For perceptive comments on the general "neglect" of the wider social dimensions in the healing ministry of the church over the centuries, see R. Kydd. *Healing Through the Centuries*, pp. xvi-xx and Chapter 1.

12. E. Allen, *et al.*, *Health, Healing and Transformation*, MARC, World Vision International, Monrovia, 1991, p. 14.

13. Cited in Allen, (et. al), p. 20.

14. "Poor Miss out on a Healthier World," *Reuters News Service*, Washington, in the "Age" No. 43087, D. Syme, Melbourne, July 8, 1993, p. 9.

15. J. Grange, "Globalisation, Health Sector Reform, and Justice," in *International Review of Mission*, WCC, Geneva, Vol. 90, Nos. 356-357, Jan-April, 2001, pp. 160-165. See also:

C. L. De Vries, "The global health situation — priorities for the churches healing ministry beyond AD 2000," pp. 149-159.

16. Australian Catholic Bishops' Conference, *Common Wealth for the Common Good*, Collins Dove, Blackburn, 1992, p. 111.

17. *Ibid.*, pp. 111, 112.

18. Christian Medical Commission, WCC, p. 1.

19. *Ibid.*, p. 2.

20. *Ibid.*, p. 3.

21. *Ibid.*, p. 4.

22. Pattison, p. 34. See also K. Luscombe (*et. al.*), Health, *Healing and Transformation*, MARC, World Vision International, Monrovia, 1991, pp. 50-51.

23. This tendency is referred to in an article by P. Borgen, "Miracles of Healing in the New Testament," in *Studia Theologica*, No. 35, 1981, pp. 91-106.

24. R. Kent Hughes, *Mark, Volume 1 — Jesus, Servant and Savior,* Crossway Books, Illinois, 1989, pp. 53, 55.

25. S. Pattison, p. 58.

26. K. L. Luscombe (et. al.), *Health, Healing and Transformation,* p. 52.

27. Pattison, p. 74.

28. Based on Christian Medical Commission, WCC, pp. 31-33.

29. *Ibid.,* p. 32.